AACN PROCEDURE MANUAL FOR CRITICAL CARE

SECOND EDITION

Editor-in-Chief

SALLY MILLAR, R.N., CCRN

Clinical Nurse Leader, Intensive Care Nursing Service,
Massachusetts General Hospital, Boston, Massachusetts

Editors

LESLIE K. SAMPSON, R.N., B.S.N., CCRN

Nurse Director — Administrative Coordinator,
Abington Memorial Hospital, Abington, Pennsylvania

SISTER MAURITA SOUKUP, R.S.M., R.N., M.S.N., CCRN

Critical Care Nursing Specialist, St. Luke's Hospital,
Cedar Rapids, Iowa; Member of Adjunct Faculty, University
of Iowa, Iowa City; Mount Mercy College, Cedar Rapids, Iowa

W. B. SAUNDERS COMPANY

Philadelphia, London, Toronto, Mexico City, Rio de Janeiro, Sydney, Tokyo

W. B. Saunders Company: West Washington Square
                           Philadelphia, PA   19105

                           1 St. Anne's Road
                           Eastbourne, East Sussex BN21 3UN, England

                           1 Goldthorne Avenue
                           Toronto, Ontario M8Z 5T9, Canada

                           Apartado 26370—Cedro 512
                           Mexico 4, D.F., Mexico

                           Rua Coronel Cabrita, 8
                           Sao Cristovao Caixa Postal 21176
                           Rio de Janeiro, Brazil

                           9 Waltham Street
                           Artarmon, N.S.W. 2064, Australia

                           Ichibancho, Central Bldg., 22-1 Ichibancho
                           Chiyoda-Ku, Tokyo 102, Japan

Library of Congress Cataloging in Publication Data
Main entry under title:

AACN procedure manual for critical care.

   Rev. ed. of: Methods in critical care/by the American Association of Critical–Care Nurses. 1980.
   Includes bibliographies and index.
   1. Intensive care nursing—Handbooks, manuals, etc.   I. Millar, Sally. II. Sampson, Leslie K. III. Soukup, Maurita. IV. American Association of Critical–Care Nurses. V. American Association of Critical–Care Nurses. Methods in critical care. VI. Title: A.A.C.N. procedure manual for critical care. [DNLM: 1. Critical Care—methods—handbooks. 2. Critical Care—methods—nurses' instruction.   WY 39 A111]
RT120.I5A43   1985   616'.028   84–23575
ISBN 0–7216–1106–0

AACN—Procedure Manual for Critical Care   ISBN   0–7216–1106–0

Last digit is the print number: 9   8   7   6   5   4   3   2

DEDICATION*

As critical care nurses we will be faced with ever-increasing automation and computerization. An important challenge will be to prevent dehumanization in patient care.

Dorothy Voorman, R.N., B.S.N., CCRN
President, AACN, 1975–1976
Heart and Lung, 5:364, 1976

*Because of our profound commitment to the human aspects of critical care, the second edition's dedication is unchanged from that of the first.

S.M.
L.S.
S.M.S.

CONTRIBUTORS

JUDITH J. (HENDERSON) BOEHM, R.N., M.S.N.

Affiliate Faculty, University of New Hampshire School of Nursing, Durham. Cardiac Clinical Nurse Specialist, Mary Hitchcock Memorial Hospital, Hanover, New Hampshire.

Invasive Site Care

ELAINE BROGDON, R.N., M.N.

Staff Nurse—Psychiatry, Providence Hospital Medical Center, Seattle, Washington.

Upper Gastrointestinal Hemorrhage, Gastric Lavage in Overdose, Paracentesis

JANICE M. CASPER, R.N., B.S.N.

Head Nurse—ICU/CCU, St. Joseph's Hospital, Milwaukee, Wisconsin.

Therapeutic Phlebotomy, Thoracentesis

CAROLYN B. CHALKLEY, R.N., M.S.N.

Clinical Instructor, School of Nursing, University of Alabama in Birmingham; Assistant Clinical Professor, Division of Nursing, Birmingham-Southern College, Birmingham; Administrative Director, Cardiovascular Medical Nursing, Brookwood Medical Center, Birmingham, Alabama.

Permanent Pacemaker Management

RITA COLLEY, R.N., B.A.

Manager of Collaborative Research/Alternative Site Therapies, Parenteral Products Division, Travenol Laboratories, Inc., Deerfield, Illinois.

Total Parenteral Nutrition, Lipid Emulsion Therapy, Enteral Nutrition Via an Enteral Feeding Tube

SHERRI DANO-ADAMS, R.N.

Renal Dialysis Educational Coordinator and Assistant Head Nurse, Dialysis and Renal Transplant Unit, University of Washington Hospital, Seattle, Washington.

Peritoneal Dialysis

RUTH M. DeLOOR, R.N., M.S.N., C.S.

Assistant District Coordinator, Medical District 9, Veterans Administration, Atlanta, Georgia.

Blood and Blood Component Administration, Transfusion Reaction, Autotransfusion, Blood Warming, Use of a Blood Pump

DIANE K. DRESSLER, R.N., M.S.N., CCRN

Clinical Nurse Specialist, Midwest Heart Surgery Institute, Milwaukee, Wisconsin.

Central Line Insertion

BARBARA FELLOWS, R.N., M.A., E.T.

Enterostomal Therapist, University of Washington Hospital, Seattle, Washington.

Peritoneal Dialysis

PENNY J. FORD, R.N., M.S.

Cardiac Clinician, Intensive Care Nursing Service, Massachusetts General Hospital, Boston, Massachusetts.

Intra-Aortic Balloon Pump Management, External Counterpressure with G-Suit, External Counterpressure with MAST Garment

BARBARA BUSS FUGLEBERG, R.N., B.S.N., CCRN

Shift Administrator, Overlake Memorial Hospital, Bellevue, Washington.

Intra-arterial Infusion for Chemotherapy, Upper Gastrointestinal Hemorrhage, Gastric Lavage in Overdose, Paracentesis, Peritoneal Lavage

KAREN C. JOHNSON, R.N., Ed.D.

Interim Chair, Department of Nursing, San Francisco State University, San Francisco, California.

Hemodynamic Monitoring

ELAINE LARSON, R.N., Ph.D., FAAN

Robert Wood Johnson Clinical Scholar in Nursing, School of Nursing, University of Pennsylvania, Philadelphia, Pennsylvania.

Peritoneal Dialysis, Infection Surveillance and Control in the Critical Care Unit

ANNA J. LAVELLE, R.N., B.S.N., M.N.

Head Nurse, Nephrology and Renal Transplant Unit, Swedish Hospital Medical Center, Seattle, Washington.

Acute Hemodialysis

ELLEN F. LENIHAN, R.N., M.S.N.

Clinical Inservice Instructor, Montefiore Medical Center, Bronx, New York.

Radiation Safety

JEANNETTE MCCANN MCHUGH, R.N., M.S.N.

Pulmonary Clinical Nurse Specialist and Instructor, Trocaire College School of Nursing, Buffalo, New York.

Airway Management, Ventilatory Management, Transcutaneous Blood Gas Monitoring, Chest Tube Management, Chest Physiotherapy

KAREN M. MILLER, R.N., M.S.N.

Clinical Director, Emergency Room/Outpatient Department, Family Hospital, Milwaukee, Wisconsin.

Venipuncture, Arterial Puncture

NORMA MOCK, R.N., B.S.N., M.S.

Director, Cardiovascular Services, Broward General Medical Center, Fort Lauderdale, Florida.

Electrocardiogram

KATHY MOSSING, R.N., M.A., M.B.A.

Assistant Director of Nursing, Saint Cabrini Hospital, Seattle, Washington.

Upper Gastrointestinal Hemorrhage, Gastric Lavage in Overdose, Paracentesis

LEONA A. MOURAD, R.N., M.S.N.

Associate Professor Emeritus, College of Nursing, Ohio State University, Columbus, Ohio.

Care of Persons in Traction

BETTY W. NORRIS, R.N., M.S.N.

Assistant Professor, School of Nursing, Samford University; Cardiovascular Clinical Nurse Specialist, Baptist Medical Center, Birmingham, Alabama.

Temporary Pacemaker Management, Electrical Safety Precautions for Patients with Direct Conduction Pathways to the Myocardium

SANDRA J. PFAFF, R.N., B.S.N.

Faculty Member, Centers for Disease Control; Infection Control Nurse, Strong Memorial Hospital, Rochester, New York.

Wound Management: Clean Wounds, Contaminated Wounds, Decubiti, Burns

REBECCA A. PRESTON, R.N., B.S.N.

Medical Student, Albany Medical College, Albany, New York.

Intra-Aortic Balloon Pump Management, External Counterpressure with G-suit

PEGGY J. REILEY, R.N., M.S.

Head Nurse—Medical Unit, Beth Israel Hospital, Boston, Massachusetts.

Organ Donation

MARILYN M. RICCI, R.N., M.S.N., CNRN

Adjunct Professor, College of Nursing, Arizona State University, Tempe; Clinical Nurse Specialist, Neurology/Neurosurgery, Barrow Neurological Institute of St. Joseph's Hospital and Medical Center, Phoenix, Arizona.

Intracranial Pressure Monitoring, Lumbar and Cisternal Punctures, Hypothermia and Hyperthermia, Skeletal Traction of the Cervical Spine

MARY JO SCHREIBER, R.N., M.S.N., CCRN

Cardiovascular Clinical Nurse Specialist, Winter Haven Hospital, Winter Haven, Florida.

Blood and Blood Component Administration, Transfusion Reaction, Autotransfusion, Blood Warming, Use of a Blood Pump

RAE NADINE SMITH, R.N., M.S.N.

Clinical Nurse Specialist; President, Medical Communicators and Associates, Los Angeles, California.

Intracompartmental Pressure Monitoring

MARTHA I. SPENCE, R.N., M.N., CCRN

Instructor, Nursing Education, Baptist Hospital of Miami, Miami, Florida.

Cardioversion, Defibrillation

KIT STAHLER-MILLER, R.N., M.S.N.

Instructor, Department of Nursing, LaSalle University, Philadelphia, Pennsylvania.

Electrical Safety for Patients and Medical Device Operators

BARBARA TABOR, R.N., B.S.N., CEN

Nurse Consultant, Northwest Emergency Physicians, Kirkland, Washington.

Upper Gastrointestinal Hemorrhage, Gastric Lavage in Overdose, Paracentesis

CAROLYN A. TAMER, R.N., E.T.

Ostomy Clinician—Stoma Service, Massachusetts General Hospital, Boston, Massachusetts.

Stoma/Fistula Management

F. MICHAEL VISLOSKY, JR., R.N.

Clinical Research Nurse, Cardiac Unit/Intensive Study Area, Massachusetts General Hospital, Boston, Massachusetts.

Intra-Aortic Balloon Pump Management, External Counterpressure with G-suit, External Counterpressure with MAST Garment

KAREN L. WHEELOCK, R.N., B.S.N., M.A.

Director of Nursing Services, St. Olaf Hospital, Austin, Minnesota.

Noninvasive Peripheral Vascular Blood Flow Measurement, Rotating Tourniquets, Pericardiocentesis

CHERYL TOMICH WYMAN, R.N., B.S.N.

Head Nurse, Lake Washington Kidney Center/Northwest Kidney Center, Bellevue, Washington.

Acute Hemodialysis

PREFACE

The American Association of Critical-Care Nurses endorses the philosophy that each critically ill person has the right to expect nursing care provided by a critical care nurse. Critical care nursing practice requires the utilization of various procedures in the prevention of and intervention in life-threatening situations.

The *AACN Procedure Manual for Critical Care* has been written to provide the critical care nurse with specific procedural guidelines that can be used rapidly in adult critical care areas. This second edition contains many new features. The most readily apparent is the title change from the first edition, *Methods in Critical Care—The AACN Manual*. The second edition uses the term "procedure" rather than "method." This change was made because "procedure" is a more universally identifiable and acceptable term for those step-by-step protocols that are followed in critical care units every day. A new chapter, The Musculoskeletal System, has been added to the second edition. Because many critical care units admit multiple trauma patients daily, it is vital that critical care nurses be able to care effectively for patients in traction and patients requiring intracompartmental pressure monitoring. Other new procedures have been added throughout the text, and outdated procedures have been deleted. All the procedures have been reviewed for currency in equipment, generally accepted nursing practices, and references.

As with the first edition, the *AACN Procedure Manual for Critical Care* can also be utilized by nurses caring for critically ill patients outside of a critical care unit. In addition, it will be valuable in teaching entry-level and continuing education courses in critical care. The *AACN Procedure Manual for Critical Care* may also be used by institutions in the preparation of their own procedural manuals or be adopted in its entirety for use in courses to fulfill licensure or accreditation requirements.

Much has been written since the advent of critical care as a specialty. This manual presents a specific part of the most pertinent information. The procedures follow a consistent format: Overview and Instrumentation (as appropriate), Objectives, Special Equipment, Procedure, Precautions,

Related Care, and Complications. Illustrations are used throughout. For the user who requires additional theoretical background information, a sampling of references from the literature is included. Finally, a list of suppliers follows each procedure. Because equipment utilized within the critical care setting is constantly changing, it is a formidable, if not impossible, task to include all the manufacturers of equipment that can be utilized in critical care areas.

In addition, there are certain expectations common to the performance of the majority of the procedures. These expectations are that the critical care nurse will:

- Read the equipment operator manuals so as to become familiar with specific controls, functions, safety devices, trouble-shooting techniques, and precautions.
- Provide patients or family or both with appropriate explanations of the procedures and make sure they understand them. Emotional and intellectual preparation may lessen anxiety and increase cooperation. In some instances, the patient or family will require more detail and an educational process will have to be completed.
- Obtain a physician's order when required by the institution.
- Obtain permits signed by the patient or person legally permitted to sign when indicated. This process must be carried out carefully in light of legal requirements for informed consent.
- Ascertain the patient's allergy history to prevent unfavorable reactions to prep solutions, anesthetic agents, or drugs.
- Collect, organize, and set up equipment and supplies necessary for the efficient completion of the procedure.
- Wash hands prior to beginning of each procedure. This is one of the most significant and effective means of preventing nosocomial infections.
- Strictly adhere to sterile technique and assume an active, assertive role in implementing it.
- Integrate emotional support into each procedure. Many of the procedures cause discomfort or anxiety and will require use of touch or contact with the patient, frequent explanations, and an understanding of responses. Premedicating patients prior to initiating some of the procedures may also lessen the discomfort or anxiety.

It is important to note that these procedures are most appropriately carried out in the critical care environment. Support personnel, supplies, and emergency equipment must be immediately available.

There are some constraints imposed on the *AACN Procedure Manual for Critical Care* by the diverse nature of critical care practice. Identification of personnel who are permitted to perform the procedures is not included here because of varying institutional and state policies and regulations. There may also be differing requirements for certification or authorization by professional organizations. In addition, specific subspecialty procedures (e.g., pediatrics, neonatology, and others) have not been included.

These procedures have been written in light of what is accepted methodology supported by current literature. However, the only constant is change, and the fields of nursing and medicine are so broad that all acceptable modalities cannot be anticipated or be presented. The user must evaluate regional or institutional variability against established, acceptable principles.

Finally, there is a risk involved in writing a book like the *AACN Procedure Manual for Critical Care*. This is a manual oriented to technical tasks. It *cannot* be considered a sole resource that, if followed, will result in competent critical care practice. These procedures are not meant to be used in a vacuum. They are only one part of the holistic approach to critical care nursing, an approach based on a specific and thorough knowledge of the interrelatedness of body systems, the dynamic nature of the life process, and a recognition and appreciation of the individual's wholeness, uniqueness, and significant social and environmental relationships.

SALLY MILLAR
LESLIE K. SAMPSON
SISTER MAURITA SOUKUP

ACKNOWLEDGMENTS

We would like to acknowledge the work on this second edition that was done by our illustrator, Steve Moskowitz, of ARRCO Medical Art and Design, Boston, Massachusetts; our typists—Joanne Ernst, of Marion, Iowa; Jody Fitzgerald, of Boston, Massachusetts; and Judy Munroe, of Norwood, Massachusetts.

CONTENTS

1

THE
CARDIOVASCULAR
SYSTEM

ELECTROCARDIOGRAM

Norma Mock, R.N., B.S.N., M.S.

Overview

Within the field of critical care, electrocardiographic (ECG) monitoring is a required competency of the multidisciplinary health team. It may be done by using serial 12-lead ECG's, an isolated but continuous ECG lead system, or a computerized system that correlates multiple physiologic parameters. Select ECG monitoring is also available for the ambulatory patient.

12-Lead Electrocardiogram. The 12-lead ECG is a graphic recording of the electrical potential generated by the electrical activity of the heart. The electrical impulses generated by the heart's conduction system produce electrical currents that diffuse throughout the body. Electrodes, placed upon the surface of the body and connected to an electrocardiographic apparatus, record the mean electrical currents of the heart and produce the ECG. The primary purpose of the 12-lead ECG is to provide data related to the patient's cardiac electrical activity to help diagnose select pathologic conditions.

The 12-lead ECG may be useful in many ways to the critical care nurse. The areas in which the 12-lead ECG is most significant are summarized below.

MAJOR AREAS	IMPORTANCE
Dysrhythmia detection	Supraventricular, ventricular, and atrioventricular block of dysrhythmias
Cardiac electrical axis	Establishing presence of left anterior hemiblock and left posterior hemiblock; pacemaker tip location
Electrical changes associated with acute myocardial infarction	Current of injury, ischemia, necrosis
Electrical changes associated with bundle-branch block	Identifying left bundle-branch block and right bundle-branch block
Electrical changes associated with hypertrophy	Identifying left ventricular hypertrophy and right ventricular hypertrophy.

Two basic 12-lead ECG recorders are commonly used, the single-channel and three-channel ECG recorders. The single-channel ECG recorder (Fig.

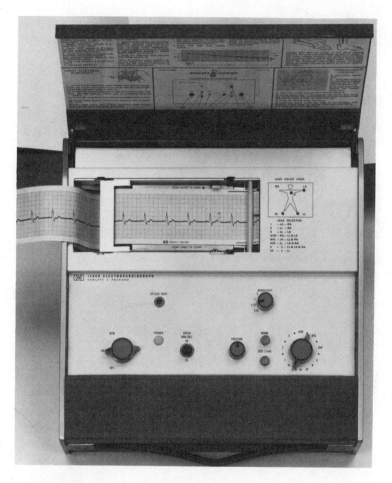

Figure 1-1. Single-channel ECG recorder. (Reprinted with permission of Hewlett-Packard Company.)

1-1) is directly controlled by the operator, thus allowing individual lead selection and variable lengths of lead recordings. The three-channel ECG recorder (Fig. 1-2) documents three consecutive leads simultaneously. Once the three-channel ECG recorder begins to operate, the 12-lead ECG is recorded without further input from the operator.

Both the single-channel and three-channel ECG recorders record 12-lead ECG's accurately; however, there are some situations in which selection of a specific recorder is advantageous. The single-channel ECG recorder is preferred when recording ECG's for uncooperative patients and arrest situations. For patients who are unable to cooperate, frequent stops and restarts may be necessary. The single-channel ECG recorder offers the operator more control over the resultant ECG. In arrest situations, paper use is voluminous. The single-lead ECG recorder minimizes this volume in comparison to that which the three-channel ECG would use, since the operator has control over the ECG machine. Use of the three-channel ECG recorder is advantageous when recording ECG's for routine 12-lead ECG's or evaluating ectopy or dysrhythmia, since the recording is obtained rapidly and one copy may be left for the patient's chart, thus omitting any delay due to mounting and interpreting. Also, simultaneous leads are advantageous in the diagnosis of difficult dysrhythmias and the determination of the origin of ventricular ectopy with more accuracy.

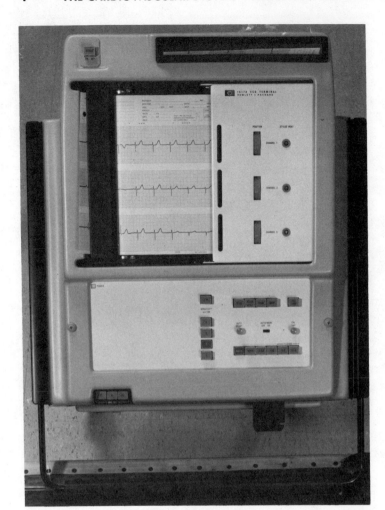

Figure 1-2. Three-channel ECG recorder. (Reprinted with permission of Hewlett-Packard Company.)

Computer analysis systems recently available as a tool to provide detailed calculated 12-lead ECG interpretation for the practitioner are helpful, particularly in emergency situations and for rapidity of readings. It should, however, be kept in mind that conditions may occur, as with computer assist analysis in bedside monitoring, producing errors of interpretation, and therefore interpretation should be regarded as "unofficial" until validated by an experienced professional.

Bedside ECG Monitoring System. The bedside ECG monitoring system (Fig. 1-3) permits observation of the ECG and relays information to the central monitoring station. An ECG lead system transmits the ECG signal from the patient's electrodes to the monitor. The location of the electrodes on the chest wall and the connecting lead system determine the QRS morphology, which is displayed on the bedside oscilloscope. While detailed instructions for specific bedside monitoring ECG systems can be found in the information manuals accompanying the system, standard components should be recognized:

Power—off/on switch.

Oscilloscope—permits direct visual observation of the ECG signal.

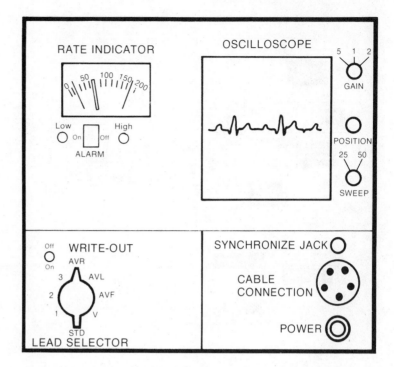

Figure 1-3. Bedside ECG monitoring.

Gain control—allows adjustment of amplitude for the QRS signal, usually set at 1 mV.

Position control—permits the ECG tracing to be adjusted to the top, bottom, or central area of the screen.

Sweep control—regulates the rate at which the ECG signal travels across the oscilloscope. The usual setting is 25 mm./second. A setting of 50 mm./second may be used to visualize the QRS morphology more adequately.

Rate indicator—averages and shows heart rate per minute, using a digital number or a rate meter.

Alarm system—integrated with the rate indicator, operates according to preset levels.

Additional components may include:

Lead selector—allows lead selection for monitoring; usually accompanies a five-lead cable system.

Synchronizer jack—used to connect to the defibrillator for cardioversion; located in the front or rear of the monitor.

Write-out—facilitates manual operation of the ECG recorder at a central nurses' station.

Central Monitoring Station.   The central monitoring station (Fig. 1-4) receives data from the bedside monitors, allows observation of several patients' ECG's at one time in a central area, provides the ability to document the ECG tracing away from the bedside automatically or manually, and reduces the number of staff members required to monitor a large number of patients' ECG recordings individually.

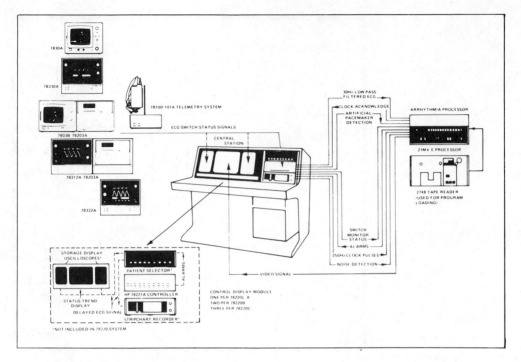

Figure 1-4. Central monitoring station. (Reprinted with permission of Hewlett-Packard Company.)

Components of the central console may include:

"Slave" oscilloscope—for continuous display of each patient's ECG rhythm, showing several patients at one time.

Direct recorder—for manual or automatic response in providing ECG recordings.

Memory tape loop—to record and later play back events immediately prior to and following an alarm situation.

Dysrhythmia detector—to "sense" QRS alternations in R-to-R intervals and institute an alarm.

Lead failure signal—to indicate *mechanical* failure in the monitoring cable system, differentiating from a patient alarm situation.

Timer-date marker—to mark the ECG tracing automatically; may also include a bed identification number.

Alarm system—to alert the staff of a patient emergency; this system is dependent upon information from the bedside monitor.

Computerized ECG Monitoring. The application of computer microprocessor techniques in the management of cardiac patients may be used for ECG monitoring in many ways. Computerized dysrhythmia systems provide periodic and demand ECG monitoring, a continuous scanning of ECG rhythms and patterns, an accumulation of data for review, and a system of audible and visual alarms in life-threatening situations. It must be borne in mind, however, that even though computers are valuable adjuncts to the nursing staff, they do not replace a staff member's ability to discern between

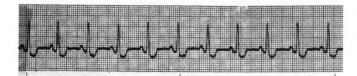 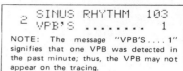

Figure 1-5. Status displays from computerized dysrhythmia system. (Reprinted with permission of Hewlett-Packard Company.)

a false alarm and a real emergency. Yet, computers do direct attention to cardiac rhythm variations that might otherwise go unnoticed. Computerized monitoring is advantageous for its processing power, which illustrates trends of the heart rate, ventricular extrasystoles, and other dysrhythmias.

Features of computerized ECG monitoring may include:

Continuous monitoring—performs an around-the-clock observation of rhythm and QRS patterns, providing a diagnosis as often as every minute.

Automatic detection of dysrhythmias—examines the morphology of the QRS as well as the rate and rhythm; detects ventricular dysrhythmias, supraventricular premature beats, and irregular rhythms.

Priority alarm system—alerts the nurse according to the severity of the condition, since alarms are coded for specific events. This also initiates operation of the strip chart recorder.

Detection of paced rhythms—displays a total number of paced and non-paced beats per minute; signals pacemaker nonfunction.

Status displays—provide continuous displays of heart rate, ectopic activity, rhythm, and monitoring status (Fig. 1-5).

Trend charts—provide instant display of significant events in a trend plot form, provided on demand (Fig. 1-6).

Telemetry. ECG telemetry allows transmission of the ECG without requiring that the patient be attached to a monitor by lead wires. It is especially practical for an ambulatory cardiac patient resuming progressive activity. Telemetry monitoring involves attaching a two-lead system to the pa-

Figure 1-6. Trend recording. (Reprinted with permission of Hewlett-Packard Company.)

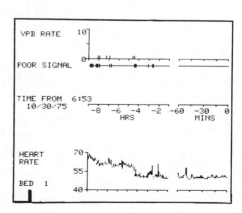

tient, connecting it to a small transmitter about the size of a small transistor radio, and securing the transmitter to the patient.

Components of a telemetry system include:

Transmitter—emits a signal to a receiver with which it is paired. (This signal may be lost or interfered with for various reasons. Check the manual or contact a service representative if this occurs.)

Antenna—usually incorporated into the lead wires. Transmission may be further enhanced by the installation of an antenna at the acute health care facility.

Receiver—usually located at a central station, along with an oscilloscope, for monitoring several patients at one time. It can pick up several transmitting signals simultaneously.

Special features offered by a telemetry system include the ability to switch from a monitor to a diagnostic trace, the ability to be converted to a regular cable or "hard wire" system, a signal indicating battery depletion, a special jack to transmit the signal over the telephone, and a delay switch to minimize false alarms.

The critical care nurse assumes multidimensional responsibility for ECG monitoring. This section describes methods for a 12-lead ECG, lead systems, and telemetry.

12–LEAD ECG

Objective

To provide data regarding the patient's electrical cardiac activity for diagnostic purposes, utilizing a single-channel or three-channel ECG recorder.

Special Equipment

ECG recorder: single-channel or
   three-channel ECG recorder
ECG recording paper
Electrode cable
Four limb electrode plates with
   electrode straps
Chest suction cup for single-channel
   ECG recorder
Six chest suction cups for three-
   channel ECG recorder
ECG electrode gel
Alcohol prep pads
Gauze pads

Procedure

ACTION

1. Prepare ECG recorder.
    A. Select single-channel or three-channel ECG recorder.
    B. Plug in grounded ECG recorder.
    C. Activate power on ECG recorder.

2. Prepare patient.
    A. Place patient in supine position in the center of the bed for adequate support to all limbs.
    B. Expose the forearms, forelegs, and chest.
    C. Check that feet do not touch foot board of bed.

3. Apply limb leads (Fig.1-7).

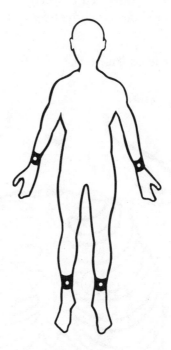

Figure 1-7.   Limb lead location for 12-lead ECG.

A. Use one ECG electrode plate for inner aspect of each forearm and for medial aspect of each lower leg.
B. Cleanse skin site with alcohol prep pad.

C. Apply electrode gel to skin site and rub onto the ECG electrode plate to ensure good contact.
D. Secure ECG electrode plates with electrode straps; check tension.

RATIONALE

A. See "Overview" for advantages.

A. The skin sites selected should ensure good contact and stabilization of the ECG electrode plate.

B. Removing oil from the skin surfaces enhances ECG electrode contact and controls for artifact.

D. Straps that are too tight may induce artifacts on tracing; electrodes should be placed so that the patient cable may be attached without bending or pulling the individual lead wires.

ACTION	**RATIONALE**
E. Attach limb lead cable wires to appropriate ECG electrodes.	E. The tip of each lead cable wire is lettered and color-coded for easy identification.

E. Attach limb lead cable wires to appropriate ECG electrodes.
  (1) Use white or RA for right arm.
  (2) Use black or LA for left arm.
  (3) Use red or LL for left leg.
  (4) Use green or RL for right leg.
  (5) Use brown or V1-6 for chest lead.

E. The tip of each lead cable wire is lettered and color-coded for easy identification.

F. Verify that each limb lead ECG electrode is positioned properly and secured on the correct extremity.

F. Avoid draping the cable over the abdomen, as this will cause a respiratory artifact.

4. Apply chest leads (Fig. 1-8).

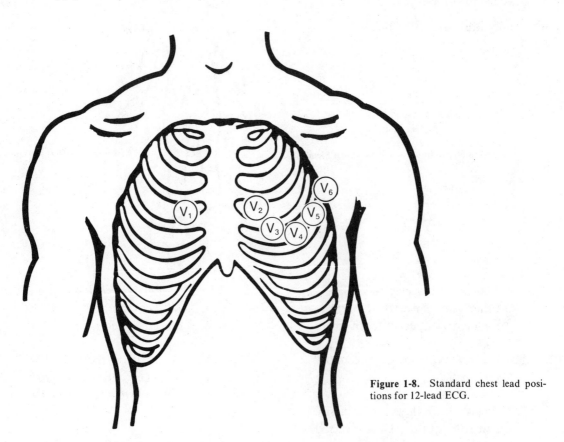

Figure 1-8. Standard chest lead positions for 12-lead ECG.

A. Single-channel ECG recorder:
  (1) Place chest suction cup electrode on brown tip of patient cable marked "C."
  (2) Cleanse sites with alcohol prep pads.

ACTION   RATIONALE

(3) Apply electrode gel to chest
    lead sites.
    (a) Use fourth intercostal
        space, right sternal
        border, for V_1.
    (b) Use fourth intercostal
        space, left sternal bord-
        er, for V_2.
    (c) Use location midway
        between V_2 and V_4 for
        V_3.
    (d) Use fifth intercostal
        space, left of sternum,
        midclavicular line, for
        V_4.
    (e) Use fifth intercostal
        space, left of sternum,
        anterior axillary line, for
        V_5.
    (f) Use fifth intercostal
        space, left of sternum,
        midaxillary line, for V_6.
(4) Secure suction cup to
    predetermined site to record
    individual chest leads.

B. Three-channel ECG recorder:
   (1) Place all six suction cups on
       appropriate six chest lead tips
       of the patient cable as
       described for single channel
       recorder.
   (2) Apply electrode gel to chest
       lead sites.
   (3) Secure all six suction cups to
       predetermined and gelled
       sites.

5. Record the ECG.
   A. Single-channel ECG recorder (Fig.
      1-9):
      (1) Turn power switch to "run."
          ECG recording paper should
          feed correctly.
      (2) Turn lead selector switch to
          "STD" (standard) position.
      (3) Center the stylus on the
          ECG paper using position
          control; adjust heat control.

ACTION   RATIONALE

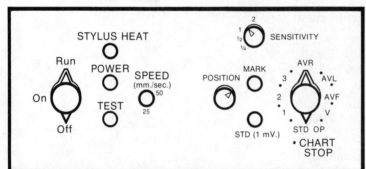

Figure 1-9. Single-channel ECG recorder.

(4) Press the STD 1 mV. button.
    (a) Check for deflection.
    (b) Adjust to 1 mV. if standardization is not correct.
(5) Press marker button; note code on lower or upper edge of ECG paper.
(6) Return power switch to "on" to stop paper flow.
(7) Place lead selector to lead I.
(8) Turn power switch to "run" and record approximately 10 beats.
(9) Mark lead I with appropriate code. Suggested code:

Lead I ___
Lead II ___ ___
Lead III ___ ___ ___
AVR _____
AVL _____ _____
AVF _____ _____ _____
V_1 _____ ___
V_2 _____ ___ ___
V_3 _____ ___ ___ ___
V_4 _____ ___ ___ ___ ___
V_5 _____ ___ ___ ___ ___ ___
V_6 _____ ___ ___ ___ ___ ___ ___

(10) Repeat steps 5 through 8 for each frontal plane lead.
(11) Return power switch to "on" and apply chest suction cups to brown chest electrode.
(12) Turn lead selector switch to "V" and record all chest leads.
(13) Apply electrode gel to the six chest lead sites.

(4) The ECG is standardized to assure that at 1 mV, the deflection will be 10 mm.; at 0.5 mV, the deflection will be 5 mm. (Each small square on the recording paper equals 1 mm.)

ACTION	RATIONALE

(14) Place the suction cup on V_1 site.

(15) Turn power switch to "run" and record.

(16) Repeat process for each chest lead, moving the suction cup appropriately.

B. Three-channel ECG recorder (Fig. 1-10):

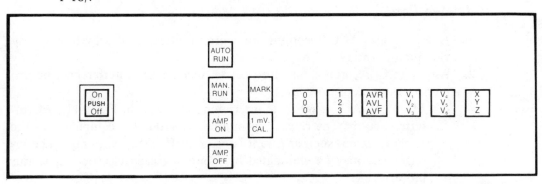

(1) Position all leads, including the six chest leads, before the recording process is started.

(2) Standardize to 1 mV.

(3) Turn paper speed to 25 mm./second.

(4) Turn on automatic marking.

(5) Depress AUTO–RUN button to record 12 leads in approximately 12 to 30 seconds.

    (a) To interrupt an ECG recording, press the reset button and AUTO–RUN for a new ECG recording.

    (b) Use manual mode as an option for further studies of select leads or for dysrhythmia recordings.

6. Turn off ECG recorder.

7. Remove ECG electrodes from patient; cleanse site and equipment.

8. Label ECG recording with patient's name, medical record number, date, and time; mount ECG recording appropriately.

Figure 1-10. Three-channel ECG recorder.

Precautions

1. Follow electrical safety guidelines. Ground ECG recorder and any electrical equipment in direct contact with patient for safety and to enhance the quality of the ECG recording.
2. Check accuracy of lead placement. Inaccurate chest lead placement may misrepresent the anterior surface of the heart. If the leads are mistakenly placed below the fifth intercostal space, a horizontal plane lead may be inadvertently transposed into a frontal plane lead.

Related Care

1. Assess 12-lead ECG recording for warning of lethal dysrhythmias; provide prompt intervention.
2. Assess ECG recording for electrical or mechanical interference, or improper electrode placement:
   A. Electrical, AC, or 60-cycle interference (as seen in Fig. 1-11); AC interference may be caused by improperly grounded equipment in the patient's room, such as a ventilator or an IV infusion pump. The interference may be eliminated by grounding each electrical apparatus properly.

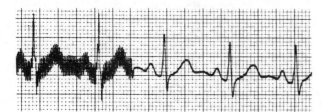

Figure 1-11.   AC interference.

   B. Mechanical interference, muscle tremor, singultus, or seizure activity activity may cause mechanical interference (as shown in Fig. 1-12). Mechanical interference may be eliminated by treating the cause; e.g., if muscle tremor is due to shivering or chilling, provide warm environment.

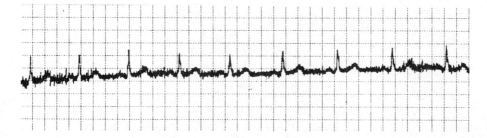

Figure 1-12.   Mechanical interference.

   C. Improper electrode placement in the limb leads is usually seen on lead I, where the left arm and the right arm may have been accidentally reversed. Lead reversal is demonstrated in Figure 1-13; correct lead placement is shown in Figure 1-14.

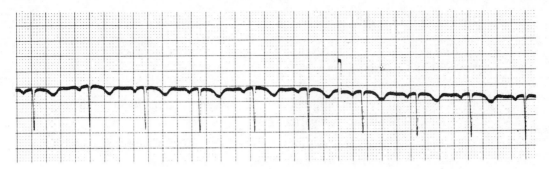

Figure 1-13. Lead reversal.

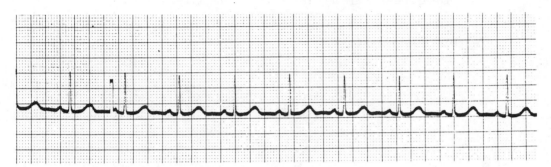

Figure 1-14. Correct lead placement.

3. Note adjustments in recordings of 0.5 or 2 mv. by providing calibration marking on 12-lead ECG.

4. Adjust paper speed to enable better examination of complexes during periods of rapid heart rate.

5. In the case of an amputee, apply electrode to stump of affected extremity.

6. Apply electrodes high on extremities for patient with involuntary trembling.

7. Use minimal suction with suction cups when patient is being anticoagulated.

Complications

Dysrhythmias
Altered skin integrity
Electromicroshock
Equipment malfunction

REFERENCES

AACN: Clinical Reference for Critical-Care Nursing (edited by M. Kinney, et al). New York, McGraw-Hill, 1981.

Andreoli, K. G., et al.: Comprehensive Cardiac Care, 4th ed. St. Louis, C.V. Mosby, 1979, pp. 87–127.

Brunner, L.F., and Suddarth, D.S.: Lippincott Manual of Nursing Practice, 3rd ed. Philadelphia: J.B. Lippincott, 1982.

Conover, M.: Understanding Electrocardiography: Physiological and Interpretive Concepts, 3rd ed. St. Louis, C.V. Mosby, 1981.

LEAD SYSTEMS

Objectives

1. To determine the appropriate ECG lead system for therapeutic ECG monitoring of selected patients.

2. To provide an adequate and stable QRS complex and signal voltage, ensuring both visual observation and optimal monitoring operation.

3. To enhance individualization and flexibility among lead selections to recognize and diagnose electrical cardiac abnormalities.

Special Equipment

ECG monitor
Electrodes (pregelled disposable or nondisposable and electrode gel)
Razor

Gauze pads
Alcohol prep pads
Computerized monitoring equipment (optional)

Procedure

ACTION	RATIONALE
1. Prepare bedside ECG monitor and central monitoring station as directed by manufacturer.	
2. Apply ECG electrodes to preselected and prepared skin sites.	2. Proper application of electrodes will enhance quality of ECG recording, with a distinct R wave.
A. Choose sites for electrode placement (see 3, below, for options).	A. Care should be taken to avoid skeletal muscle by using the hollow of the clavicles and the lower sides of the thoracic cage.
B. Shave a 4- X 4-inch square site for each electrode.	B. Removal of hair will minimize patient discomfort and facilitate conduction.
C. Clean areas with alcohol prep pad, rubbing dry with gauze pads and abrading the skin lightly.	C. Removal of skin oils and debris reduces the barrier to electrical flow.
D. Connect electrode to lead wire.	
E. Apply gel-coated electrode to predetermined sites, pressing firmly in a circular pattern.	E. Pressure applied on electrode may cause disbursement of gel with poor adhesive contact.
3. Select lead system (options).	

ACTION	RATIONALE

A.   Three-lead system:

(1)   Lead II (Fig. 1-15):

  (a)   Apply negative electrode to first intercostal space, right sternal border.

  (b)   Apply positive electrode to fourth intercostal space, left midclavicular line.

  (c)   Apply ground electrode at fourth intercostal space, right sternal border.

(1)   This is best utilized for a positive and tall QRS complex and normally has a good positive P wave. Also, this may be used for observation of QRS axis change denoting left anterior hemiblock.

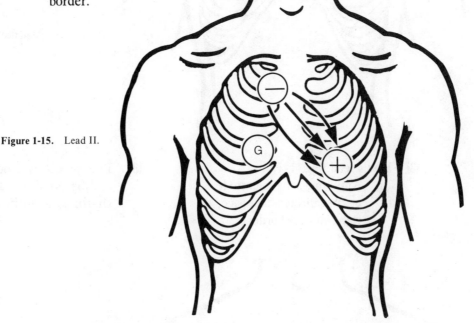

Figure 1-15.   Lead II.

(2) MCL_1 (modified chest lead V_1) (Fig. 1-16):

  (a)   Apply negative electrode just inferior to left clavicle, midclavicular line.

  (b)   Apply positive electrode at fourth intercostal space, right sternal border.

  (c)   Apply ground electrode just inferior to right clavicle, midclavicular line.

(2)   This is an excellent lead for identifying left or right bundle-branch block, the differential diagnosis of ventricular ectopy, and a shift in pacing catheter electrode sites. It produces variable P-wave polarity and a negative QRS complex.

ACTION   RATIONALE

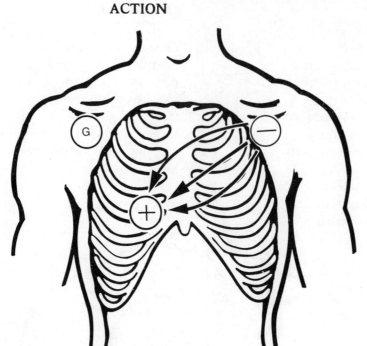

Figure 1-16.   Modified chest Lead I.

(3) Lewis lead (Fig. 1-17):
     (a) Apply negative electrode
          at first intercostal space,
          right sternal border.

(3) This produces good P waves
     and is used in atrial dys-
     rhythmia identification.

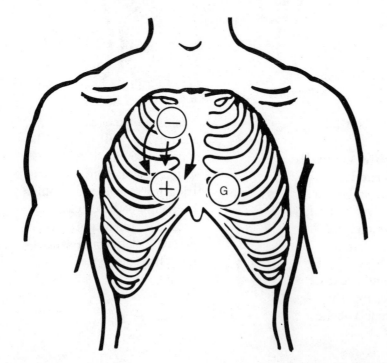

Figure 1-17.   Lewis Lead.

ACTION	RATIONALE

(b) Apply positive electrode at fourth intercostal space, right sternal border.

(c) Apply ground electrode at the fourth intercostal space, left sternal border.

(4) MCL$_3$ (modified chest lead III) (Fig. 1-18):

   (a) Apply negative electrode just inferior to left clavicle, midclavicular line.

   (b) Apply positive electrode on last left intercostal space, midclavicular line.

   (c) Apply ground electrode inferior to right clavicle, midclavicular line.

(4) This offers another lead position for a positive QRS complex.

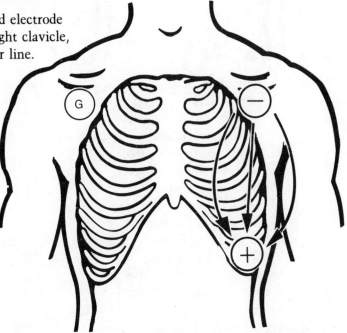

Figure 1-18. Modified Lead III.

(5) MCL$_6$ (modified chest lead V$_6$) (Fig. 1-19):

   (a) Apply negative electrode inferior to left clavicle, midclavicular line.

   (b) Apply positive electrode to fifth intercostal space, midclavicular line.

   (c) Apply ground electrode inferior to right clavicle, midclavicular line.

(5) This is used frequently for patients with median sternotomy incisions and for telemetry monitoring. A tall QRS complex, ST- and T-wave changes, and left ventricular ectopy and right bundle-branch block can be identified.

ACTION   RATIONALE

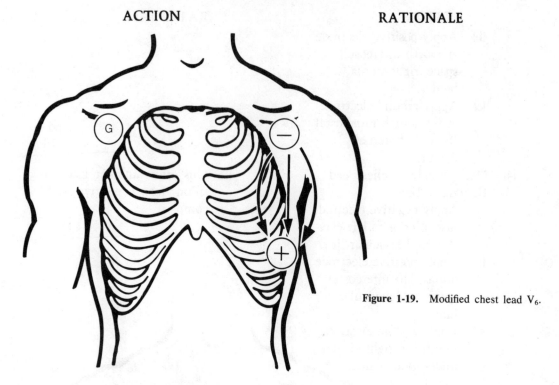

Figure 1-19.   Modified chest lead V_6.

(6) Marriott MCL_6 lead:
   (a) Apply negative electrode inferior to right clavicle, midclavicular line.
   (b) Apply positive electrode to fifth intercostal space, midclavicular line.
   (c) Apply ground electrode inferior to left clavicle, midclavicular line.

B. Five-lead system (Fig. 1-20):
   (1) Apply RA electrode inferior to right clavicle, midclavicular line.
   (2) Apply LA electrode inferior to left clavicle, midclavicular line.
   (3) Apply RL electrode on sixth intercostal space, right midclavicular line.
   (4) Apply LL electrode on sixth intercostal space, left midclavicular line.
   (5) Apply chest lead electrode on selected chest sites V_1, V_2, V_3, V_4, V_5, or V_6 position.

(6) This lead system offers the feasibility of switching from MCL_1 to MCL_6 by moving only the positive electrode.

B. The five-lead system facilitates rapid ECG monitoring from select sites. It should not be used as a complete 12-lead ECG for diagnostic purposes.

ACTION

RATIONALE

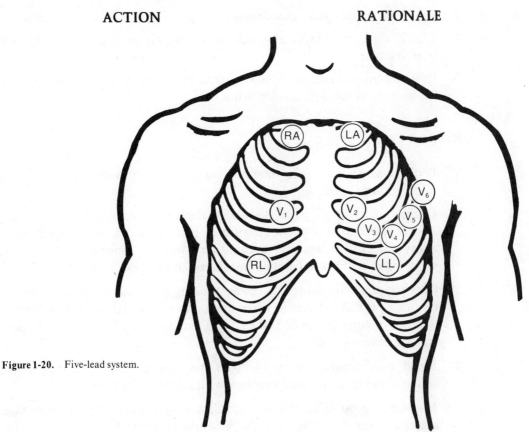

Figure 1-20.   Five-lead system.

(a)   Place V electrode in an
      insulating material if
      not used on patient's
      chest.

(6)   Activate ECG lead selector
      for desired lead; record.

4.   Examine ECG recording; verify quali-
     ty of R wave.

5.   Set rate alarms.

6.   Label recording for the lead system
     selected.

7.   Enter into computerized dysrhythmia
     system as directed by manufacturer.

(a)   This maintains electrical
      patient isolation.

4.   The R wave should be approximately
     twice the height of the wave form
     components to assure proper ECG
     triggering.

Precautions

1.   Check that alarms are always on.

2.   Provide defibrillator, emergency cart, and medications for immediate use
     as necessary.

3. Follow electrical safety guidelines.

4. Check tension of ECG electrode wires, which may contribute to lead wire fractures.

5. Integrate monitoring with observation and care of the cardiac patient. Monitoring is one tool among many.

Related Care

1. Perform continuous ECG monitor surveillance; provide prompt nursing intervention as necessary.

2. Check quality of pregelled disposable electrodes. Since quality and adhesion characteristics vary, a mixture of brands should not be used. Also, always check the disc after opening for sufficient moist gel; loss of ECG gel or paste will cause baseline instability and motion artifact.

3. Check contact of electrodes, using thorough site cleansing and application of new ECG electrode when appropriate. For excessive perspiration, tincture of benzoin applied to electrode adhesive sites may help to maintain an adhesive bond.

4. Assess skin integrity every 24 hours; rotate electrode sites. Skin allergy or sensitivity is a potential problem with adhesive bonding.

5. Maintain a good ECG monitor recording with a good QRS signal voltage, a stable clear baseline, and the absence of artifact or distortion (Fig. 1–21).

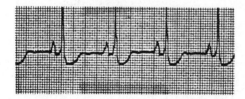

Figure 1-21. Good quality QRS signal, stable clear baseline, absence of artifact.

6. Check for potential source of false alarm triggering.
    A. High rate alarm may be due to:
        (1) Excessive gain, causing the T wave to be "sensed" by the monitor as well as the R wave, thus doubling the rate.
        (2) Excessive muscle artifact, caused by patient movement.
        (3) Insufficient increase in high rate alarm setting above the patient's own rate.
    B. Low rate alarm may be due to:
        (1) Insufficient gain setting.
        (2) Presence of a wandering baseline, with not all signals being sensed.
        (3) Decrease of R wave signal on a particular lead, caused by axis shift.
        (4) Insufficient decrease in low rate alarm setting below the patient's own rate.

C. Other causes of false alarm triggering may be due to a loose lead, dried electrode gel, patient movement, muscle tremor due to shivering or seizure, damaged cable or leads, or AC interference.

7. Check quality of electrode contact for patients with temporary or permanent pacemakers; electrodes should be changed every 24 hours. (Minute charge build-up in electrode may occur, producing pacer inhibition).

8. Identify alterations in ECG monitor recordings.
    A. Low voltage signal (Fig. 1–22):

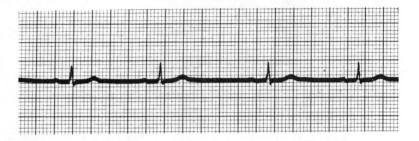

Figure 1-22. Low voltage signal.

(1) Potential causes:
    (a) Low gain setting on the ECG monitor.
    (b) Poor electrode contact or disconnected electrode.
    (c) Disconnected or broken lead wire.
    (d) Loose cable connection from the monitor.
    (e) Loss of amplitude of QRS signal.
(2) Significance: Will trigger false low rate alarm.
(3) Intervention:
    (a) Check connections of lead wires and cable.
    (b) Reapply electrode as required.
    (c) Increase the gain.
    (d) Trouble-shoot for specific lead problem.

    B. Excessive artifact (Fig. 1–23):

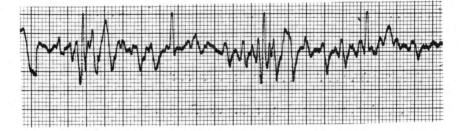

Figure 1-23. Excessive artifact.

(1) Potential causes:
    (a) Patient movement
    (b) Dry or loose electrode.
    (c) Intermittent electrical interference.
(2) Significance:
    (a) Excessive artifact may cause irregular oscillations on the ECG trace.

(b)   May allow dysrhythmias to go unnoticed.

(c)   May trigger the false high rate alarm.

(3)   Intervention:

(a)   Check electrode contact.

(b)   Reposition electrodes to an area with less skeletal muscle.

(c)   Check lead wires for stress on patient movement.

C.   Electrical interference (Fig. 1-24):

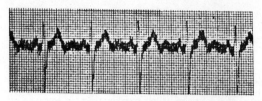

Figure 1-24.   Electrical interference.

(1)   Potential causes:

(a)   Improper electrical equipment grounding.

(b)   X-ray or diathermy equipment in operation.

(c)   Exposed broken lead wires or cables.

(2)   Significance: (a) ECG trace may be distorted by the production of 60 cycle per second artifact; (b) Presents a potential hazard to the patient.

(3)   Intervention: The source may be isolated by disconnecting pieces of electrical equipment surrounding the patient one at a time, while checking for the elimination of the problem.

D.   Wandering ECG baseline (Fig. 1-25):

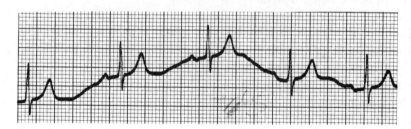

Figure 1-25.   Wandering baseline.

(1)   Potential causes:

(a)   Poor electrode contact or too much gel.

(b)   Tension on electrode and lead wires.

(c)   Movement of the cable with respiration.

(2)   Significance:

(a)   Provides a tracing difficult to interpret for rhythm.

(b)   May trigger alarms, since not all beats will be sensed by the monitor.

(3)   Intervention:

(a)   Check tension on lead wires and cable.

(b)   Reposition the patient cable to the side of the chest or wherever there is the least movement.

(c)   Replace electrodes as required.

E.   Poor quality ECG recordings in select leads:

(1)   Intervention: Isolate cause to select ECG lead; correct.

Poor ECG Recordings in: *Potential Source:*

Leads I, II, III   RL electrode/lead wire
Leads II, III   LL electrode/lead wire
Leads I, II   RA electrode/lead wire
Leads I, III   LA electrode/lead wire
Lead V   Lead wire

Complications

Dysrhythmias   Altered skin integrity
Cardiac arrest   Equipment malfunction
Electromicroshock

Suppliers

Abbott   Hewlett-Packard
American Optical   Lexington
Datascope   Midwest Analog and Digital
Electrodyne   Siemens
Electronics-for-Medicine   Telemed

REFERENCES

AACN: Clinical Reference for Critical-Care Nursing, (edited by M. Kinney et al.), New York, McGraw-Hill, 1981.

Andreoli, K.G., et al.: Comprehensive Cardiac Care, 4th ed. St. Louis, C.V. Mosby, 1979.

Brunner, L.F., and Suddarth, S.D.: Lippincott Manual of Nursing Practice, 3rd ed. Philadelphia, J.B. Lippincott, 1982.

Conover, M.: Understanding Electrocardiography: Physiological and Interpretive Concepts, 3rd ed. St. Louis, C.V. Mosby, 1980.

TELEMETRY _____

Objective

To maintain continuous ECG monitoring utilizing a select lead-to-transmitter system for patients requiring progressive ambulatory activity and freedom from lead-to-monitor cable attachment.

Special Equipment

Telemetry unit   ECG electrodes
Battery   Alcohol prep pads
Patient cable

Procedure

ACTION	RATIONALE
1. Prepare display control console.	1. This enters patient into system for continuous ECG surveillance.

2. Apply electrodes to patient's chest for desired lead system.
   A. Lead II (Fig. 1-26):

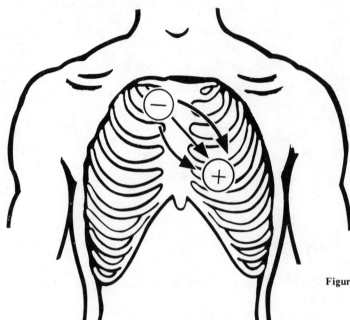

Figure 1-26.   Lead II. Telemetry monitoring.

   (1) Apply negative electrode to first intercostal space, right of sternal border.
   (2) Apply positive electrode at fourth intercostal space, left of midclavicular line.
   B. MCL$_1$ (Fig. 1-27);
   (1) Apply negative electrode left of midclavicular line, below clavicle.
   (2) Apply positive electrode at fourth intercostal space, right of sternal border.

3. Place battery in telemetry unit; check battery position for positive (+) and negative (−) poles.

4. Place ECG cable from telemetry unit to corresponding ECG electrodes for desired lead system.

ACTION   RATIONALE

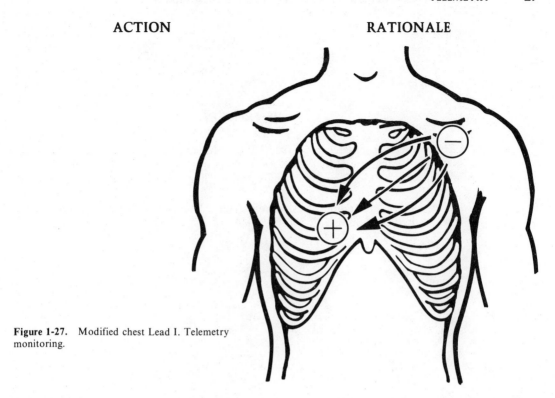

Figure 1-27.   Modified chest Lead I. Telemetry
monitoring.

5.   Check ECG pattern on display control
     oscilloscope; set rate alarms.

Precautions

1.   Check for proper ECG electrode placement and security.
2.   Monitor patient's activity location for prompt intervention should dys-
     rhythmias occur.
3.   Provide defibrillator, emergency cart, and medications for immediate use
     as necessary.

Related Care

1.   Observe for dysrhythmias; provide appropriate nursing intervention.
2.   Protect transmitter from direct trauma by securing in a gown pocket or
     in a pouch around the neck, or on a belt designed with a pocket.
3.   Change battery for telemetry unit as necessary, utilizing indicator light.
4.   Reposition ECG electrodes and assess skin integrity every 24 hours.

Complications

Dysrhythmias
Altered skin integrity
Equipment malfunctions

Suppliers

Abbott
Hewlett-Packard

REFERENCES

AACN: Clinical Reference for Critical-Care Nursing (edited by M. Kinney et al.). New York, McGraw-Hill, 1981.

Andreoli, K.G., et al.: Comprehensive Cardiac Care, 4th ed. St. Louis, C.V. Mosby, 1974.

Conover, M. Understanding Electrocardiography: Physiological and Interpretive Concepts, 3rd ed. St. Louis, C.V. Mosby, 1974.

CARDIOVERSION

Martha I. Spence, R.N., M.N., CCRN

Overview

Cardioversion is an elective therapy to terminate tachydysrhythmias by delivering a synchronized direct current charge. This charge simultaneously depolarizes the entire myocardium, thereby interrupting reentry circuits and establishing electrical homogeneity. As a result, the sinoatrial node resumes control of the rhythm. Synchronization with QRS complex permits timing the electrical discharge so that it appears outside the vulnerable period of the T wave of the ECG.

Cardioversion is often effective in terminating atrial tachycardia, atrial flutter, atrial fibrillation, and ventricular tachycardia. Dysrhythmias associated with digitalis toxicity should not be terminated electrically because of the possibility of initiating complex ventricular ectopic rhythms after cardioversion. Digitalis is usually discontinued for 2 or more days prior to elective cardioversion, depending upon the specific glycoside preparation being used. Premedication with antiarrhythmic drugs is a common practice for ensuring maintenance of postconversion rhythms.

Objective

To convert select supraventricular and ventricular tachydysrhythmias to sinus rhythm.

Special Equipment

Cardioverter/defibrillator capable of delivering a synchronized shock
Paddles: anterior-posterior or transverse
ECG monitor and recorder
Conductive medium or conductive pads
Oxygen therapy equipment
Airway
Resuscitator bag
Emergency pacing equipment
Emergency cart and medications

Procedure

ACTION	RATIONALE
1. Obtain a 12-lead ECG.	1. Recording of the precardioversion rhythm provides a baseline to be compared with that of postcardioversion ECG.

ACTION	RATIONALE
2. Secure patient's IV line.	2. This provides an access route for administration of medications, anesthetic, or both.
3. Place patient in supine position.	3. The supine position facilitates a clear ECG recording, proper placement of paddles, easier access for resuscitation, and greater relaxation with limb support.
4. Administer oxygen as prescribed *prior* to cardioversion; discontinue at the moment of cardioversion.	4. Unless contraindicated, oxygen therapy 5 to 10 minutes before cardioversion promotes myocardial oxygenation. In the presence of electrical arcing, oxygen may support combustion.
5. Assess patient, including vital signs, cardiac rhythm, peripheral pulses, and mentation level.	5. These data will serve as a baseline for postcardioversion evaluation.
6. Remove dentures or dental prosthesis as appropriate.	6. This reduces the risk of airway obstruction. Removal of dentures is not always appropriate; airway support is sometimes enhanced by dentures.
7. Prepare cardioversion equipment.	
A. Attach the patient to the ECG monitor, selecting a lead with a distinct tall R wave and a T wave of small magnitude or in a direction opposite to the R wave.	A. The synchronizer times the electrical current to be delivered only on the patient's R wave. Improper synchronization can lead to discharge on the T wave and result in ventricular fibrillation.
(1) Check monitor for artifact; change leads if artifact is present.	(1) Proper electrode placement and contact are critical, since artifact could result in the electrical current being delivered at an improper time during the cardiac cycle.
B. Plug grounded equipment into electrical outlet.	B. Proper grounding will prevent current leaks, microshocks, or accidental electrocution.
C. Turn power switch on several minutes prior to use.	C. Most equipment requires a warm-up period.
D. Turn synchronizer switch on.	D. In the synchronizing mode, the machine will sense an R wave and discharge the preset electrical

ACTION

RATIONALE

current. If the synchronizing mode is not activated, discharge occurs at the instant the paddle buttons are depressed, regardless of the phase of the cardiac cycle.

E. Monitor or test, or both, for synchronization.
   (1) Use manual synchronization button to determine the proper timing of the electrical charge. (Optional, depending upon equipment.)
   (2) Observe that charge release appears on the downslope of the R wave or within the S wave.

E. This will ensure proper synchronization of charge to QRS and charge release outside of vulnerable period.

8. Administer medication as ordered.

8. Electrical shocks vary from being uncomfortable to being painful, depending upon the patient and the voltage used. If a short-acting anesthetic agent is administered, it is recommended that an anesthesiologist or nurse anesthetist be present for respiratory support.

9. Prepare paddles by applying conductive medium to metal surface of paddles or conductive pads to chest surface.

9. Conductive medium reduces resistance of skin to current flow, Adequate coverage of metal surfaces will prevent skin burns and allow for optimal flow to the myocardium. Excess conducting medium contributes to skin burns and electrical arcing. The use of conductive pads greatly reduces the possibility of arcing as well as skin burns.

10. Charge cardioversion machine to prescribed voltage.
   A. Check that power switch is on and synchronizer mode is activated.
   B. Turn selector dial to the prescribed number of watt-seconds.

B. The current level is prescribed by the physician according to the patient's body weight, ECG rhythm, and precardioversion medication(s). Normally a low watt-seconds selection is used initially (5 to 25 joules or watt-

ACTION	RATIONALE
	seconds); this is then increased in small increments as prescribed by the physician. For emergency cardioversion, A.H.A. recommends 200 joules (watt-seconds) be used initially. Many dysrhythmias will convert with low voltages. The larger the voltage, the more tissue trauma and the greater discomfort to the patient.

C.   Activate charge button.

11. Place paddles firmly into position against the chest, using approximately 25 to 30 lb. of pressure (Fig. 1-28).

11. Firm pressure establishes good contact. Current should flow across axis of cardiac muscle mass, regardless of paddle position used.

ANTERIOR-POSTERIOR

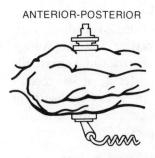

TRANSVERSE

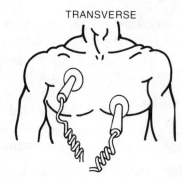

Figure 1-28.   Placement of paddles on chest.

A.   Transverse position:
   (1)   Place one paddle at second intercostal space, to the right of sternum.
   (2)   Place second paddle at fifth intercostal space midclavicular line, to the left of sternum.

B.   Anterior-posterior position:
   (1)   Place one paddle at anterior-precordial area.
   (2)   Place second paddle at posterior-intrascapular area.

B.   Anterior-posterior position may decrease amount of current required.

12. Check ECG rhythm on monitor.

12. ECG rhythm may change prior to cardioversion.

13. Activate ECG recorder.

13. ECG rhythm may change prior to cardioversion.

14. Check for synchronization indication superimposed on the patient's R wave as presented on the ECG oscilloscope.

14. This ensures proper synchronization.

ACTION	RATIONALE
15. Stand clear of bed and give command to stand clear.	15. Electrical current follows the path of least resistance; this measure reduces risk of accidental microshock or macroshock.
16. Depress discharge buttons on the two paddles simultaneously; keep both firmly depressed until the electrical current is delivered.	16. Premature release of discharge buttons may result in failure of the machine to discharge energy.
17. Assess ECG rhythm to ascertain postcardioversion ECG rhythm (Figs. 1-29 and 1-30).	17. Cardioversion may convert original ECG rhythm, have no effect, or produce a lethal disrhythmia.

LEAD II

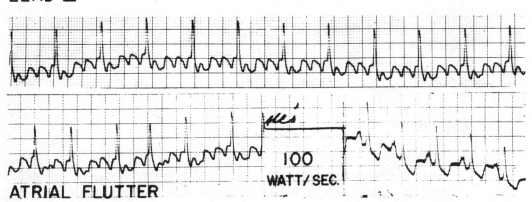

ATRIAL FLUTTER

100 WATT/SEC.

Figure 1-29. Cardioversion of atrial flutter.

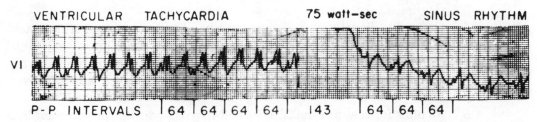

VENTRICULAR TACHYCARDIA   75 watt-sec   SINUS RHYTHM

VI

P-P INTERVALS | 64 | 64 | 64 | 64 | 143 | 64 | 64 | 64 |

Figure 1-30. Cardioversion of ventricular tachycardia.

ACTION	RATIONALE
18. Repeat procedure as prescribed to terminate tachydysrhythmia.	18. Repeated cardioversion therapy is given by increasing current in small increments as prescribed by the physician and separating each attempt by approximately 3 minutes.

ACTION	RATIONALE

19. Perform postcardioversion care:

A. Assess the patient, especially the level of consciousness and respiratory status, immediately after cardioversion:
   (1) Airway patency.
   (2) Respiratory rate and depth.
   (3) Lung sounds.
   (4) Need for supplemental oxygen.

A. Sedation may contribute to respiratory depression and decreased level of consciousness.

   (1) Airway support is commonly required for a short time after cardioversion.

B. Record ECG rhythm by a 12-lead ECG.

B. This validates effects of cardioversion and allows assessment of myocardial damage.

C. Monitor the patient's ECG rhythm continuously for the next 2 hours.

D. Observe skin of chest wall for presence of burns.

E. Reorient and support patient as necessary.

Precautions

1. Check that cardioversion is performed in a setting where resuscitation and respiratory support are immediately available. It is recommended that an anesthesiologist or nurse anesthetist be immediately available.
2. Check that equipment being used is properly grounded to prevent current leakage.
3. Determine serum potassium levels prior to cardioversion. Hypokalemia enhances electrical instability and thus may increase postconversion dysrhythmias.
4. Determine digitalis level, if time permits. Defer cardioversion if digitalis toxicity is suspected because of risk of lethal dysrhythmias. Set initial energy level at 5 watt-seconds, and, if this low energy level results in frequent premature ventricular contractions, do not proceed with cardioversion.
5. Monitor for acid-base imbalances and hypoxia prior to cardioversion by a baseline blood gas determination.
6. Observe for respiratory depression due to premedication.
7. Turn off synchronizer if ventricular fibrillation occurs. Since there are no R waves in ventricular fibrillation, the unit will fail to discharge in the synchronized mode.

Related Care

1. Give patient nothing by mouth for 6 to 12 hours prior to elective cardioversion.

2. Obtain signed consent according to hospital policy.
3. Check for availability of emergency cardiac medications at bedside (i.e., lidocaine, atropine and the like).
4. Check potential causes for failure to convert:
    A. Faulty equipment or frayed wires.
    B. Debris on paddles.
    C. Nonsynchronized mode.
    D. Artifact interference.
    E. Battery failure, if unit is portable.
    F. Inadequate paddle pressure to chest wall during elective cardioversion.
5. Document sequence of therapy, including voltage delivered with each attempt and postcardioversion ECG rhythm.

Complications

Cardiac arrest (asystole, ventricular fibrillation)
Respiratory depression or arrest
Dysrhythmias
Pulmonary or systemic emboli
Skin burns
Equipment malfunction

Suppliers

Abbott
Datascope
Hewlett-Packard
Physiocontrol

REFERENCES

Desilva, R.A., et al.: Cardioversion and defibrillation. Am. Heart J. *100*:881-895, 1980.
Fisher, J.D., et al.: The sparkling joules of internal cardiac stimulation: Cardioversion, defibrillation, and ablation. Am. Heart J., *103*:177-181, 1982.
McIntyre, K.M., and Lewis, A.J. (eds.): Textbook of Advanced Cardiac Life Support. Dallas, American Heart Association, 1981.
Vinsant, M.D., and Spence, J.I.: A Common Sense Approach to Coronary Care, 3rd ed. St. Louis, C.V. Mosby, 1981, pp. 329-332.
Weaver, W.D., et al.: Ventricular defibrillation—A comparative trial using 175-J and 320-J shocks. N. Eng. J. Med., *307*:1101-1105, 1982.

DEFIBRILLATION

Martha I. Spence, R.N., M.N., CCRN

Overview

Defibrillation is emergency therapy in which a nonsynchronized direct current charge is delivered to the myocardium to terminate ventricular fibrillation. Complete depolarization of the myocardium simultaneously disrupts all electrical circuits responsible for ventricular fibrillation, allowing the sinoatrial node or another potential pacemaker to regain control of the heart rhythm. The charge is delivered via metal paddles, either to the external chest wall or directly to the myocaradium during cardiac surgery.

Careful assessment of the clinical state of the patient and ECG patterns is necessary predefibrillation and postdefibrillation. Cardiopulmonary support measures and pharmacologic therapy are integral components of treatment. Success in patient survival depends upon early recognition and rapid treatment of lethal dysrhythmias.

Objective

To terminate ventricular fibrillation immediately, facilitating the establishment of an effective cardiac rhythm.

Special Equipment

Defibrillator with external paddles/ internal paddles (sterilized)
ECG monitor and recorder
Conductive pads or conductive medium

Emergency cart and medications
Oxygen therapy equipment
Airway
Resuscitator bag
Emergency pacing equipment

Procedure

ACTION	RATIONALE
1. Verify ventricular fibrillation by ECG; correlate with the clinical state of the patient.	1. Ventricular fibrillation may be mistaken for artifact on ECG.
2. Prepare to defibrillate.	2. Assess the situation. If a second person is getting the defibrillator, establish an airway and begin ventilation and external cardiac massage.
A. Plug grounded defibrillator into electrical outlet, if necessary.	

ACTION	RATIONALE
B. Turn power on.	
C. Prepare defibrillator paddles. Options:	C. Conductive pads on chest or conductive medium on entire metal surfaces reduces resistance of skin to current flow, prevents skin burns, and allows for optimal current flow to the myocardium.
(1) Place conductive pads in desired position on chest.	
(2) Cover entire metal surface of paddles with conductive medium.	
D. Dial 200 to 300 joules (watt-seconds) for an adult.	D. Current levels needed to convert ventricular fibrillation are related to body size. Initial voltage of 200 to 300 joules (watt-seconds) is currently recommended by the A.H.A.
E. Activate charge button.	E. This will charge unit with electrical current.
F. Check that defibrillation unit is in the nonsynchronized mode.	F. In the synchronized mode the machine will not fire, owing to the absence of R waves in ventricular fibrillation.
G. Place paddles firmly into position against the chest, using approximately 25 to 30 lb. pressure (see Fig. 1-28 for illustration of transverse and anterior-posterior positions).	G. Firm pressure establishes good contact and reduces transthoracic resistance.
(1) Transverse position:	
(a) Place one paddle at second intercostal space, right of sternum.	
(b) Place the second paddle at fifth intercostal space, midclavicular line, left of sternum.	
(2) Anterior-posterior position:	(2) Anterior-posterior position may decrease amount of current required.
(a) Place one paddle at anterior-precordial area.	
(b) Place the second paddle at posterior-infrascapular area.	
3. Stand clear of bed; give command to stand clear prior to defibrillation. Visually check to see that personnel are standing away from bed.	3. Electrical current follows the path of least resistance. This measure reduces the risk of accidental microshock or macroshock.

ACTION	RATIONALE
4. Recheck ECG rhythm on monitor to ascertain ventricular fibrillation.	4. ECG rhythm may change prior to defibrillation.
5. Depress the discharge buttons on the two paddles simultaneously; continue keeping both firmly depressed until the electrical current is delivered.	5. Premature release of the discharge buttons may result in failure of the machine to discharge energy.
6. Determine effects of defibrillation by checking the postdefibrillation ECG rhythm (Fig. 1–31).	

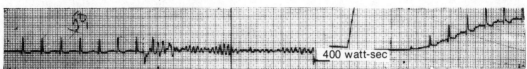

Figure 1-31.   Defibrillation of pacer-induced ventricular fibrillation.

A. Prepare paddles and defibrillator for immediate reuse if ventricular fibrillation persists.	
B. Continue cardiopulmonary resuscitation during preparation of equipment.	
C. Assess patient status and precipating factors to prevent further decompensation of the patient.	
7. Perform postdefibrillation care:	
A. Monitor ECG rhythm.	A. This establishes data for subsequent therapy.
B. Validate IV patency.	B. This may be needed to administer medications.
C. Assess patient status and precipitating factors to prevent further decompensation of the patient. (3) Skin temperature, moisture, color.	
D. Monitor vital signs till stable.	
E. Discuss with physician need for antidysrhythmic medication.	E. Recurrence of ventricular fibrillation may be prevented by drugs that reestablish electrical homogeneity. (See ACLS guidelines in McIntyre and Lewis.)
F. Monitor adequacy of oxygenation via blood gas data.	F. Cardiac arrest may result in sustained hypoxia and lactic acidosis. Shifts in pH may further compromise effects of drug therapy. Pulmonary gas transport may

ACTION	RATIONALE
	also be compromised because of respiratory dysfunction resulting in hypoxemia.
G. Obtain a 12-lead ECG.	G. These data assist in assessing for myocardial damage and ECG rhythm.
H. Assess skin of chest wall for presence of burns.	H. Burns are a common complication of defibrillation. Steroid or lanolin-based creams may be prescribed.

Precautions

1. Check that all equipment is properly grounded to prevent current leakage.
2. Disconnect ungrounded electrical equipment. Defibrillation may result in damage to the equipment.
3. Avoid excessive conductive gel on paddles to prevent arcing of current with decreased flow to patient.
4. Clear defibrillator of remaining electrical current immediately after use; never set charged defibrillator paddles down. Prepare equipment for future use.

Related Care

1. Resume cardiopulmonary resucitation (CPR) immediately if initial defibrillation attempt is unsuccessful. Recharge machine and prepare for subsequent countershocks according to A.H.A. ACLS protocols (McIntyre and Lewis).

2. Check possible causes of failure to convert ventricular fibrillation:
    A. Defibrillator on *synchronized* rather than *nonsynchronized* mode.
    B. Debris on paddles, which impairs conductivity.
    C. Low amplitude fibrillatory waves, which can be associated with long-standing ventricular fibrillation, acidosis, and hypoxia; this may require cardiopulmonary resuscitative measures and pharmacologic intervention prior to defibrillation.
    D. Frayed wires and faulty equipment.
    E. Inadequate paddle pressure to chest wall during defibrillation.

3. Record predefibrillation ECG rhythm, number of times defibrillation was attempted, voltage used with each attempt, postdefibrillation ECG rhythm, and multisubsystem status.

4. Support patient and family as necessary.

5. Recognize the following differences for internal defibrillation:
    A. Use sterile internal defibrillation paddles.

B. Use sterile, saline-moistened gauze pads between the myocardium and defibrillation paddles.

C. Charge defibrillator to prescribed voltage; a significantly lower 15 to 30 joules (watt-seconds) energy level is used.

6. Recognize the following changes for pacemaker defibrillation:

A. Avoid placing defibrillator paddles over permanent pulse generator or electrode (Fig. 1-32).

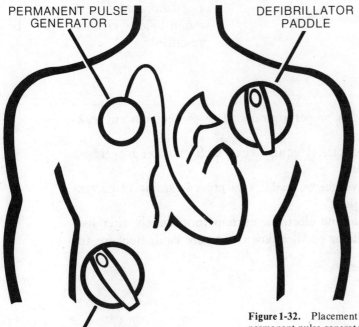

PERMANENT PULSE GENERATOR

DEFIBRILLATOR PADDLE

DEFIBRILLATOR PADDLE

Figure 1-32.   Placement of defibrillator paddles on patient with a permanent pulse generator.

Complications

Equipment malfunction   Skin or chest wall burns
Myocardial necrosis

Suppliers

Abbott   Hewlett-Packard
Datascope   Physiocontrol

REFERENCES

Desilva, R.A., et al.: Cardioversion and defibrillation. Am. Heart J., *100*:881–895, 1980.

Fisher, J.D., et al.: The sparkling joules of internal cardiac stimulation: Cardioversion, defibrillation, and ablation. Am. Heart J., *103*:177–181, 1982.

McIntyre, K.M., and Lewis, A.J. (eds.): Textbook of Advanced Cardiac Life Support. Dallas, American Heart Association, 1981.

Vinsant, M.D., and Spence, J.I.: A Common Sense Approach to Coronary Care, 3rd ed. St.Louis, C.V. Mosby, 1981, pp. 329–332.

Weaver, W.D., et al.: Ventricular defibrillation—A comparative trial using 175-J and 320-J shocks. N. Engl. J. Med. *307*:1101–1105, 1982.

VASCULAR INVASIVE
TECHNIQUES

Overview

Venipuncture, central line insertion (assisting with), and arterial puncture are common vascular invasive techniques used by the critical care nurse. Securing and maintaining a patent venous route is of high priority for the critically ill patient or the patient who is a "high" risk for dysrhythmias or a medical emergency. Catheterization of a central vein provides a reliable route for fluid and blood administration, obtaining venous samples, measurement of right-sided cardiac filling pressures, and administration of hyperosmolar and irritating solutions. A single arterial puncture is performed selectively to obtain an arterial blood sample for immediate gas analysis in such instances as cardiopulmonary arrest, suspected altered respiratory function, or monitoring of oxygen therapy.

This section presents procedures for performing a venipuncture, using two types of indwelling catheters; central line insertion (assisting with); and a single arterial puncture.

VENIPUNCTURE

Karen M. Miller, R.N., M.S.N.

Instrumentation

Combination disposable catheter needles are widely used in the care of the critically ill; they are available in various lengths and lumen sizes. A "catheter-over-the-needle" set consists of an external catheter and internal needle, with the bevel point extending beyond the catheter tip (Fig. 1–33). The needle serves as a stylus during the venipuncture, after which it is withdrawn and discarded. A primed IV administration set is connected directly to the adapter. A "catheter-through-the-needle" set consists of a catheter enclosed within a needle and catheter guard sleeve (Fig. 1–34). Following a successful venipuncture, the catheter is threaded into the vein, the stylus removed, and primed IV administration set connected directly to the adapter. This catheter set requires the needle to be withdrawn and protectively secured externally, utilizing the needle bevel cover and proper connection at the adapter point.

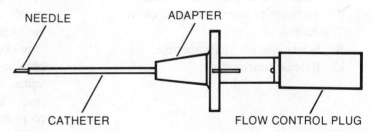

NEEDLE   ADAPTER

Figure 1-33. Components of the catheter-over-the-needle type insertion set.

CATHETER   FLOW CONTROL PLUG

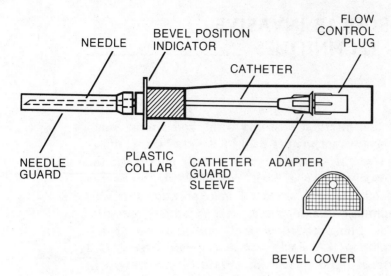

Figure 1-34. Components of the catheter-through-the-needle type insertion set.

Objectives

1. To provide a route for administration of IV fluid, medication, blood, and blood components.
2. To provide nutritional supplement and hydration for patients unable to obtain them by other means.

Special Equipment

IV fluid	Sterile gauze dressings
IV administration set	Povidone-iodine ointment
Infusion needle (catheter-over-the-needle or catheter-through-the-needle)	Povidone-iodine prep pads or swabs
	Alcohol prep pads
	Tape
Tourniquet	Arm board
Depilatory or razor	

Procedure

ACTION	RATIONALE
1. Determine appropriate venipuncture site (Fig. 1–35):	
A. Apply tourniquet with enough pressure to impede venous circulation.	A. Tourniquet should not impede arterial circulation. Extreme or prolonged pressure may make the vein become tortuous. Minimal pressure is required for sclerosed veins; in these cases a tourniquet may make venipuncture even more difficult.
B. Select site for venipuncture.	
C. Release tourniquet.	

ACTION   RATIONALE

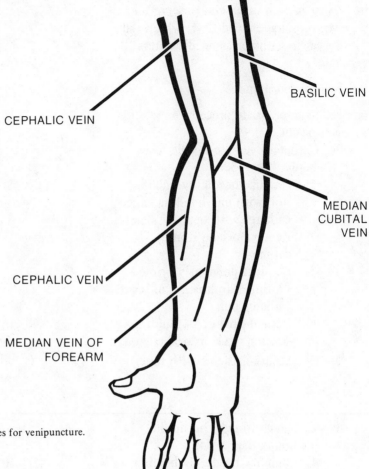

CEPHALIC VEIN

BASILIC VEIN

MEDIAN CUBITAL VEIN

CEPHALIC VEIN

MEDIAN VEIN OF FOREARM

Figure 1-35. Anatomic sites for venipuncture.

2. Prepare selected site for venipuncture.
   A. Trim or remove hair with depilatory or razor.

   B. Reapply tourniquet immediately prior to venipuncture.
   C. Cleanse site with povidone-iodine prep pad or swab; allow to dry.
   D. Remove povidone-iodine solution with alcohol prep pad if vein cannot be visualized.

3. Puncture skin with needle at a 45-degree angle; bevel should be upward and lateral to the vein.

A. Shaving can cause abrasions that may lead to infection. Shaving and hair removal remain controversial.

3. This causes the least amount of discomfort for the patient.

ACTION	RATIONALE
4. Reduce angle of the needle and insert ⅛ to ¼ inch into vein; observe for free retrograde blood flow, which will appear in catheter as needle enters the vein.	
5. Release tourniquet.	
6. Follow appropriate procedure for infusion needle. A. Catheter-over-the-needle technique (Fig. 1–33):	
(1) Stabilize needle by holding hub with one hand; advance catheter with opposite hand.	(1) Stabilization of the needle prevents posterior puncturing of the vein.
(2) Remove needle from catheter.	
(3) Connect previously primed IV fluid administration set to catheter hub.	
(4) Initiate flow of IV fluid; assess for signs of local edema.	(4) If the catheter has punctured the vein completely, fluid will infuse into surrounding tissue, as evidenced by edema.
(5) Secure catheter with tape.	
B. Catheter-through-the-needle technique (Fig. 1–34): (1) Stabilize needle by holding hub; advance catheter by applying pressure at base of catheter in plastic sleeve.	(1) It is preferable to thread the catheter until catheter and hub of the needle are engaged. The catheter should be advanced a minimum of 4 inches; when the catheter cannot be advanced at least 4 inches, the needle and catheter must be removed simultaneously and a new site located.
(2) Engage needle hub into catheter hub.	(2) If catheter is inserted at least 4 inches, but less than its full length, it is necessary to pull needle back until it engages the catheter hub.

ACTION	RATIONALE
(3) Apply slight pressure above puncture site with one hand; use opposite hand to withdraw needle from vein until 1½ inches of the catheter are exposed.	(3) The application of pressure should eliminate excessive bleeding or trauma.
(4) Remove catheter guard sleeve, holding catheter hub securely.	(4) Holding catheter hub securely prevents its accidental removal.
(5) Remove flow control plug and stylet.	
(6) Connect previously primed IV fluid administration set to catheter hub.	
(7) Initiate flow of IV fluid.	
(8) Apply needle guard securely over tip of needle.	(8) The guard will protect the catheter from being pierced by the needle inadvertently. Needle and catheter should lie firmly in the groove of the needle guard before it is closed. If the catheter is not in the groove, infusion will cease when the guard is closed.
(9) Secure with tape.	

7. Apply povidone-iodine ointment at catheter insertion site; secure with gauze dressings and tape.

8. Adjust IV infusion rate.

9. Record type of catheter (gauge and length) inserted and site used.

Precautions

1. Select the type of infusion needle with the following considerations:
   A. Type of solution—fluids with higher viscosity may require a larger-bore needle.
   B. Location of the vein.
   C. Phlebitis related to antibiotic infusion is less likely to result if larger, deeper veins are used.

2. Select the vein with the following considerations:
   A. Activity/flexibility needed by the patient.
   B. Hand orientation of the patient (right- or left-handed).
   C. Condition of the vein.

    D. Type of solution or medication for which the infusion is required.

    E. Anticipated duration of therapy.

3. Monitor length of time catheter is in place; recommended duration is 72 hours.

Related Care

1. Use a sterile catheter for each venipuncture.
2. Label dressing with type of infusion needle and gauge, date, and time of insertion.
3. Perform site care with povidone-iodine ointment and sterile gauze dressings every 24 hours (see "Short Venous and Arterial Indwelling Catheter Site Care" and "Long Venous and Arterial Indwelling Catheter Site Care").
4. Maintain catheter patency.
5. Monitor IV fluid infusion rate.
6. Observe for development of phlebitis.

Complications

Thrombus formation	Tissue sloughing related to local fluid infiltration
Phlebitis	Local or systemic infection
Hematoma	Nerve injuries

Suppliers

Abbott	Deseret
Argyle	Sorenson
Becton-Dickinson	

REFERENCES

Kaye, W.: Invasive monitoring techniques: Arterial cannulation, bedside pulmonary artery catheterization, and arterial puncture. Heart Lung 12:395–427, 1983.

McIntyre, K.M., and Lewis, A.J. (eds.): Textbook of Advanced Cardiac Life Support. Dallas, American Heart Association, 1981.

CENTRAL LINE INSERTION (ASSISTING WITH) _____

Diane K. Dressler, R.N., M.S.N., CCRN

Instrumentation

Central venous catheterization is generally performed via the subclavian, internal jugular, median basilic, or femoral vein. The catheter is threaded through the vein until its tip lies in the superior vena cava (Fig. 1–36), or inferior vena cava when the femoral site is used.

The site that is selected for an individual patient may be determined by anatomic or clinical indications:

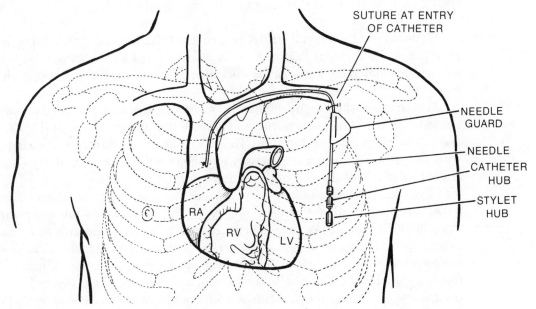

Figure 1-36.   Anatomic catheter placement.

Subclavian. The subclavian vein begins as a continuation of the axillary vein. It crosses over the first rib and passes in front of the anterior scalene muscle, which separates it from the subclavian artery. It continues under the inner third of the clavicle.

The subclavian route may be preferred for prolonged catheterization since it does not interfere with patient mobility. It may be selected for emergency access to the venous circulation when peripheral veins are collapsed. This site has a slightly higher incidence of pneumothorax and subclavian artery puncture.

Jugular. The internal jugular vein lies adjacent to the internal and common carotid artery and to the sternocleidomastoid muscle. It may be selected for emergency access to the venous circulation when peripheral veins are collapsed. It has a lower incidence of catheter-related complications than the subclavian site but may be a more difficult site to enter. Complications such as pneumothorax and carotid artery puncture are rare; however, patients may report limited mobility of the neck and neck tenderness.

When the jugular site is chosen, the right jugular vein is often preferred because there is a more direct line to the right atrium and there is less danger of puncturing the dome of the lung or thoracic duct.

Antecubital (Median Basilic).   The median vein of the forearm bifurcates into a Y in the antecubital fossa, becoming the median cephalic vein laterally and the median basilic vein medially. A peripheral site for central venous catheterization may be desirable during cardiac arrest so that cardiopulmonary resuscitation (CPR) does not have to be interrupted; the median basilic vein is frequently chosen. However, the peripheral veins may be collapsed and difficult to catheterize. These lines are associated with a somewhat higher incidence of thrombophlebitis and infection.

Femoral.   The femoral vein lies medial to the femoral artery immediately below the inguinal ligament. It is easily located in the patient with a palpable femoral pulse but can be difficult to locate when this pulse is absent.

The femoral site may be preferred in certain situations. It may be more accessible in the obese patient and may also be first choice of site during cardiac arrest to avoid interrupting CPR. The main disadvantages associated with this site are related to decreased mobility of the patient and an increased incidence of thrombophlebitis and infection.

Two insertion techniques may be used to insert a central line. An indwelling plastic catheter may be inserted through a hollow needle following venipuncture. The needle is then retracted and a needle guard attached. An alternative technique is to use a guidewire (Seldinger technique). Following venipuncture with a needle, a flexible-tipped or J-tipped guidewire is inserted through the needle. The needle is removed, and the catheter is inserted over the guidewire. When the catheter is properly placed the guidewire is withdrawn. Guidewires are also used to introduce a dilator and sheath for insertion of an intracardiac catheter.

Objectives

1. To rapidly administer blood or fluids.
2. To obtain venous access when peripheral veins are small, thrombosed, or difficult to find.
3. To measure right-sided cardiac filling pressures and serve as a guide to fluid replacement.
4. To administer drugs that should not be given through peripheral veins.
5. To place temporary cardiac pacemaker or pulmonary artery pressure catheter.
6. To obtain venous blood samples.
7. To permit access for hemodialysis.

Special Equipment

Jugular-subclavian catheter set (14-gauge);
    24-inch or 36-inch intra-catheter
10-ml. syringe
Suture (3-0 silk)
Needle holder
Suture scissors
Sterile field:
    Sterile sponges   Cap
    Povidone-iodine solution   Gown
    Draping towels and towel clips   Sterile gloves
    Mask
3-ml syringe, 23-gauge needle, and local anesthetic
IV solution, administration set and stand
Sterile dressing
Guidewires
Sterile hemostat } for use with Seldinger technique
Vessel dilators

Procedure

ACTION	RATIONALE
1. Assemble appropriate equipment and prime IV tubing.	1. Depending on the site chosen, a jugular-subclavian catheter set or a 24- or 36-inch intracatheter may be used. Special catheters are used for hemodialysis access and for combinations of pacemaker and pulmonary artery pressure measurements along with central line access.
2. Position the patient: A. Subclavian and jugular: (1) Place the patient in a Trendelenburg position of at least 15 degrees.	(1) This distends the subclavian and jugular veins and lessens the risk of air embolus during insertion.
(2) Place a rolled sheet under the patient's shoulder if desired by the physician.	
(3) Turn the patient's head opposite the side of entry.	(3) This aids in exposing the jugular vein; during subclavian catheter insertion this prevents the catheter from advancing up the internal jugular vein.

ACTION	RATIONALE
B. Antecubital:	
(1) Place the patient in supine position.	(1) This lessens the risk of air embolism and provides a straighter path for the intra-catheter.
(2) Extend the arm and position it at a right angle to the body.	
C. Femoral:	
(1) Place the patient in supine position.	(1) This aids in exposing the site and provides a straight path for the intracatheter.
3. Prepare the insertion site for veni-puncture.	
A. Trim or remove hair with depila-tory or razor as necessary.	A. This facilitates aseptic technique during insertion and with subse-quent dressing changes.
B. Mask all persons in the immedi-ate area; provide gown, cap, and gloves for the person performing catheter insertion.	B. Optimum sterile technique is recommended since many of these catheters remain in place longer than 48 hours.
C. Scrub the area around the inser-tion site with povidone-iodine solution.	
D. Apply a tourniquet to the arm if an antecubital vein will be used.	
E. Drape a sterile field.	
F. Provide local anesthesia.	F. In patients who are awake, the area is anesthetized prior to inser-tion of the catheterization needle.
4. Monitor the patient during insertion.	
A. Assist the patient in remaining immobile during needle insertion.	A. Tissue damage or shearing of the catheter may occur if the patient moves.
B. Facilitate the use of various nee-dle guidewires and catheters dur-ing the catheterization.	B. See also the procedure for "Vas-cular Invasive Techniques" for more information on catheter-through-the-needle insertion.
(1) When blood return is ob-tained from the catheteriza-tion needle, provide the phy-sician with the intracatheter.	(1) The intracatheter will be threaded through the needle and advanced into the super-ior or inferior vena cava. Fol-lowing this the catheter-ization needle and catheter are withdrawn as a unit to prevent shearing of the catheter.

ACTION	RATIONALE
(2) Connect the primed IV tubing to the catheter and check for patency of flow by lowering the IV bag below the level of the heart.	(2) Blood flow back into the tubing assists in confirming catheter placement. Do not infuse blood or hypertonic solution until catheter placement is confirmed by x-ray.
(3) Administer IV fluids per physician's order.	

5. Secure the central catheter.
   A. Facilitate applying needle guard when appropriate.
   B. Facilitate securing with suture (preferred) or taping.

        B. The catheter must be secured to the skin to prevent accidental withdrawal.

6. Provide site care and dressing.
   A. Cleanse site with sterile gauze pads.

        A. Aseptic technique is maintained because of potential catheter-related sepsis. (See "Long Venous and Arterial Indwelling Catheter Site Care" and "Insertion of a Subclavian Total Parenteral Nutrition Catheter (Assisting With).")

        B. Apply povidone-iodine ointment to insertion site, emerging catheter, and sutures.
   C. Apply tincture of benzoin to help secure a sterile gauze and tape dressing. Alternatively a self-adhering wound dressing may be used.

7. Elevate head of bed and prepare patient for chest x-ray.

Precautions

1. Inform the physician if the patient is receiving anticoagulants or if the patient has a bleeding disorder.

2. Select site most appropriate for the patient. In patients with severe respiratory dysfunction, a site other than the subclavian vein may be preferred because a pneumothorax can be fatal. Patients receiving mechanical ventilation or positive end expiratory pressure (PEEP) are also at greater risk for pneumothorax.

Related Care

1. Assess and monitor the patient:
   A. Check the chest x-ray for catheter position and evidence of a pneumothorax or hemothorax.
   B. Auscultate the lung fields for symmetric breath sounds.

2. Maintain catheter asepsis: change the dressing according to institutional protocol (usually every 48 hours). See "Long Venous and Arterial Indwelling Catheter Care." If fever occurs, obtain an order for blood cultures.

3. Label the dressing with type of catheter and size, date, and time of insertion.

4. Reposition the patient following catheter insertion; elevate the head of the bed. Place the patient in the recumbent position for central venous pressure readings or when the IV tubing is disconnected from the catheter to minimize risk of air embolus.

5. Monitor IV flow rate at frequent intervals as IV flow rate may fluctuate with position and other variables. Use of an IV flow controller is helpful in maintaining a steady flow through central lines.

6. Facilitate catheter removal when appropriate and:
   A. Remove the sutures.
   B. Pull the catheter back slowly and steadily.
   C. Culture the catheter tip if infection is suspected.
   D. Apply pressure to the area to prevent bleeding.
   E. Apply a sterile occlusive dressing.
   F. Inspect the catheter to make sure it is intact.
   G. Assess the patient and monitor for complications after catheter removal.

Complications

Pneumothorax
Hemothorax related to subclavian or innominate artery puncture
Hematoma at the puncture site
Myocardial perforation related to the catheter advancement
Infection
Phlebitis
Thrombosis
Air embolism
Mediastinal fluid infusion or hydrothorax
Catheter shearing and embolism
Brachial plexus injury during subclavian insertion
Osteomyelitis related to subclavian insertion

Suppliers

Bard-Parker
Becton-Dickinson
Deseret
Jelco

REFERENCES

Brunner, L.F., and Suddarth, D.S.: Lippincott Manual of Nursing Practice. Philadelphia, J.B. Lippincott, 1982.
Cowley, R.A., and Dunham, C.M. (eds.): Shock Trauma/Critical Care Manual. Baltimore, University Park Press, 1982.
McIntyre, K.M., and Lewis, A.J. (eds.): Textbook of Advanced Cardiac Life Support. Dallas, American Heart Association, 1981.
Suratt, P.M., and Givson, R.S. (eds.): Manual of Medical Procedures. St. Louis, C.V. Mosby, 1982.

ARTERIAL PUNCTURE _____

Karen M. Miller, R.N., M.S.N.

Instrumentation

Disposable arterial puncture kits are available with various gauges and lengths of needles, plastic or glass syringes, and multiple syringe sizes. These prepackaged kits are especially useful in critical care units and emergency carts for cardiopulmonary arrest situation.

The sites commonly used for arterial puncture include radial artery, brachial artery, and femoral artery. If serial arterial blood specimens are needed, arterial cannulation should be performed. (See "Hemodynamic Monitoring.")

Objectives

1. To obtain a blood specimen for analysis of arterial pH, oxygen tension (PO_2), carbon dioxide tension (PCO_2), oxygen saturation, and acid-base balance.
2. To aid in management of hypoxic states, acid-base balance, oxygen therapy, respiratory failure, and continuous ventilatory assistance.

Special Equipment

Arterial blood gas kit (disposable):
   One 5-ml. glass or plastic syringe with rubber stopper or cap
   One 22-gauge x 1-inch needle (short bevel)
   One 20-gauge x 1½-inch needle
   Two sterile gauze pads
   Two alcohol prep pads
   One adhesive bandage
   One patient label
   One sterile field
   Povidone-iodine prep swabs
   One plastic bag or container with crushed ice
One 1-ml. ampule sodium heparin
Local anesthetic (optional)
1-ml. syringe with 25-gauge needle (optional)
Laboratory requisition

Procedure

ACTION	RATIONALE
1. Instruct patient regarding purpose, procedure, and responsibilities.	1. Information may alleviate hyperventilation that, when present, might alter arterial blood gas values.

ACTION	RATIONALE

2. Select site.
   A. Radial artery (Fig. 1-37):
      (1) Use as first choice, except in the case of multiple radial artery punctures, hematoma, occlusion of ulnar artery, history of circulatory impairment to extremity, or cardiac arrest.

      (1) The radial artery is a small artery; however, it is easily stabilized as it passes over a bone groove, located at the wrist. The percutaneous puncture and pressure control are enhanced by the anatomical landmark.

      (2) Perform the Allen test or modified Allen test (see "Related Care"), or use a Doppler instrument to determine ulnar and radial artery patency.

      (2) Collateral circulation to hand is provided by the ulnar artery; the Allen test assesses for ulnar artery patency.

   B. Brachial artery (Fig. 1-37):
      (1) Use as second choice, except in the case of poor pulsation due to shock, obesity, or sclerotic vessel.

      (1) The brachial artery is larger than the radial artery. Pres-

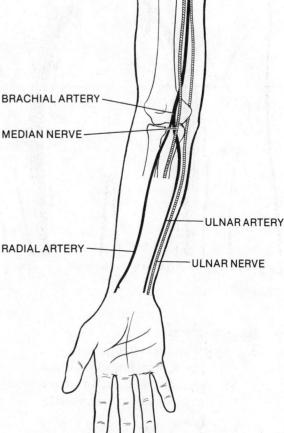

Figure 1-37. Anatomic landmarks for radial and brachial arterial punctures.

BRACHIAL ARTERY

MEDIAN NERVE

ULNAR ARTERY

RADIAL ARTERY

ULNAR NERVE

ACTION

RATIONALE

sure control after percutaneous puncture is enhanced by its proximity to bone if entry point is approximately 1½ inches above antecubital fossa.

C. Femoral artery (Fig. 1-38):
   (1) Use as third choice, except in the case of cardiac arrest or altered perfusion to upper extremity arteries.

(1) The femoral artery is a large artery; however, there is no collateral circulation available if it is injured. Because the femoral artery is located in proximity to the femoral vein, there is potential for false pH, PO_2, and PCO_2 values related to venous blood contamination or arteriovenous fistulas. Hemorrhage/hematomas are possible since bleeding is more difficult to control.

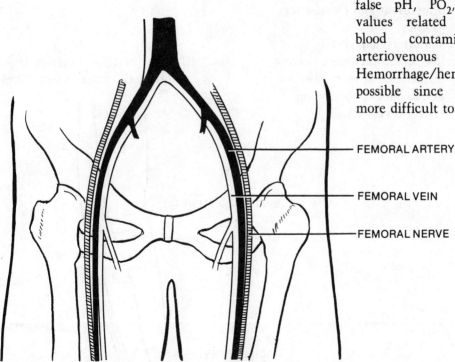

FEMORAL ARTERY

FEMORAL VEIN

FEMORAL NERVE

Figure 1-38.   Anatomic landmarks for femoral arterial puncture.

3. Position patient.
   A. Radial arterial puncture:
      (1) Use semirecumbent position.
      (2) Elevate and dorsiflex patient's wrist slightly, using a small pillow.
      (3) Rotate patient's hand until pulse is palpable.

(2) Dorsiflexion of the wrist moves the artery closer to the skin surface, making the artery easier to palpate.

ACTION	RATIONALE

B. Brachial arterial puncture:
  (1) Use semirecumbent position.
  (2) Elevate and hyperextend patient's arm, supporting with pillow, until pulse is palpable.
  (3) Rotate patient's arm until pulse is palpable.
C. Femoral arterial puncture:
  (1) Use supine position with leg straight.

4. Heparinize syringe and needle.

A. Assemble 22-gauge short-bevel needle on syringe.

    A. A short-bevel needle diminishes the risk of overshooting the artery during entry.

B. Prime syringe and needle with heparin, leaving only enough heparin to fill the dead space.

    B. Priming the syringe with heparin prevents specimen coagulation. However, any heparin in excess of that needed to fill the dead space will lower the pH and PCO_2 of arterial blood.

C. Eject all air bubbles from syringe.

    C. All air must be ejected to maintain accuracy of blood gas values.

5. Prep site and fingers used to palpate site.

A. Cleanse selected site in circular motion outward with povidone-iodine prep swabs; allow to dry.

    A. Drying of povidone-iodine solution reduces risk of local infection or systemic sepsis.

B. Cleanse site with alcohol swab; allow to dry.

    B. Alcohol removes povidone-iodine coloring from site and thereby increases visibility. Puncturing through a moist alcohol-prepared site can increase pain.

6. Locally anesthetize site (optional).

A. Use 1-ml. syringe with 25-gauge needle and lidocaine (Xylocaine) 1%.

B. Aspirate prior to injecting local anesthetic to ascertain that a blood vessel has not been entered.

C. Inject intradermally and then with full infiltration around artery, using approximately 0.2 to 0.3 ml. for an adult.

7. Perform percutaneous puncture of selected artery.

A. Locate pulsating artery.

ACTION	RATIONALE
B. Stabilize artery by pulling skin taut and bracketing the area of maximum pulsation with finger-tips of free hand.	
C. Puncture skin slowly, holding syringe like pencil; advance nee-dle slowly with bevel upward at approximately a 45- to 60-degree angle to the radial or brachial ar-tery (Fig.1-39). For femoral ar-terial puncture a 90-degree angle is used.	C. A slow gradual thrust will pro-mote arterial entry without pass-ing directly through it. Enter at angle comfortable for stabilizing your hand. Certainty of position is more important than entry an-gle.

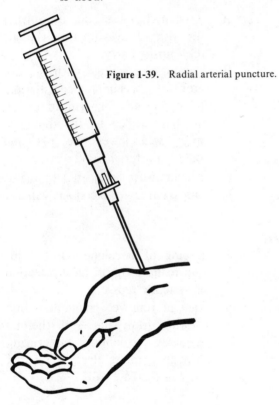

Figure 1-39. Radial arterial puncture.

D. Observe syringe for flashback of arterial blood.	D. Pulsation of blood into the syringe verifies that the artery has been punctured. Flashback occurs readily with a glass syringe. Gentle aspiration may be necessary with a plastic syringe.
E. If puncture is unsuccessful, with-draw needle to skin level, angle slightly toward artery, and re-advance.	
8. Obtain a 3- to 5-ml. specimen.	8. This amount allows for rechecking and additional studies, if necessary.

ACTION	RATIONALE
9. Withdraw needle while stabilizing barrel of syringe.	9. This prevents inadvertent aspiration of air during withdrawal when using a glass syringe.

10. Apply firm continuous pressure to arterial puncture site for 5 minutes or until bleeding stops.
   A. Apply firm pressure for 10 minutes if the patient has a history of increased coagulation time.
   B. Apply ice pack to help decrease persistant bleeding.
	10. Hematomas following an arterial puncture can cause circulatory impedance, discomfort or can predispose to infection.

11. Protect blood sample.
   A. Hold syringe upright; express any air bubbles rapidly.
   B. Seal needle immediately, using rubber stopper or cap.
   C. Roll the syringe gently to mix blood and heparin.
   D. Immerse blood sample in enough ice for transport to laboratory.
	A. Air bubbles may alter laboratory test results.
	B. Specimen must be kept airtight to prevent alteration of test results.
	
	D. The use of ice reduces temperature of the sample to below 4°C. and slows the metabolism of oxygen. A delay longer than 2 minutes alters values.

E. Label specimen; complete appropriate laboratory requisition. Note the percentage of O_2 therapy, if applicable, the temperature, especially if elevated, and the time specimen was drawn. F. Expedite immediate laboratory services.	E. Specific information related to sample collections enhances accurate analysis of results. F. No test results for any specimen, even if chilled, can be accepted as reliable if sample is tested more than 15 to 30 minutes after arterial puncture.

Precautions

1. Avoid femoral arterial punctures in patients with a history of aorto-femoral synthetic grafts.

2. Check for medication allergies if local anesthetic is utilized.

3. Alternate sites for serial arterial blood gas punctures.

Related Care

1. Consider arterial line placement to facilitate obtaining serial arterial blood gas samples.

2. Perform Allen test (or modified Allen test) prior to radial artery puncture.
   A. Instruct patient to form a tight fist or raise arm above heart level for several seconds to force blood from hand.
   B. Apply direct pressure on radial and ulnar arteries to obstruct arterial blood flow to hand while patient opens and closes fist rapidly several times.
   C. Instruct patient to open hand or keep arm above heart level with radial artery compressed.
   D. Examine palmar surface for an erythematous blush or pallor within 6 seconds. An erythematous blush indicates ulnar artery patency and is interpreted as a positive Allen test. Pallor indicates occlusion of the ulnar artery and is interpreted as a negative Allen's test. With a negative Allen's test the radial arterial puncture should be avoided.

3. Monitor arterial puncture site.
   A. Maintain continuous firm pressure on puncture site for 5 to 10 minutes after needle withdrawal; length of time varies with patient's age, health, medical history, and anticoagulation therapy.
   B. Check site for delayed hematoma formation and circulation to extremity every 5 minutes times 6. Circulatory impairment can occur for various reasons. A medical history of arteriosclerosis increases the risk of thrombosis, especially in the femoral artery. Large or small arterial occlusions due to thrombosis, intramural hemorrhage, or emboli may produce symptoms such as cold extremities, absence of pulses, or petechiae. In this event, protect the extremity from future punctures at the same site. Also, local edema not attributed to local anesthesia injection usually indicates internal hemorrhage that can be controlled by direct compression.

4. Assess results of arterial blood gas tests.

5. Record temperature of patient, oxygen percentage and method of delivery, site of arterial puncture, ease of puncture, time length of applied pressure, site assessment, and circulation assessment after arterial puncture.

Complications

Hematoma (major)	Impaired circulation to extemity
Intraluminal clotting	Arterial spasm
Nerve injury	Thrombosis (after repeated punctures)
Hemorrhage	Arteriovenous fistulas

Suppliers

Argyle
Bard-Parker
Travenol

REFERENCES

Kaye, W.: Invasive monitoring techniques: Arterial cannulation, bedside pulmonary artery catheterization, and arterial puncture. Heart Lung, *12*:395–427, 1983.

McIntyre, K.M., and Lewis, A.J. (eds.): Textbook of Advanced Cardiac Life Support. Dallas, American Heart Association, 1981.

INTRA-ARTERIAL INFUSION
FOR CHEMOTHERAPY

Barbara Buss Fugleberg, R.N., B.S.N., CCRN

Overview

Antineoplastic drugs can be infused directly into a tumor through a catheter placed into a major artery. The artery chosen is determined by the location of the tumor. This procedure allows a concentrated solution of the drug to reach the tumor with minimal dilution by the circulatory system and before the drug is metabolized by the liver or kidneys. The intra-arterial catheter is inserted surgically or by fluoroscopic guidance. The administration of chemotherapeutic agents may last several days.

Objective

To administer chemotherapy directly into the tumor.

Special Equipment

> Volumetric infusion pump and administration tubing
> Three-way stopcock
> Gloves
> Tape
> Sterile transparent dressing
> Chemotherapy drug in solution
> Heparinized IV saline solution (if needed)

Procedure

ACTION	RATIONALE
1. Monitor patient response while intra-arterial catheter is inserted under fluoroscopy.	1. Visualization is necessary to ensure placement of catheter near the tumor.
2. Don gloves prior to preparing the chemotherapeutic drug.	2. This prevents absorption of drug through the nurse's skin.
3. Prime IV administration tubing and infusion pump with ordered solution or chemotherapy agent.	
4. Administer heparinized saline solution if chemotherapy is not ordered to begin at time of insertion.	4. This prevents clotting in the catheter.

ACTION	RATIONALE
5. Place stopcock between infusion pump tubing and the intra-arterial catheter.	5. This prevents backflow of blood when changing the tubing or solution.
6. Tape all connections	6. This prevents accidental separation of tubing.
7. Start infusion pump to deliver at ordered rate.	7. An infusion pump is necessary to maintain an accurate flow and to overcome the arterial pressure.
8. Place sterile occlusive dressing over the catheter site.	8. This anchors the catheter as well as providing a barrier against infection.

9. Monitor patient for signs of catheter displacement.
  A. Monitor daily x-ray reports.
  B. Watch for changes in catheter length.
  C. Assess patient for symptoms of pain, dyspepsia, severe nausea, diarrhea, and vomiting.
  D. Observe the site for bleeding, hematoma, or edema.
	9. If catheter becomes displaced it must be repositioned or removed.

10. Administer anticoagulants as ordered. A. Maintain partial thromboplastin 1½ times the normal value by administering 10,000 to 30,000 units of heparin intra-arterially every 24 hours per physician's order.	10. This prevents potential complications of embolus or thrombus.
B. Administer 650 mg. of aspirin twice daily per physician's order.	B. This decreases platelet aggregation.
11. Change the tubing and solution every 24 hours.	11. This decreases the incidence of infection.

Precautions

1. Check the tubing frequently for patency.
2. Observe for signs of catheter displacement. Do not irrigate the catheter if it becomes occluded.
3. Do not irrigate the catheter if it becomes occluded.
4. Review the actions, dose, and side effects for all medications administered.

Related Care

1. Record the drug and fluid infused.

2. Assess the catheter site and change the dressing every 24 hours. (See "Long Venous and Arterial Indwelling Catheter Site Care.")

Complications

Thrombus formation   Bleeding at the insertion site
Emboli   Drug reactions
Infection   Shock

REFERENCES

Johnson, S.: Caring for the patient on intraarterial chemotherapy...Are you ready? Nursing 81, 11:108–112, 1981.

Newton, M.: Intraarterial Administration. Giving Medications—The Nursing Photobook. Horsham, Pa., Intermed Communications, 1980, pp. 95–97.

Tourigan, R.: Intra-arterial Infusion. Procedures: The Nurse's Reference Library, Springhouse, PA, Intermed Communication Book Division, 1983, pp. 358–360.

HEMODYNAMIC MONITORING

Karen C. Johnson, R.N., Ed.D.

Overview

Hemodynamic monitoring includes both invasive and noninvasive assessment techniques, and ranges from simple measurement using a blood pressure cuff to measurement of intracardiac pressures directly. Pressure measurement is critical for patient assessment; modern biomedical engineering has produced sophisticated equipment to monitor pressure continuously at the bedside. This is invaluable when caring for the critically ill patient in whom changes can occur rapidly.

Manifestations of Altered Hemodynamics. Signs and symptoms can vary from those of cardiac dysfunction, leading to pulmonary or systemic congestion with rales, pulmonary edema, increased jugular venous distention, and peripheral edema, to those of acute cardiovascular collapse and profound shock. These symptoms include weakness, pallor, confusion, cold clammy skin, diminished pulses to absence of pulses, cardiac dysrhythmias, low arterial blood pressure and decreased cardiac output. Also, new murmurs, rubs, and extra heart sounds may develop.

Fluid Challenge. Further evaluation of left ventricular performance can be obtained by altering therapy according to pressure measurements; this is known as fluid challenge. Fluid volume expansion causes an increase in myocardial end-diastolic fiber length. According to the Starling principle this increases the force of ventricular contraction. In uncomplicated hypovolemia, fluids may be pushed until adequate *central venous pressure* (CVP) and *pulmonary artery wedge pressures* (PAWP) are reached, returning the patient to a normal volemic state. If the CVP and PAWP rise with the fluid challenge but the patient remains hypotensive, then the possibility of heart failure must be considered.

Preload and Afterload. Preload may be defined briefly as end-diastolic fiber length (PAWP). Afterload is the resistance to ventricular ejection (aortic pressure). Cardiac function may be improved by increasing preload to increase the length of fiber stretch, thereby increasing myocardial contractility, and decreasing afterload, thereby increasing cardiac output. There are both mechanical and pharmaceutical agents that accomplish this. A common method is to administer dopamine to increase preload while simultaneously titrating sodium nitroprusside (Nipride) to decrease afterload. This careful balance of vasotonic agents may assist the failing heart.

Assessment of Altered Hemodynamics. Multiple hemodynamic parameters are used in subsystem assessment of the critically ill patient.

Physiologic monitoring can include measurement of central venous, pulmonary artery, pulmonary artery wedge, left atrial, and arterial pressures, and cardiac output or cardiac index determination or both.

Central Venous Pressure. The CVP indicates the pressure in the right atrium and is also known as RAP; this directly reflects right ventricular diastolic pressure, or the ability of the right side of the heart to pump blood. In patients with normal cardiac reserve and normal pulmonary vascular resistance, the CVP can be valuable for assessing the dynamic interrelationships among cardiac action, vascular tone, and blood volume. The CVP is especially useful in monitoring the overall fluid dynamics of noncardiac patients such as one with gastrointestinal bleeding. CVP is not an accurate index of left ventricular function and may, indeed, be one of the last parameters to change. However, it is a valuable diagnostic tool for many patients in whom fluid status is of concern. Fluid replacement or restriction can be prescribed more judiciously on the basis of the CVP findings. A normal CVP ranged from 5 to 10 cm. of water or 6 to 12 mm. Hg.

Pulmonary Artery Wedge Pressure. The flow-directed pulmonary artery catheter makes possible indirect measurements of left-sided heart pres-

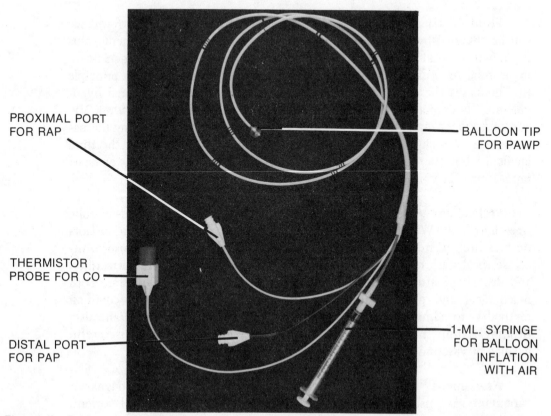

PROXIMAL PORT
FOR RAP

BALLOON TIP
FOR PAWP

THERMISTOR
PROBE FOR CO

DISTAL PORT
FOR PAP

1-ML. SYRINGE
FOR BALLOON
INFLATION
WITH AIR

Figure 1-40. Pulmonary artery catheter.

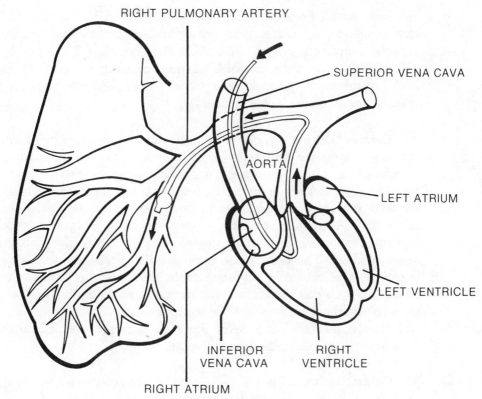

Figure 1-41.   Pulmonary artery catheter and balloon inflation.

sures at the bedside (Fig. 1-40). A small balloon at the end of the catheter becomes buoyant when inflated and passes through the cardiac chambers in the direction of blood flow. Thus, when the catheter is inserted into a large intrathoracic vein it passes into the right atrium, through the tricuspid valve into the right ventricle, and through the pulmonary valve into the pulmonary artery (PA), where it finally wedges itself in a smaller lumen of the artery (Fig. 1-41). The opening of the catheter beyond the inflated balloon reflects pressures distal to the PA, that is, the passive runoff of pulmonary venous blood into the left atrium. This PAWP, then, measures left ventricular function indirectly, since the mean PAWP ($\overline{\text{PAWP}}$) and left atrial pressure ($\overline{\text{LAP}}$) closely approximate left ventricular end-diastolic pressure (LVEDP) in patients with normal left ventricular and mitral valve function. When the balloon is deflated, the catheter measures PA pressure (PAP) directly.

PA catheters are available in multiple sizes and with assorted features. These include a single-lumen catheter for PAP, a double-lumen catheter for PAP and PAWP, a triple-lumen catheter for PAP, PAWP, and CVP, a quadri-lumen catheter for PAP, PAWP, and CVP, and a thermistor probe for cardiac output studies. In addition, some catheters feature an additional side-arm port for IV infusion, and some feature a double lumen into the right atrium itself so that continuous noninterrupted CVP monitoring and IV infusion into the right atrium may occur simultaneously. Finally, some catheters feature a pacing electrode.

Left Atrial Pressure.   This is measured by a left atrial (LA) catheter that is inserted by the surgeon during cardiac surgery and connected to a pressure transducer system. Mean left atrial pressure (LAP) closely reflects LVEDP in patients with normal LV and mitral valve function. Patients with LAP monitoring are potential risks for air emboli; security of all connections must be checked closely and frequently.

Cardiac Output.   This is the product of heart rate times stroke volume, in liters per minute. Normal resting cardiac output is about 4 to 8 liters/minute. Unless an intracardiac shunt is present, the cardiac output of both the right and left ventricles is essentially the same. Monitoring cardiac output is important in assessment of cardiac status and the patient's response to therapy. A low resting cardiac output may be due to poor ventricular filling from hypovolemia, valvular stenosis, or poor ventricular emptying, as in aortic stenosis. The usual cause is myocardial dysfunction. A high cardiac output may be caused by hypermetabolic states such as hyperthyroidism or by anxiety. Cardiac output may be increased by increasing preload and decreasing afterload. There are three basic methods for measuring cardiac output—the method based upon the Fick principle, the indicator-dilution method, and the thermodilution technique.

Cardiac Index.   This is the patient's cardiac output per square meter of body surface area (BSA). Normal cardiac index is 2.5 to 4.0 liters/minute/m.^{2} and is calculated by dividing the cardiac output in liters per minute by the BSA is square meters. The BSA is obtained from the Dubois Body Surface Chart (Fig. 1–42).
Relating cardiac output to body size provides more accurate measurement than cardiac output alone, because it takes into consideration the needs of an individual's tissues according to his or her actual body size.

Techniques of Hemodynamic Monitoring.   Arterial pressure monitoring may be obtained by continuous pressure monitoring, intermittent and automatic indirect techniques, or cuff pressure technique.

Direct Monitoring.   In direct arterial monitoring the arterial wave form should be sharp, with a rapid upstroke (anacrotic limb), clear systolic peak, definite dicrotic notch, and definite end-diastolic component. The recorded wave forms may be delayed from the corresponding electrical event of the cardiac cycle because of recording pressure delay of events when using a long catheter.

Noninvasive Automated Systems.   Automatic blood pressure measurements are generally programmed so that the frequency of blood pressure determinations may be selected; determinations may be made as often as every minute or as infrequently as every 8½ minutes. On many models, once a determination is completed, the values are given on a digital display(s) until a new determination is made. The results of the most recent determinations are then shown on the face of the blood pressure unit. Equipment

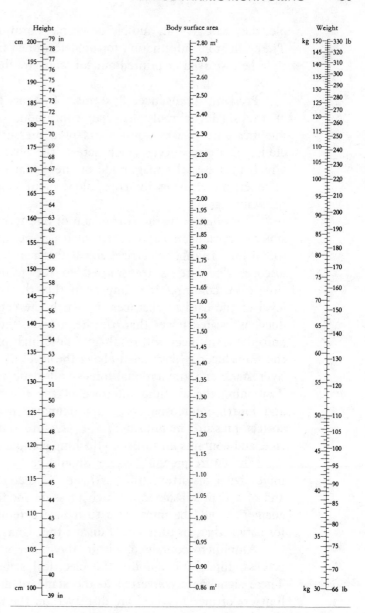

Figure 1-42. Dubois body surface chart. Find the patient's height in either feet or centimeters in the left column and the patient's weight in pounds or kilograms in the right column. Connect these two points with a ruler. The BSA is indicated at the point where the ruler crosses the middle column.

varies according to the automatic blood pressure device utilized. Some have external transducers or microphones; others may include only the automated blood pressure apparatus, an ordinary blood pressure cuff, and two pneumatic hoses between the cuff and blood pressure machine. Many different automatic blood pressure monitoring models are being utilized to measure arterial blood pressure noninvasively with or without heart rate. Some models record Korotkoff's sounds electronically during automatic inflation and deflation of the cuff; others use ultrasound to measure arterial wall movement during automatic cuff deflation and inflation. Noninvasive automated systems can be programmed to detect changes in preset parameters. For example, they can give an audible or visible alarm, or both, when changes occur. They can store information for predetermined times, and the information can then be displayed or printed out for study by the health care team.

Pressure Transducer Systems.   Systems for bedside utilization can be of the single or multiple type, continuous or intermittent, with various modifications. Basic components of a pressure monitoring system can include: (1) a transducer, which detects the physiologic event; (2) an amplifier, which increases the magnitude of the signal from the transducer; and (3) a recorder, meter, or oscilloscope, alone or in combination, which displays the resultant signal.

Transduction is the conversion of one form of energy into another. Physiologic transducers can convert such parameters as pressure, temperature, or sound into a usable electrical signal that can be displayed on a bedside oscilloscope. Pressure is transmitted to the transducer diaphragm through a fluid-filled column. It is important that the transducer be positioned at the level of the cardiac chamber in which the catheter is placed. If the transducer is located lower than the heart level, the force of hydrostatic pressure onto the transducer will result in a false high pressure reading. Conversely, if the transducer is positioned above the level of the heart, the combination of hydrostatic and gravitational forces will result in a false low pressure reading. Positioning the air-fluid interface of the transducer to the midaxillary line and fourth intercostal space approximates heart level most accurately for correct pressure monitoring. The pressure transducer system is closed, air-free, and contains an infusion/flushing component.

The entire pressure system should be kept simple and compact to eliminate signal distortion from artifact. Catheters and tubing should be short and of a firm substance for high pressure monitoring. Use of stopcocks and adapters should be minimized to reduce potential sources of air leaks or clot formation that, in turn, could distort the signal.

Amplifiers contained within the monitor may simply amplify or may process, filter, and amplify the electrical signals sent from the transducer. These signals are converted to the standard measurement for pressure, millimeters of mercury, and are displayed on the meters or digital component of the bedside pressure module. The pressure wave form can be displayed on a device such as an oscilloscope or chart recorder. These are mandatory for viewing the pressure wave form as a function of time.

Precautions.   The same electrical equipment that is invaluable in critical care monitoring and resuscitation also may be a potential risk to the patient; the most hazardous is ventricular fibrillation. Respect of electrical and safety monitoring guidelines is crucial. (See "Electrical Safety," pp. 552). A defibrillator, emergency cart, and medications must be readily accessible.

This section will present procedures for pressure transducer systems, select hemodynamic pressure monitoring, and automatic blood pressure measurements.

SINGLE PRESSURE TRANSDUCER SYSTEM _____

Objective

To monitor one pressure continuously, using a single pressure system (Fig. 1-43).

Special Equipment

Pressure transducer
Hemodynamic single monitoring system set-up (preassembled, sterile, disposable components customized to hospital needs):
Continuous flush device (1)
Macrodrip IV set (1)
Three-way stopcocks (2)
Pressure monitoring tube (72 inches) with male/female connectors (1)
Pressure monitoring tube (12 inches) with male/female connectors (1)
Male dead end protectors (2)
Transducer dome (1)
One-way stopcock (1)

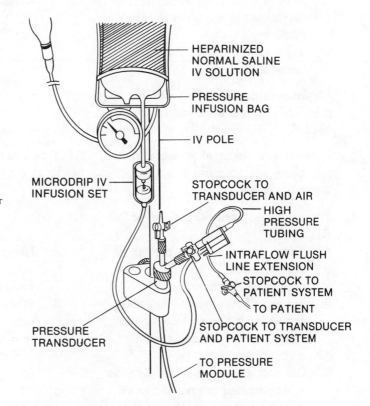

Figure 1-43. Single pressure transducer system.

Transducer mount or manifold (1)
Manifold mount
IV Pole
Normal saline (0.9% sodium chloride) IV solution (bag)
Sodium heparin for normal saline IV solution: 1 unit/ml. of
    fluid (or as ordered by physician)
Inflatable pressure cuff
Sterile water to prime transducer

For single pressure system with direct patient mounting, substitute:
    Transducer (sterile)
    Pressure monitor tubing (6 inches)
    Transducer mounting clip
    Inflatable pressure cuff (for arterial only)

Procedure

ACTION	RATIONALE
1. Prepare transducer dome.	
A. Remove protective dome from transducer.	
B. Hold the transducer level and place several drops of sterile bacteriostatic water on the transducer head.	B. Use sterile water, since saline solution may cause rust.
C. Screw on the sterile disposable transducer dome.	
2. Mount transducer on IV pole; use manifold and manifold mount, if needed.	
3. Connect transducer to pressure monitor; allow 5 to 10 minutes as a warm-up period.	3. This ensures accurate transducer calibration.
4. Prepare heparinized normal saline IV solution.	
A. Add 1 unit of heparin per ml. of normal saline IV solution, or as prescribed by physician.	A. Heparinized normal saline IV solution prevents clotting and embolic complications.
B. Extract all air from IV solution bag through the medication port, using a sterile 22-gauge needle and syringe.	B. If all air is not removed from IV solution bag, air may be forced into patient when the IV solution is depleted.
C. Connect microdrip IV infusion set to heparinized normal saline IV solution; clamp-on IV infusion set should be in "closed" position.	

ACTION	RATIONALE
5. Attach pressure cuff over heparinized normal saline IV solution bag; inflate to approximately 50 mm. Hg.	
6. Tighten all adapter connections.	6. Small leaks can allow blood to back up into catheter.
7. Prime preassembled, sterile, hemo-dynamic pressure monitoring system and transducer dome, using sterile technique and per manufacturer's guidelines.	
8. Pressurize heparinized IV solution bag cuff to 300 mm. Hg; observe that IV drip chamber does not completely fill during pressurization.	8. Pressure should be above the systolic pressure of the patient to ensure the forward and continuous IV solution flush at a rate of approximately 2 to 3 ml./hour.
9. Replace vented caps on stopcocks with sterile dead caps.	
10. Check for air-free system.	10. Air bubbles trapped within system may dampen pressure tracing, posing a potential risk for air emboli.

11. Connect pressure line to catheter.
  A. Activate flush device until heparinized IV solution fills connecting hub completely.
  B. Hold catheter hub in a vertical position, allowing blood to prime the catheter hub retrogradely.
  C. Connect pressure line to catheter; secure connecting site.
  D. Activate flush device to clear blood from line.	

12. Using single pressure transducer system with "direct patient mounting":
  A. Attach primed IV tubing system to intraflow (see steps 4 and 5 above).
  B. Connect sterile transducer to transducer mounting clip; turn power on; allow 10 to 15 minutes as a warm-up period.
  C. Attach three-way stopcock to male end of intraflow; close to intraflow.
  D. Prime intraflow.
	B. This ensures accurate calibration.

ACTION	RATIONALE
E. Attach primed transducer with sterile dome to female end of intraflow.	E. Air bubbles trapped within system may dampen pressure tracing and pose a risk for air emboli.
F. Position transducer to level of patient's right atrium; secure with transducer mounting clip.	F. This will ensure accuracy of pressure determinations.
G. Connect pressure monitoring tubing to stopcock of intraflow; prime tubing.	
H. Attach pressure monitoring tubing to stopcock at patient's catheter.	

13. Perform "zero-reference" (or balance) check:
    A. Select appropriate ranges on monitor pressure module.
    B. Close stopcock to transducer and patient system (Fig. 1-43).
    C. Open transducer stopcock to transducer and air (Fig. 1-43).

D. Balance to zero reading according to manufacturer's instructions.	D. Transducer must be adjusted to zero at room air conditions for proper balancing.
E. Proceed with calibration; or leave transducer stopcock open to air if transducer will not be connected directly to patient for a time; or close stopcock to transducer and air and open stopcock to transducer and patient system (Fig. 1-43).	E. Leaving the transducer open to air while waiting for an indefinite period prevents pressure build-up and inaccurate readings.

14. Perform electrical calibration check according to range selected. A. Balance to zero. B. Adjust calibration dial to correct number that has been preassigned for selected ranges according to manufacturer's instructions. C. Close stopcock to transducer and air (Fig. 1-43). D. Open stopcock to transducer and patient system (Fig. 1-43).	14. This involves checking the monitor system's built-in electrical calibration that has a known pressure valve (see "Related Care").

ACTION	RATIONALE
15. Rebalance and recalibrate 30 minutes after connecting system to patient and leveling to right atrial position.	15. This ensures proper calibration.

Precautions

1. Maintain sterile technique throughout preparation of system.
2. Disconnect transducer from patient during defibrillation or cardioversion to prevent damage to the transducer.
3. Check for accurate readings; rebalance and recalibrate as necessary. Be sure that fluid-air interface is at the level of the patient's right atrium during pressure system connection.
4. Check that all connections are secure and dome is free from cracks.
5. Ascertain that all stopcocks are in the proper position.
6. Free all tubing and cables from potential pressure or kinking points.
7. Respect electrical safety guidelines for invasive monitoring; see also "Electrical Safety."
8. Maintain 300 mm. Hg pressure in inflatable pressure cuff during pressure monitoring. (The desired flow rate will generally be approximately 2 to 4 ml./hour. If the continuous flow rate is not within the desired range it may be adjusted by changing the IV solution pressure. Higher IV solution pressure will increase the flow rate, and lower IV solution pressure will decrease it.)
9. Set alarm limits.
10. Control for artifact by minimizing the number of electrical items in use, patient movement, and faulty transducers. Transducers that have been dropped, cleaned improperly, or exposed to even minimal diaphragm surface scratching are potential sources of erroneous readings or equipment artifact.

Related Care

1. Calibrate each transducer prior to hemodynamic monitoring. Transducers are sensitive and can be easily damaged. The biomedical electronics department often performs these checks per manufacturer's guidelines.
2. Observe IV drip chamber after each fast flush; monitor to verify that the continuous flow rate is in the desired range.
3. Locate stopcocks used in the collection of blood samples as near to the catheter connection site as possible to avoid withdrawal from the patient of a larger blood sample volume than needed or the subsequent flushing of a large fluid volume or both.
4. Check trace position or correct range pressure curve when pressure curve is positioned off the oscilloscope.
5. Change single pressure system every 24 hours.

Complications

Hemorrhage	Tubing separation
Sepsis	Electromicroshock
Air emboli	Equipment malfunction

Suppliers

Pharmaseal
Sorenson

REFERENCES

Daily, E.K., and Schroeder. J.: Techniques in Bedside Hemodynamic Monitoring, 2nd ed. St. Louis, C.V. Mosby, 1981.

Kaye, W.: Invasive monitoring techniques: Arterial cannulation, bedside pulmonary artery catheterization, and arterial puncture. Heart Lung, 12:395–427, 1983.

MULTIPLE PRESSURE TRANSDUCER SYSTEM _____

Objective

To monitor two or more pressures, using a multiple pressure system or modified single transducer systems (Fig. 1-44).

Special Equipment

MULTIPLE PRESSURE SYSTEM

Pressure transducer; (one for each pressure being monitored)
Hemodynamic multiple monitoring system setup (preassembled, sterile, disposable components customized to hospital needs)
    Five-gang manifold (1)
    Transducer domes (2)
    Continuous flush device (1)
    Three-way stopcocks (6)
    Pressure monitoring tubes (72 inches)
        with male/female connectors (2)
    Male vented protectors (5)

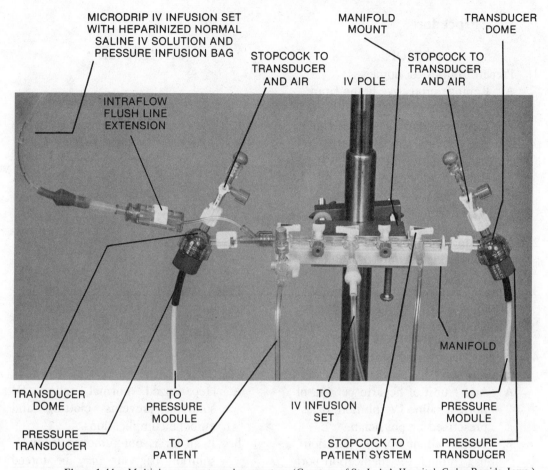

Figure 1-44. Multiple pressure transducer system. (Courtesy of St. Luke's Hospital, Cedar Rapids, Iowa.)

Male dead end protectors (9)
Manifold mount
IV pole
Normal saline (0.9% sodium chloride) IV solution bag
Sodium heparin for normal saline IV solution:
    1 unit ml. of fluid (or as ordered by physician)
Inflatable pressure cuff
Sterile water to prime transducer
Monitor capable of two or more pressures

SINGLE PRESSURE SYSTEM WITH SEPARATE TRANSDUCERS

See "Single Pressure Transducer System" and
    double or triple the equipment listed.

Procedure

ACTION	RATIONALE

1. Prepare transducer domes.
   A. Remove protective dome from transducer.
   B. Hold the transducer level and place several drops of sterile bacteriostatic water on the transducer head.
   C. Screw on the sterile disposable transducer dome.
	B. Use sterile water, since saline solution may cause rust.

2. Mount manifold on IV pole, using manifold holder; secure transducers.	
3. Connect transducer to pressure monitor; allow 5 to 10 minutes as a warm-up period.	3. This ensures accurate transducer calibration.

4. Prepare heparinized normal saline IV solution.
   A. Add 1 unit of heparin per ml. of normal saline IV solution, or as prescribed by physician.
   B. Extract all air from IV solution bag through the medication port, using a sterile 22-gauge needle and syringe.
   C. Connect microdrip IV infusion sets to heparinized normal saline IV solution; clamps on IV infusion sets should be in "closed" position.
	A. Heparinized normal saline IV solution prevents clotting and embolic complications.
	B. If all air is not removed from IV solution bag, air may be forced into patient when the IV solution is depleted.

5. Attach pressure cuff over heparinized normal saline IV solution bag; inflate to approximately 50 mm. Hg.	
6. Tighten all adapter connections.	6. Small leaks can allow blood to back up into catheter.
7. Prime preassembled, sterile, hemodynamic pressure monitoring system and transducer dome, using sterile technique and per manufacturer's guidelines.	

ACTION	RATIONALE
8. Pressurize heparinized IV solution bag cuff to 300 mm. Hg; observe that IV drip chamber does not completely fill during pressurization.	8. Pressure should be greater than the systolic pressure of the patient to ensure the forward and continuous IV solution flush at a rate of approximately 2 to 3 ml./hour.
9. Replace vented caps on stopcocks with sterile dead caps.	
10. Check for air-free system.	10. Air bubbles trapped within system may dampen pressure tracing, posing a potential risk for air emboli.
11. Perform "zero-reference" (or balance) check: A. Select appropriate ranges on monitor pressure module for each system. B. Close manifold stopcocks to transducer and patient system (Fig. 1-44). C. Open transducer stopcock to transducer and air (Fig. 1-44). D. Balance to zero reading according to manufacturer's instructions. E. Proceed with calibration; or leave transducer stopcock open to air if transducer will not be connected directly to patient for an indefinite time; or close transducer stopcock to transducer and air and open manifold stopcocks to transducer and patient systems (Fig. 1-44).	D. Transducer must be adjusted to a zero reading at room temperature for proper balancing. E. Leaving the transducer open to air while waiting for an indefinite time prevents pressure build-up and inaccurate readings.
12. Perform electrical calibration check according to range selected. A. Balance to zero. B. Adjust calibration dial to correct number that has been preassigned for selected ranges. C. Close transducer to stopcock to transducer and air (Fig. 1-44). D. Open manifold stopcock to transducer and patient system (Fig. 1-44).	12. This involves checking the monitor system's built-in electrical calibration that has a known pressure value (see "Related Care" step 1).

ACTION	RATIONALE

13. Rebalance and recalibrate 30 minutes after connecting multiple pressure systems to the patient and leveling to right atrial position.

Precautions

1. Maintain sterile technique throughout preparation of system.
2. Disconnect transducer from patient during defibrillation or cardioversion to prevent damage to the transducer.
3. Check for accurate readings; rebalance and recalibrate as necessary. Be sure that fluid-air interface is at the level of the patient's right atrium during pressure system connection.
4. Check that all connections are secure and dome is free from cracks.
5. Ascertain that all stopcocks are in the proper position.
6. Free all tubing and cables from potential pressure or kinking points.
7. Respect electrical safety guidelines for invasive monitoring (see "Electrical Safety").
8. Maintain 300 mm. Hg pressure in inflatable pressure cuff during pressure monitoring. (The desired flow rate will generally be approximately 2 to 4 ml./hour. If the continuous flow rate is not within the desired range it may be adjusted by changing the IV solution pressure. Higher IV solution pressure will increase the flow rate, and lower IV solution pressure will decrease the flow rate.)
9. Set alarm limits.
10. Control for artifact by minimizing the number of electrical items in use, patient movement, and faulty transducers. Transducers that have been dropped, cleaned improperly, or exposed to even minimal diaphragm surface scratching are potential sources of erroneous readings or equipment artifact.

Related Care

1. Calibrate each transducer prior to hemodynamic monitoring. Transducers are sensitive and can be easily damaged. The biomedical electronics department often performs these checks per manufacturer's guidelines.
2. Observe IV drip chamber after each fast flush; monitor to verify that the continuous flow rate is in the desired range.
3. Locate stopcocks used in the collection of blood samples as near to the catheter connection site as possible to avoid withdrawal from the patient of a larger blood sample volume than needed or the subsequent flushing of a large fluid volume.
4. Check trace position or correct range pressure curve when pressure curve is positioned off the oscilloscope.
5. Change multiple pressure system every 24 hours.

Complications

Hemorrhage   Tubing separation
Sepsis   Electromicroshock
Air emboli   Equipment malfunction

Suppliers

Pharmaseal
Sorenson

REFERENCES

Daily, E., and Schroeder, J.: Techniques in Bedside Hemodynamic Monitoring, 2nd ed. St Louis, C.V. Mosby, 1981.
Kaye, W.: Invasive monitoring techniques: Arterial cannulation, bedside pulmonary artery catheterization, and arterial puncture. Heart Lung, *12*:395–427, 1983.

CENTRAL VENOUS PRESSURE _____

Objectives

1. To obtain intermittent or continuous CVP to assist in assessing the hemodynamic profile or clinical evaluation, or both, of a patient.
2. To assess fluid replacement for selected patients, such as the postoperative patient, the patient who is actively bleeding, or the patient in whom volume status is questioned.
3. To obtain frequent blood samples without discomfort to the patient.

Special Equipment

CONTINUOUS PRESSURE MONITORING

Single or multiple pressure transducer system setup
ECG and pressure monitor and recorder
Central venous line

INTERMITTENT READINGS WITH A WATER MANOMETER

CVP manometer
Three-way stopcock
Central venous catheter
IV solution (as prescribed)
IV administration set

Procedure

CONTINUOUS PRESSURE MONITORING

ACTION

1. Prepare a pressurized monitoring system (see "Single Pressure Transducer System" or "Multiple Pressure Transducer System").

2. Connect pressure monitoring system to indwelling CVP catheter (see "Single Pressure Transducer System" or "Multiple Pressure Transducer System").

3. Level the air-fluid interface of the transducer with the patient's RA.
   A. Use the 90-degree angle port of the transducer dome stopcock as the air-fluid interface.
   B. Use midaxillary line, fourth intercostal space, as a landmark for the patient's right atrium.

4. Rebalance and recalibrate the transducer (see "Single Pressure Transducer System" or "Multiple Pressure Transducer System").

5. Monitor CVP pressure.
   A. Place monitor pressure selector on "venous."
   B. Check wave form (Fig. 1–45). CVP or right atrial wave forms show an *a, c,* and *v* wave with an *x* and *y* descent. Atrial contraction produces the *a* wave. Closing of the tricuspid valve produces the *c* wave. Pressure changes in the RA produce the *v* wave. Normal valve for CVP is 1 to 6 mm. Hg.

RATIONALE

3. Pressures reflect pressure changes or a movable diaphragm through a fluid-filled column. A transducer lower than heart level will reflect false high pressures because of hydrostatic and gravitational forces. Conversely, a transducer higher than heart level will reflect a false low pressure.

4. Variations in room temperature and withdrawal of blood may cause the transducer to drift; recalibration will ensure accuracy.

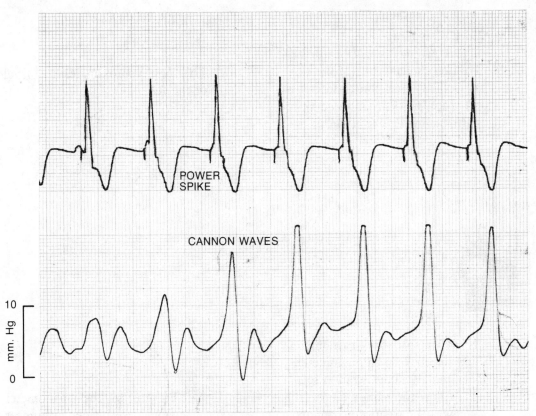

Figure 1-45. Central venous pressure; normal is 1 to 6 mm. Hg. The wave forms are delayed from the electrodynamic components owing to the time factor when recording pressure events through a long catheter. Note: Cannon waves occur as a result of atrial contraction against a closed tricuspid valve.

INTERMITTENT READINGS WITH A WATER MANOMETER

ACTION	RATIONALE
1. Prepare CVP equipment.	
A. Connect IV administration set to prescribed IV solution. Normal saline solutions are recommended; however, these may be contraindicated in certain patients.	
B. Connect CVP manometer to IV solution administration set.	
C. Use a connecting tubing between the CVP catheter and CVP manometer tubing (optional).	C. This may be necessary for ease of patient movement, measurement, and the like.
D. Prime system; check that all air has been removed.	D. Air entrapped within the tubing poses a risk of air emboli.
2. Connect air-free CVP catheter to prepared system.	

ACTION	RATIONALE

3. Obtain CVP reading.
   A. Check patency of CVP catheter.
   B. Position the zero line of the midaxillary line, fourth intercostal space; mark location on skin.
   C. Fill manometer (Fig. 1–46).

B. This best approximates the level of the RA.

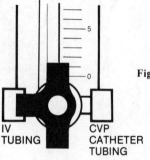

Figure 1-46.   Position for filling CVP manometer.

IV
TUBING

CVP
CATHETER
TUBING

   (1) Turn three-way manometer stopcock on to manometer and IV administration set.
   (2) Allow the manometer to fill with IV solution to approximately 10 to 20 cm. H_2O above the anticipated pressure reading.
   D. Establish fluid flow for CVP measurement (Fig. 1–47).

(2) Preventing the manometer from overfilling minimizes the possibility of contamination.

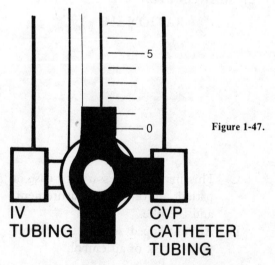

Figure 1-47.   Position for CVP measurement.

IV
TUBING

CVP
CATHETER
TUBING

   (1) Turn three-way manometer stopcock on to manometer and CVP catheter.

ACTION	RATIONALE
(2) Observe the falling fluid column in the manometer; check for respiratory fluctuations in the fluid column.	(2) For accuracy, there must be a free fall of fluid, pulsations with each heartbeat, and fluctuation of approximately 1 cm. H_2O with each respiration. Respiratory fluctuations reflect changes in intrathoracic pressures during the respiratory cycle.
E. Identify CVP measurement when the fluid level stops falling. Normal value of CVP is 3 to 15 cm. H_2O.	

4. Resume IV fluid administration to patient; check for prescribed infusion rate and CVP line patency (Fig. 1–48).

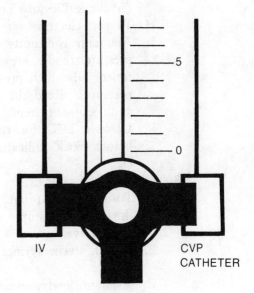

Figure 1-48. Position for IV fluid administration.

Precautions

1. Maintain patency of CVP line; aspirate before irrigating.
2. Monitor CVP line for absence of air or clots, and check that all connections are secure.
3. See also the precautions for the "Single Pressure Transducer System" or "Multiple Pressure Transducer System".

Related Care

1. Facilitate preinsertion responsibilities:
   A. Maintain aseptic technique.
   B. Place patient in Trendelenburg position during subclavian CVP insertion approach to prevent air emboli and facilitate gravitational filling of vessel.
   C. Choose proper length of catheter, depending upon insertion site.

2. Facilitate postinsertion responsiblities.
   A. Order chest x-ray to confirm catheter position and to rule out a pneumothorax.
   B. Perform dressing change and site assessment. (See "Long Venous and Arterial Indwelling Catheter Site Care").
   C. Obtain CVP measurement from same zero-reference point to ensure continuity and validity of data.
   D. Monitor CVP hourly, or as ordered by the physician. Observe for significant changes, CVP line obstruction, or potential sources for emboli.
   E. Change system every 24 hours.
   F. Recheck calibration of the transducer at least every 8 hours.
   G. See the related care for the "Single Pressure Transducer System" or "Multiple Pressure Transducer System."
   H. Respect electrical safety guidelines.
   I. Maintain continuity in pressure readings and observe changes in pressure trends. Pressures taken with the patient on a ventilator will reflect false high pressure readings because of positive intrathoracic pressures. Read the pressures consistently on or off the ventilator and document them.
   J. Observe ECG for right ventricular dysrhythmias or left bundle-branch block, indicating CVP catheter positioning in the right ventricle.

3. Obtain blood samples.
   A. Position patient flat to prevent air from entering the bloodstream during blood sample withdrawal from the internal, external jugular, or subclavian vein.
   B. Attach sterile syringe to CVP stopcock; open to CVP catheter and syringe.
   C. Aspirate slowly; amount will vary according to length of CVP line.
   D. Turn stopcock to halfway position to close to all ports; remove syringe and attach syringe for blood sample. Open to CVP catheter and syringe; obtain blood sample. Close to halfway position and remove syringe.
   E. Connect sterile syringe; open stopcock to syringe and IV fluid administration set. Clear stopcock and port of blood. Open stopcock to IV fluid administration and CVP catheter; resume IV infusion to clear line.
   F. Connect protective cap to stopcock; check prescribed fluid rate.

4. Remove CVP line.
   A. Position patient in a Trendelenburg position to prevent air emboli during catheter removal from the internal, external jugular, or subclavian vein.
   B. Expose site; culture as necessary.
   C. Clean incision with povidone-iodine prep swabs.

D. Remove catheter slowly, noting ease of withdrawal and effect on patient.
E. Check CVP catheter length; culture tip.
F. Apply pressure to site until bleeding is controlled.
G. Apply povidone-iodine ointment to site and secure sterile occlusive pressure dressing for 24 hours.
H. Observe site for hematoma or delayed bleeding.
I. Facilitate suture removal after 72 hours.

Complications

Pulmonary emboli
Phlebitis
Vein trauma
Pneumothorax
Infection (local, systemic, or both)
Malposition of catheter into jugular system
Dysrhythmias

Nonpatent CVP line
Fluid overload
Air emboli
Altered skin integrity
Inaccurate pressures
Equipment malfunction
Electromicroshock

REFERENCES

AACN: Clinical Reference for Critical-Care Nursing (edited by M. Kinney et al.). New York, McGraw-Hill, 1981.

Daily, E., and Schroeder, J.: Techniques in Bedside Hemodynamic Monitoring, 2nd ed. St. Louis, C.V. Mosby, 1981.

Kaye, W.: Invasive monitoring techniques: Arterial cannulation, bedside pulmonary artery catheterization, and Arterial Puncture. Heart Lung, 12:395–427, 1983.

PULMONARY ARTERY PRESSURE

Objectives

1. To assess the LVEDP indirectly when mitral valve function is normal.
2. To determine precisely the hemodynamic response of the patient to fluid therapy, medication, or other treatment.
3. To obtain accurate central vascular pressures in the presence of low cardiac output.
4. To obtain mixed venous blood samples.
5. To measure cardiac output directly or indirectly.

Special Equipment

Single or multiple pressure transducer system monitor
Recorder
Pulmonary artery catheter (single lumen, double lumen, triple lumen, quadruple lumen)
10-ml. syringe
1-ml. syringe
Sterile basin containing normal saline solution
Flouroscopy table and equipment, if ordered
Defibrillator
Emergency cart and medications
Sterile gauze pads
Povidone-iodine ointment
Sterile occlusive dressing
Pressure dressing

Procedure

ACTION	RATIONALE
1. Obtain vital signs and ECG recording.	1. This serves as baseline data.
2. Check security and position of ECG electrodes.	
3. Prepare a pressurized monitoring system (see "Single Pressure Transducer System" or "Multiple Pressure Transducer System"). A. Balance transducer. B. Calibrate.	
4. Level air-fluid interface of the transducer with the patient's RA. A. Use 90-degree angle port of the transducer dome stopcock as the air-fluid interface. B. Use midaxillary line, fourth intercostal space, as a landmark for the patient's RA.	4. Pressures reflect pressure changes or a movable diaphragm through a fluid-filled coumn. A transducer lower than heart level will reflect false high pressures with the addition of hydrostatic and gravitational forces. Conversely, a transducer higher than heart level reflects false low pressures.
5. Monitor patient's response during PA catheter insertion. A. Perform site care; drape. B. Test PA catheter balloon for air leaks by submerging into a sterile basin of normal saline solution while inflating the balloon with 1.0 to 1.5 ml. of air.	

ACTION	RATIONALE
C. Attach a primed and calibrated monitoring system to PA and RA ports; prime catheter lumens.	
D. Antecubital site is anesthetized and cutdown is performed by physician. PA catheter is advanced until the RA wave form appears on the monitor.	
(1) Instruct patient to cough; observe wave form for RA pressure and fluctuation.	(1) Coughing produces fluctuation in RA wave.
(2) Inflate PA balloon with 1.0 ml. of air to enhance passage to PA.	
(a) Observe ECG for premature ventricular contractions (PVC's) during right ventricle (RV) passage.	(a) Ventricular irritability may occur during catheter passage.
(b) Ready bolus of local anesthetic.	
E. Observe wave forms; record pressures.	
(1) RAP (Fig. 1–49). RAP has *a*, *c*, and *v* waves and an *x* and *y* descent. The *a* wave	(1) Elevated RAP may indicate volume overload, RV failure, tricuspid stenosis or

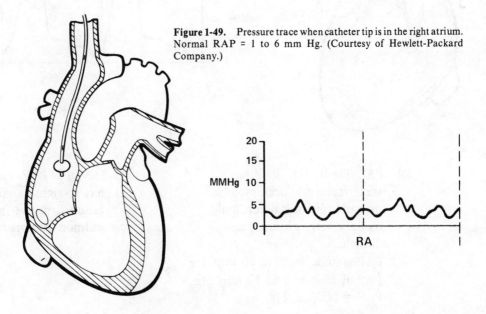

Figure 1-49. Pressure trace when catheter tip is in the right atrium. Normal RAP = 1 to 6 mm Hg. (Courtesy of Hewlett-Packard Company.)

ACTION	RATIONALE
represents atrial systole; the *c* wave represents closure of the semilunar valve; the *v* wave represents ventricular systole. The *x* descent follows atrial systole; the *y* descent represents atrioventricular (AV) opening. $\overline{RAP}$ = 1 to 6 mm. Hg.	regurgitation, pulmonary hypertension, LV failure, or constrictive pericarditis.
(2) RVP (Fig.1–50). RVP has three components: peak systolic pressure, early diastole, and late diastole. Ventricular end-diastolic pressure is read in late diastole. RVP systolic = 20 to 30 mm. Hg RVP diastolic = 0 to 5 mm. Hg.	(2) Elevated RVP may indicate pulmonary hypertension, RV failure, constrictive pericarditis, chronic congestive heart failure, ventricular septal defect, or hypoxemia.

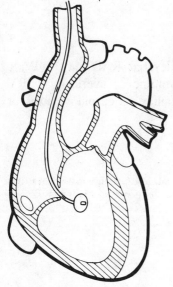

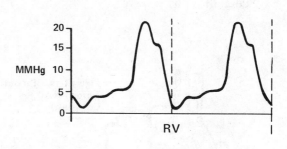

Figure 1-50. Pressure trace when catheter tip is in the right ventricle. Normal RVP = (20-30)/(0-5) mm Hg. (Courtesy of Hewlett-Packard Company.)

ACTION	RATIONALE
(3) PAP (Fig. 1–51). PAP has three features: peak systolic pressure, dicrotic notch (pulmonary valve closure), and diastole. $\overline{PAP}$ systolic = 20 to 30 mm. Hg $\overline{PAP}$ diastole = 1 to 10 mm. Hg $\overline{PAP}$ = 20 mm. Hg	(3) Elevated PAP may indicate left-to-right shunt, LV failure, mitral stenosis, or pulmonary hypertension.

ACTION

RATIONALE

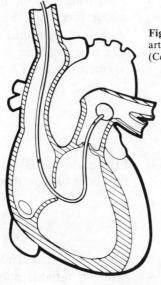

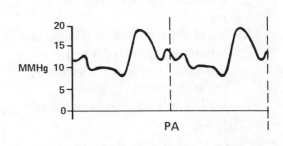

Figure 1-51. Pressure trace when catheter tip is in the pumonary artery. Normal/PAP = PAP/20 mm Hg = (20-30)/(0-10) mm Hg. (Courtesy of Hewlett-Packard Company.)

(4) PAWP (Fig. 1–52). PAWP has *a*, *c*, and *v* waves. The *a* wave occurs during atrial systole; it is absent in atrial fibrillation. The *c* wave represents closure of the A-V valves. The *v* wave is high during systolic regurgitation. $\overline{PAWP}$ = 4 to 12 mm. Hg

(4) Elevated PAWP may be an indication of LV failure, mitral insufficiency, or mitral stenosis.

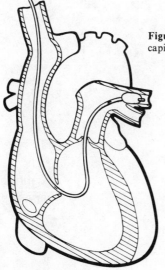

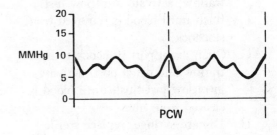

Figure 1-52. Pressure trace when catheter tip is in the pulmonary capillary wedge position. (Courtesy of Hewlett-Packard Company.)

ACTION	RATIONALE
F. Deflate balloon by removing syringe from balloon stopcock; allow balloon to deflate passively. Ensure deflation by proper PA tracing.	F. Aspirating balloon manually may cause premature balloon rupture. A balloon left inflated can cause pressure ischemia and necrosis of segments of the PA.

6. Wedge balloon.
   A. Rebalance and recalibrate transducer.
   B. Ascertain that balloon is deflated.
   C. Inflate slowly with 0.8 to 1.5 ml. air; make sure that wedge is tracing on recorder.
   D. Deflate balloon; leave syringe in place.

    C. Inflate slowly to prevent overinflation or balloon rupture.

7. Obtain blood sample of mixed venous blood by aspirating from distal port with balloon deflated.
   A. Attach a 10–ml. sterile syringe to distal port stopcock.
   B. Open stopcock to syringe and distal port; aspirate to clear line and ascertain purity of sample.
   C. Close stopcock to the halfway position; remove syringe and maintain sterile technique.
   D. Attach blood sample syringe to distal port stopcock; open stopcock to syringe and distal port; aspirate blood sample.
   E. Turn distal port stopcock to halfway position and remove blood sample syringe.
   F. Attach sterile syringe; open distal port stopcock to syringe and intraflow; activate intraflow fast flush until blood is removed from stopcock.
   G. Open distal port stopcock to intraflow and distal port; activate intraflow fast flush until blood is cleared from line.
   H. Discard syringe; replace sterile protective cap to distal port stopcock.

7. Balloon must be deflated; aspiration with balloon inflated may cause sample to become partially contaminated with arterial blood and not be a mixed venous sample.
   B. Amount of blood aspirated will vary because of tubing and catheter length. It is critical to obtain a pure sample.

ACTION	RATIONALE
8. Monitor PAP and PAWP.	
A. Integrate data with hemodynamic profile and clinical assessment of patient.	A. Isolated and absolute levels are not as important as *trend alterations* and the *effects of these alterations on the patient.*
B. Make sure that no other IV infusion is administered through the PA line.	B. Pulmonary extraversion is a potential risk.
C. Obtain chest x-ray to ascertain catheter position.	
D. Assess circulation to extremity.	
9. Prepare for removal of PA line.	
A. Close intraflow stopcocks to patient on all ports; open transducer stopcock to air; disconnect transducer from monitor.	A. These safety measures are to protect the patient and transducer.
B. Assess circulation to extremity prior to removal.	
C. Obtain vital signs.	C. These serve as baseline data.
D. Monitor patient while physician removes catheter.	
(1) Observe for dysrhythmias.	
(2) Anticipate that balloon will be inflated with approximately 0.3 to 0.5 ml. of air until the catheter has been withdrawn to the RA position.	(2) This prevents ventricular trauma to the chordae tendinae and valves.
E. Apply firm pressure until bleeding stops; apply povidone-iodine ointment and sterile occlusive dressing.	
F. Perform circulation assessment to extremity and site inspection every 5 minutes times 2; then every 15 minutes times 2; remove pressure dressing in 8 hours postbleeding at site.	

Precautions

1. See also the precautions for the "Single Pressure Transducer System" or "Multiple Pressure Transducer System."
2. Set alarms at all times, approximately 20 mm. above and below the pressure readings.

3. Monitor entire system for absence of air or clots and check security of all connections.

4. Observe PAP wave form for potential of catheter slipping into RV. Notify physician *immediately* because of risk of ventricular irritability or trauma.

5. Check for catheter wedge position. Move the patient's arm, have patient cough and deep breathe, and reposition patient. Notify the physician *immediately* if unable to dislodge a wedged catheter.

6. Use PAP line with caution for obtaining blood samples; monitor IV infusions, since pulmonary extravasation is a potential risk.

7. Ready defibrillator, emergency cart, and medications during insertion and removal of catheter.

8. Respect electrical safety guidelines.

Related Care

1. Record pressures hourly or as ordered by the physician; monitor continuously. Observe for significant changes or potential sources of emboli.

2. Perform site care. (See "Long Venous and Arterial Indwelling Catheter Site Care").

3. Change pressure transducer system every 24 hours.

4. Recheck calibration every 4 hours.

5. See related care for the "Single Pressure Transducer System" or "Multiple Pressure Transducer System."

6. Assess circulation to extremity every 2 to 4 hours.

7. Monitor $\overline{PAWP}$ every 2 to 4 hours; check integrity of balloon by using correct amount of air for balloon inflation and feeling for resistance during inflation. Keep syringe attached to catheter with correct amount of air.

Complications

Air emboli	Hemothorax
Thromboembolism	Cardiac tamponade
Cardiac arrest	Loss of balloon integrity
Dyshythmias	Balloon rupture
Catheter displacement/ dislodgment	Lung ischemia
	PA rupture
Infection	Pulmonary extravasation,
Electromicroshock	hemorrhage, or infarction
Altered skin integrity	Altered circulation to extremities
Inaccurate pressures	Frank hemorrhage
Equipment malfunction	Altered hemodynamics

Suppliers (of Pulmonary Artery Catheters)

American Electrocatheter Company
Electrocatheter Company
Swan Ganz–Edwards Laboratories

REFERENCES

AACN: Clinical Reference for Critical-Care Nursing (edited by M. Kinney et al.). New York, McGraw-Hill, 1981.
Daily, E., and Schroeder, J.: Techniques in Bedside Hemodynamic Monitoring, 2nd ed. St. Louis, C.V. Mosby, 1981.
Kaye, W.: Invasive monitoring techniques: Arterial cannulation, bedside pulmonary artery catheterization, and arterial puncture. Heart Lung, 12:395–427, 1983.

ARTERIAL PRESSURE

Objectives

1. To provide accurate, continuous, and objective data regarding a patient's altered hemodynamic status due to *high risk* for dysrhythmias, excessive vasoconstriction, low output, or unstable condition.
2. To obtain continuous blood pressure readings during the administration of potent vasoactive and vasodilating medications to measure the trends and effects of therapeutic interventions.
3. To obtain frequent blood gas determinations without discomfort to the patient and without disturbing the steady state.

Special Equipment

Single or multiple pressure transducer system
ECG and pressure monitor and recorder
Arterial line
10-ml. sterile syringe

Procedure

ACTION	RATIONALE
1. Prepare a pressurized monitoring system (see "Single Pressure Transducer System" or "Multiple Pressure Transducer System").	

ACTION	RATIONALE
2. Connect pressure monitoring system to indwelling arterial line (see "Single Pressure Transducer System" or "Multiple Pressure Transducer System").	
3. Level the air-fluid interface of the transducer with the patient's RA. A. Use the 90-degree angle port of the transducer dome stopcock as the air-fluid interface. B. Use midaxillary line, fourth intercostal space, as a landmark for the patient's RA.	3. Pressures reflect pressure changes on a movable diaphragm through a fluid-filled column. A transducer lower than heart level will reflect false high pressures with the addition of hydrostatic and gravitational forces. Conversely, a transducer higher than heart level will reflect false low pressures.
4. Rebalance and recalibrate the transducer (see "Single Pressure Transducer System" or "Multiple Pressure Transducer System").	4. Variations in room temperature and withdrawal of blood may cause the transducer to drift; recalibration will ensure accuracy.

5. Monitor arterial pressure.
  A. Place monitor pressure selector on "systolic," "diastolic," or "mean"; read meter or digital display reading.
  B. Check wave form (Fig. 1–53). Appearance of the arterial wave form is important data. Normal arterial pressure is 120/80, with a mean of 83 mm. Hg.
	A. Changes in systolic, diastolic, or mean arterial pressure require select assessment respective of trending and effect on patient.
	  B. Location of the dicrotic notch should be one-third or greater the height of the systolic peak; otherwise, suspect reduced cardiac output. A delay in the rapid rising anacrotic limb suggests a decrease in myocardial contractility, aortic

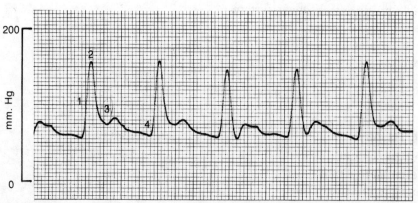

Figure 1-53. Arterial pressure tracing. 1, Anacrotic limb; 2, systolic peak; 3, dicrotic notch (Note: low due to hypovolemic status); 4, diastolic pressure.

ACTION	RATIONALE
	stenosis, or dampened pressure movement secondary to catheter position or clot formation.
C. Check wave form for various physiologic effects (Fig. 1–54).	C. Variations in arterial curves are due to increases in tachypnea, hypotension, or irregular ventricular rates such as atrial fibrillation or PVC's.

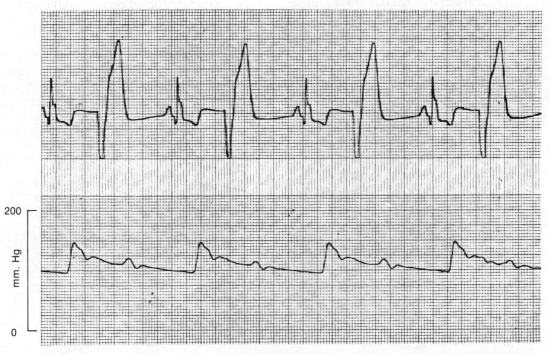

Figure 1-54. Arterial pressure tracing showing effect of bigeminy PVC's.

D. Notify the physician of significant pressure changes.	
E. Maintain patency of arterial line; control infusion rate of 3 to 4 ml./hour.	E. This prevents the potential of emboli.
F. Integrate arterial pressure data with hemodynamic profile and clinical assessment of patient.	F. Isolated and absolute values are not as important as *trend alterations* and the *effects of these alterations on the patient*.
6. Obtain a blood sample.	
A. Attach 10–ml. sterile syringe to arterial catheter stopcock.	
B. Open stopcock to syringe and arterial catheter; aspirate to clear the line and check for purity of arterial sample.	B. Amount of blood aspirated will vary because of tubing and catheter length. It is critical to obtain a *pure* sample.

ACTION	RATIONALE
C. Close stopcock to the halfway position; remove syringe and maintain sterile technique.	
D. Attach blood sample syringe to arterial catheter stopcock; open stopcock to syringe and arterial catheter; aspirate blood sample.	
E. Turn stopcock to halfway position and remove arterial blood sample syringe.	E. To prevent loss of blood from the system the stopcock should be in a halfway position.
F. Eject all air bubbles from arterial blood sample, cap immediately, and put on ice.	
G. Attach sterile syringe; open arterial catheter stopcock to syringe and intraflow; activate intraflow fast flush until blood is removed from stopcock and port.	
H. Open stopcock to intraflow and arterial line; flush using intraflow fast flush device.	
I. Discard syringe; replace sterile protective cap to arterial catheter stopcock.	
7. Prepare for removal of arterial line.	
A. Close arterial catheter stopcock to patient; open transducer stopcock to air; disconnect transducer from monitor.	A. These are safety measures to protect the patient and the transducer.
B. Expose arterial line site.	
C. Gently remove catheter from artery and place sterile gauze pads over the insertion site; apply direct pressure for a minimum of 5 minutes or until bleeding stops.	C. Direct pressure assists in sealing the puncture site; heparinized solution decreases clotting ability.
D. Apply povidone-iodine ointment, sterile gauze pads, and pressure dressing.	
E. Assess circulation to extremity.	
F. Assess circulation and dressing every 5 minutes times 2; then every 15 minutes times 2; remove pressure dressing in 8 hours postbleeding at site.	

Precautions

1. See the precautions for the "Single Pressure Transducer System" or "Multiple Pressure Transducer Sytem."
2. Set alarms at all times, approximately 20 mm. above and below the pressure readings.
3. Monitor arterial line for absence of air or clots and check security of all connections.
4. Maintain patency of arterial line; flush arterial lines after blood samples are drawn or tracing becomes dampened. Avoid excessive pressure when flushing or withdrawing samples from line; this prevents arteriospasms. If tracing dampens more often than every 30 miniutes, suspect clotting and notify physician. Correct dampened pressure tracing by repositioning catheter, straightening extremity, or aspirating with a syringe as necessary; flush line slowly with heparinized saline solution.
5. Perform the Allen test or modified Allen test prior to arterial line insertion.
6. Respect electrical safety guidelines.

Related Care

1. Monitor arterial pressure hourly or as ordered by the physician. Observe for significant changes or potential sources of emboli.
2. Perform arterial line site care (see "Long Venous and Arterial Indwelling Catheter Site Care").
3. Change pressure transducer system setup every 24 hours.
4. Recheck calibration at least every 8 hours.
5. See related care for the "Single Pressure Transducer System" or "Multiple Pressure Transducer System."
6. Assess circulation to extremity every 2 to 4 hours.

Complications

Air emboli	Electromicroshock
Thromboembolism	Altered skin integrity
Dysrhythmias	Inaccurate pressures
Altered hemodynamics	Equipment malfunction
Catheter displacement/dislodgment	Frank hemorrhage
Infection	Impaired circulation to extremities

REFERENCES

AACN: Clinical Reference for Critical-Care Nursing (edited by M. Kinney et al.). New York, McGraw-Hill, 1981.

Daily, E., and Schroeder, J.: Techniques in Bedside Hemodynamic Monitoring, 2nd ed. St. Louis, C.V. Mosby, 1981.

Kaye, W.: Invasive monitoring techniques: Arterial cannulation, bedside pulmonary artery catheterization, and arterial puncture. Heart Lung, 12:395–427, 1983.

LEFT ATRIAL PRESSURE _____

Objectives

1. To determine the LVEDP indirectly when mitral valve function is normal.
2. To determine precisely the hemodynamic response of the central vascular system to fluid therapy, medication, or other treatment.
3. To obtain accurate and continuous central vascular pressures in the presence of low cardiac output.

Special Equipment

Single or multiple pressure transducer system
Monitor
Recorder
Left atrial line
Air filter
10-ml. sterile syringe

Procedure

ACTION	RATIONALE
1. Prepare a pressurized monitoring system with an air filter.	
A. Select the procedure for a "Single Pressure Transducer System" or "Multiple Pressure Transducer System."	
B. Attach air filter to pressurized monitoring line.	
C. Prime air filter, using intraflow fast flush.	
D. Check that entire pressure transducer system and line with air filter are free from air.	D. LA line offers a high risk for air emboli.
2. Connect pressure monitoring system to patient (see "Single Pressure Transducer System" or "Multiple Pressure Transducer System").	

ACTION	**RATIONALE**
3. Level the air-fluid interface of the transducer with the patient's RA.	3. Pressures reflect pressure changes on a movable diaphragm through a fluid-filled column. A transducer lower than heart level will reflect false high pressures with the addition of hydrostatic and gravitational forces. Conversely, a transducer higher than the heart level reflects false low pressures.
A. Use the 90-degree angle port of the transducer dome stopcock as the air-fluid interface.	
B. Use midaxillary line, fourth intercostal space, as a landmark for patient's RA.	
4. Rebalance and recalibrate the transducer (see "Single Pressure Transducer System" or "Multiple Pressure Transducer System").	4. Variations in room temperature and withdrawal of blood may cause the transducer to drift; recalibration will ensure accuracy.
5. Monitor $\overline{LAP}$.	
A. Place monitor pressure selector on "mean."	A. Pressure changes between systolic and diastolic are insignificant.
B. Check wave form and $\overline{LAP}$ (Fig. 1–55). Normal $\overline{LAP}$ is 4 to 12 mm. Hg.	B. Appearance of wave form is important in assessing left ventricular function and accuracy of displayed pressures. $\overline{LAP}$ is increased in pulmonary edema, left **ventricular failure, mitral stenosis, and mitral insufficiency.**
C. Notify the physician of significant pressure changes.	

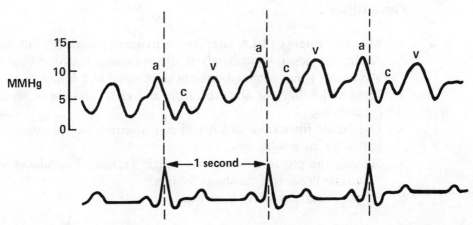

Figure 1-55.   Left atrial pressure, with a, c, and v waves. (Courtesy of Hewlett-Packard Company.)

D. Maintain patency of LA line; control infusion rate of 3 to 4 ml. per hour.	D. This prevents the potential of emboli.
E. Be sure that no other IV infusion is administered through LA line.	E. Constant entering of the closed system increases risk for air emboli or infection or both.

ACTION	RATIONALE
F. Integrate $\overline{\text{LAP}}$ data with hemo-dynamic profile and clinical assessment of the patient.	F. Isolated and absolute levels are not as important as *trend alterations* and the *effects of these alterations* on the patient.

6. Prepare for removal of LA line.

ACTION	RATIONALE
A. Close stopcock to patient; open transducer stopcock to air; disconnect transducer from monitor.	A. These safety measures protect the patient and transducer.
B. Don sterile gloves.	B. This reduces the risks of electromicroshock and infection.
C. Expose LA line site.	
D. Assess patient as physician removes LA line.	
E. Perform site care.	
F. Observe for increased bloody drainage at site or through chest tubes.	F. Cardiac tamponade is a potential complication.
G. Obtain chest x-ray 1 hour after removal of LA line.	G. This measure assists in ruling out hemothorax or cardiac tamponade. In the absence of bleeding, the chest tube may be removed.

Precautions

1. Maintain patency of LA line; do not irrigate or flush LA line manually.
2. Notify physician *immediately* if the system is nonfunctional or a good wave form is not obtained; anticipate removal of LA line.
3. Monitor LA line for absence of air and clots, and check security of all connections.
4. Use an air filter close to LA catheter insertion site to minimize the potential for air emobli.
5. See also the precautions for the "Single Pressure Transducer System" or "Multiple Pressure Transducer System."
6. Respect electrical safety guidelines.

Related Care

1. Monitor the $\overline{\text{LAP}}$ hourly, or as ordered by the physician. Observe for significant changes, LA line obstruction, or potential sources for air emboli.
2. Perform LA line insertion site care (see "Long Venous and Arterial Indwelling Catheter Site Care").

3. Change pressure transducer system setup every 24 hours.
4. Recheck calibration at least every 8 hours.
5. See related care for the "Single Pressure Transducer System" or "Multiple Pressure Transducer System."

Complications

Air emboli	Electromicroshock
Thromboembolism	Altered skin integrity
Cardiac arrest	Inaccurate pressures
Dysrhythmias	Equipment malfunction
Catheter displacement/dislodgment	Hemothorax
Infection	Cardiac tamponade

REFERENCES

AACN: Clinical Reference for Critical-Care Nursing (edited by M. Kinney et al.). New York, McGraw-Hill, 1981.

Daily, E., and Schroeder, J.: Techniques in Bedside Hemodynamic Monitoring, 2nd ed. St. Louis, C.V. Mosby, 1981.

Kaye, W.: Invasive monitoring techniques: Arterial cannulation, bedside pulmonary artery catheterization, and arterial puncture. Heart Lung, 12:395–427, 1983.

CARDIAC OUTPUT

Objectives

1. To measure cardiac output indirectly to determine overall hemodynamic status and assess patient's response to therapy.
2. To provide data for determining the cardiac index, which is cardiac output per square meter of body surface area.

Special Equipment

FICK METHOD

Heparinized syringes (2)	Volume meter
Douglas bag for collection of expired gases	Gas analyzer
	Stopwatch
Nose clip	Blood oxygen saturation analyzer
Mouthpiece	Calculator

INDICATOR-DILUTION METHOD

Densitometer	Arterial and venous catheter lines
Dye injection/flush system	Recording apparatus
Optical dye	

THERMODILUTION METHOD

Thermodilution catheter	10-ml. sterile syringe
1-ml syringe for balloon inflation	Iced normal saline IV solution at known temperature (between 0° and 5°C).
Thermodilution cardiac output computer	

Procedure

ACTION	RATIONALE
1. Monitor patient during cardiac output determination.	
2. Select appropriate procedure. Normal cardiac output at rest is 4 to 8 liters/minute. Normal cardiac index at rest is 2.5 to 4.0 liters/minute/m².	
A. Fick method. This procedure is based upon the principle of oxygen uptake per unit of blood as it flows through the lungs.	A. This method requires a stable patient and is respected for accuracy even in low cardiac output, shunts, or valvular insufficiency.
(1) Collect expired air sample.	
(a) Prepare and assess patient for an airtight system, using nose clip, mouthpiece, and Douglas bag.	
(b) Turn three-way stopcock to facilitate expelling expired air while patient breathes with the system for approximately 2 to 5 minutes.	(b) This enhances patient adjustment to the breathing system and primes the total system with the patient's expired air.
(c) Turn three-way stopcock to faciliate collection of expired air from the patient into the Douglas bag while simultaneously starting the stopwatch.	

ACTION	RATIONALE

(d) Collect expired air for approximately 2 minutes; then obtain blood samples.

(1) Collect a 10-ml. pure arterial blood sample slowly from arterial line.

(1) Controlled, slow withdrawal is important for a timed study.

(2) Collect a 10-ml. pure venous blood sample slowly from PA line.

(e) Continue collection of expired air for 5 to 6 minutes.

(e) This varies with bag size and patient variables.

(f) Turn off stopcock to the Douglas bag.

(g) Record time of collection stopped, using stopwatch.

(h) Facilitate blood and gas analysis; calculate cardiac output using Fick formula:

$$CO \text{ (ml./min.)} = \frac{O_2 \text{ consumption (ml./min.)}}{\text{arterial } O_2 \text{ content} - \text{venous } O_2 \text{ content (vol. \%)}}$$

B. Indicator-dilution method. This procedure utilizes a time-based dye concentration curve. A select amount of dye indicator is injected into the RA and concentrations are measured during arterial blood withdrawal.

B. By utilizing a computer, the results are made known immediately. This method is not affected by oxygen administration.

(1) Attach syringe containing known amount of dye to venous catheter.

(2) Attach precalibrated recording densitometer to arterial catheter.

(3) Simultaneously inject dye while steadily withdrawing an arterial sample through the densitometer.

(3) This records time-concentration curve as the dye passes through one circulation.

ACTION	RATIONALE
(4) Observe for dye reaction symptoms.	
(5) Remove syringe; flush IV lines and densitometer system.	(5) This prevents clot formation.
(6) Compute CO from dye concentration curve.	
(a) Use computer.	
(b) Calculate mean concentration in milligrams per liter.	
C. Thermodilution method. This procedure records a temperature-time curve.	C. It can be performed rapidly by one person. Inaccuracies may occur in low cardiac output, shunts, or valvular insufficiencies.
(1) Check that thermodilution catheter is positioned properly in the pulmonary artery and that balloon is deflated.	(1) There is a possibility of ventricular dysrhythmias because of current leakage if thermister probe is in right ventricle and connected to computer.
(2) Attach pretested thermodilution catheter thermistor port to precalibrated thermodilution computer; allow 5 minutes warm-up time for computer (Fig. 1–56).	

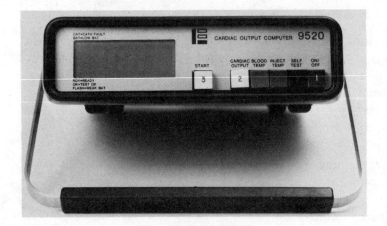

Figure 1-56. Thermodilution cardiac output computer. (Courtesy of Edwards Laboratories)

(3) Take patient's temperature rectally; dial into computer.	(3) Certain computers calculate the body temperature from the blood temperature; others do not.

ACTION	RATIONALE
(4) Rapidly inject known quantity of known temperature (cold; temperature of the injectate must be between 0° and 5° C.) sterile normal saline IV solution through proximal port (RA) of thermodilution catheter. Follow specific computer instructions.	(4) The injectate must be completely infused within 10 seconds after removal from ice bath so as not to alter temperature. Thermistor located at distal end of catheter reads temperature change in PA.
(5) Read CO from computer.	(5) Computer calculates temperature change into cardiac output.
(6) Obtain average of three sequential thermodilution readings. Remove syringe from proximal port of thermal dilution catheter; resume IV infusion.	
(7) Disconnect thermodilution computer.	

3. Check IV infusion rate and assess patient status.

Precautions

1. Maintain strict aseptic technique.
2. Follow electrical safety guidelines.
3. Observe for lethal dysrhythmias.
4. Check for proper position of the thermodilution catheter into PA before connecting to computer.
5. Also see precautions for "Pulmonary Artery Pressure."

Related Care

1. Fick method.
   A. Assess patient for hyperventilation, which can contribute to a false high reading of the respiratory quotient; repeat the expired air collection.
   B. Determine if the patient has a health history of perforated eardrums, which can contribute to expired air leakage. Cover external auditory canal tightly.
2. Indicator-dilution method: Monitor for variation in results due to dye recirculation, curve interpretation or catheter position.

3. Thermodilution method. Monitor for curve distortion due to catheter malposition, temperature change of injectate, or time delay in injection technique.
4. Provide defibrillator, emergency cart, and medications for immediate use, as necessary.

Complications

Dysrhythmias	Air emboli
Cardiac arrest	Electrical microshock
Dye reaction	or macroshock
Pulmonary emboli or	Infection
infarction	Equipment malfunction

REFERENCES

AACN: Clinical Reference for Critical-Care Nursing (edited by M. Kinney et al.). New York, McGraw-Hill, 1981.

Daily, E., and Schroeder, J.: Techniques in Bedside Hemodynamic Monitoring, 2nd ed. St. Louis, C.V. Mosby, 1981.

Kaye, W.: Invasive monitoring techniques: Arterial cannulation, bedside pulmonary artery catheterization, and arterial puncture. Heart Lung, 12:395–427, 1983.

NONINVASIVE AUTOMATIC BLOOD PRESSURE MONITORING

Objective

To monitor systolic, diastolic, and mean arterial pressures indirectly and noninvasively by automatic means.

Special Equipment

Automatic blood pressure monitoring device (equipment specific to model)
Trend Recorder (optional)

Procedure

ACTION	RATIONALE

1. Prepare automatic blood pressure monitoring equipment (Fig. 1–57).
  A. Place blood pressure device on rigid surface.
  B. Insert plug into proper voltage outlet.
  C. Arrange pneumatic hoses for free air flow and tube patency.	

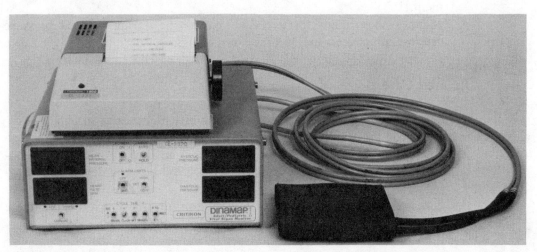

Figure 1-57. Noninvasive automatic blood pressure monitor and trend recorder. (Courtesy of St. Luke's Hospital, Cedar Rapids, Iowa)

ACTION	RATIONALE
2. Wrap deflated cuff (appropriate size) around selected extremity.	
3. Position patient's extremity at heart level and in such a way that external contact will be avoided.	
4. Turn on automatic blood pressure monitoring equipment; set alarm.	
5. Instruct patient to remain as motionless as possible during blood pressure readings. Cuff inflation will be felt; patient must remain motionless until cuff is deflated and blood pressure values recorded.	5. Excessive motion will cause altered readings.
6. Set frequency of blood pressure readings.	
7. Activate trend recorder (optional).	

Precautions

1. Avoid attaching the blood pressure cuffs to an extremity being used for IV infusion; this will result in cutting off the infusion while the cuff is being inflated. If the IV catheter is inserted in a marginal position, the increased pressure during inflation may potentiate infiltration.
2. Provide adequate ventilation around equipment console; rear of machine should be unobstructed so that heat generated by internal components is allowed to escape through the rear panel.
3. Restrict fluid placement around equipment console area; this contributes to electrical safety precautions for the patient and helps to protect equipment.
4. Monitor the patient for excessive movement during a blood pressure determination to ensure accuracy of readings.

Related Care

1. Check frequently for correct positioning of patient's arm to obtain accurate blood pressure readings.
2. Check for incorrect cuff connections, leaks in the system, kinks or obstructions in the system, or failure of the blood pressure device itself during an alarm alert.
3. Observe extremity for altered circulation or altered skin integrity; rotate extremity as needed.

Complications

Inaccurate blood pressure readings
Electrical shock
Altered skin integrity
Equipment malfunction

Suppliers

Applied Medical Research
Omega
Physiocontrol
Roche

REFERENCES

AACN: Clinical Reference for Critical-Care Nursing (edited by M. Kinney et al.). New York, McGraw-Hill, 1981.

——— CIRCULATORY ASSIST DEVICES ———

INTRA-AORTIC BALLOON PUMP
MANAGEMENT _____

Penny J. Ford, R.N., M.S.,
Rebecca A. Preston, R.N., B.S.N.,
and
F. Michael Vislosky, Jr., R.N.

Overview

The intra-aortic balloon pump (IABP) is a form of temporary circulatory assistance that has been used in (1) cardiogenic shock, (2) mechanical defects after myocardial infarction, (3) refractory cardiac ischemia, and (4) failure to wean from cardiopulmonary bypass. The balloon, mounted on a catheter, is usually threaded retrograde into the descending thoracic aorta through a femoral arteriotomy or percutaneous puncture. The catheter is connected to an external control console.

The balloon is inflated and deflated with gas in synchrony with the mechanical events of the cardiac cycle. Balloon inflation occurs during diastole, with deflation occurring during systole. Balloon inflation during diastole produces augmentation of arterial pressure, improving coronary artery and systemic perfusion. Balloon deflation occurs just prior to ventricular ejection, lowering resistance to left ventricular ejection, and thereby reducing afterload and consequently cardiac work. Typically the R-wave of the ECG is utilized as the triggering stimulus for synchronization of balloon and cardiac action.

The standard balloon catheter consists of semiflexible tubing with a single gas lumen. A double-lumen catheter with a hollow central lumen (which may be utilized for wire-guide passage, injection of contrast, or pressure monitoring) is also available. Both catheters are approximately 3 feet in length; the balloon is mounted on the distal 10 inches. The surface of both the balloon and catheter is antithrombogenic to minimize clot formation.

Two balloon designs are widely used at present. The first type consists of a single cylindrical chamber and is most commonly used for percutaneous balloon insertion. A mechanism for wrapping the balloon tightly around the catheter prior to insertion is incorporated into the balloon assembly. The second type has three segments. Inflation of the middle segment occurs first, followed by inflation of the end segments (Fig. 1–58). Balloon capacity is variable, ranging from 8 to 40 ml. Balloon size is selected according to total body surface area and size of the femoral artery.

The IABP external control console performs three important functions.

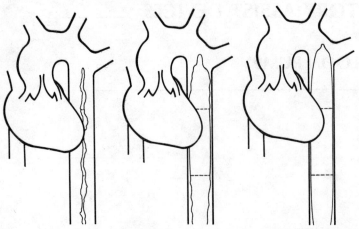

Figure 1-58. Trisegment omnidirectional balloon.

BALLOON DEFLATED   BALLOON INFLATING   BALLOON FULLY INFLATED

First, the ECG sensing circuitry within the unit permits synchronization of balloon and cardiac action. Second, the console contains the pneumatic controls that activate balloon inflation and deflation with either helium or carbon dioxide gas. Finally, automated alarms and safety features are incorporated into the design of all units. In the event of console malfunction or unsafe pumping conditions, the unit shuts down to a safe, inoperative mode with the balloon deflated. Patient transport during balloon pumping is made possible by switching the power source from wall current to battery power.

Objectives

1. To reduce cardiac work by decreasing afterload.
2. To increase cardiac output by decreasing the resistance to ventricular ejection.
3. To improve coronary artery perfusion by elevating diastolic pressure.
4. To improve myocardial oxygenation by reducing oxygen demand and increasing oxygen supply.
5. To maintain systemic perfusion.

Special Equipment

MEDICATIONS

Vasopressor mix
Colloid
Dextran 40 (Rheomacrodex) infusion
Local anesthetic bolus

Heparin bolus
Analgesics/sedatives
Atropine bolus
Antibiotic mix

STANDARD EQUIPMENT

IABP console
Fluoroscopic bed
  (if available)
IV poles
Standard IV solutions
Infusion pump
Pacemaker
Defibrillator
Multichannel monitor and
  recorder

Pressure transducers and flush
  systems
Intubation equipment
Urinary drainage system
Sterile dressing
Tape
Prep solutions
Antibiotic ointment
Sterile masks, gowns, drapes
Operating room light or head
  light

SURGICAL EQUIPMENT

Balloon catheter for surgical insertion
Surgical instrument tray
Continuous suction

PERCUTANEOUS EQUIPMENT

Percutaneous insertion kit
  (includes balloon catheter)
Silk sutures
Knife blade with handle
Umbilical tapes

Suture set
Sterile basin with heparinized
  saline
Contrast material (optional)

Procedure

ACTION	RATIONALE
1. Provide patient/family teaching after assessment of individual learning needs/readiness.	1. Pertinent teaching prior to insertion serves to diminish patient anxiety, reduce fear of the unknown, and increase patient cooperation during insertion.
2. Prepare equipment in patient cubicle for easy access and patient safety.	2. Arrangement of cubicle and preparation of equipment must be meticulous prior to insertion. Omission of these steps can be catastrophic during insertion, when the cubicle is crowded and the draped patient is relatively inaccessible.

ACTION	RATIONALE

A. Prepare bedside ECG and pressure modules for accurate recording (see "Hemodynamic Monitoring").

B. Plug in IABP console; turn on. Check gas supply and function of controls.

C. Check function of additional equipment: suction, oxygen, operating room light, pacemaker.

D. Prepare standby medications: vasopressor mix, colloid, dextran 40, local anesthetic, heparin, atropine, analgesics/sedatives, antibiotic mix.

3. Establish ECG on bedside monitor upon admission of patient.

4. Administer oxygen as prescribed.

5. Record baseline vital signs, including peripheral pulses, and 12-lead ECG. Mark peripheral pulses.

    5. Preinsertion pulses are essential for evaluating peripheral vascular disease that might preclude or complicate insertion and for comparison after insertion.

6. Assess hematologic profile.

    6. Hematologic studies are important, since heparin may be administered during insertion and platelet reduction can occur during pumping. Blood must be available during insertion in the event of arterial trauma and bleeding.

7. Sedate the patient, as necessary.

8. Establish ECG input to IABP console, either directly via patient cable or indirectly via the bedside monitor.

    8. The ECG is the triggering stimulus for balloon activation.

A. Position patient electrodes to obtain ECG configuration with maximal R-wave amplitude and minimal amplitude of all other waves and artifact.

    A. The sensing circuitry within the console utilizes wave amplitude as the primary criterion for R-wave detection.

B. Select desired sweep speed.

ACTION	RATIONALE
C. Using appropriate controls, ensure that the console is sensing the R wave consistently. Trigger light should flash once for each R wave.	C. Sensing of ECG components other than the R wave will disrupt IABP and cardiac synchrony.

9. Assist with the insertion of hemodynamic and intravenous catheters, as indicated.

ACTION	RATIONALE
A. Connect radial artery catheter, preferably in left wrist, to pressure transducer and continuous flush system.	A. IABP timing is adjusted, utilizing the arterial trace. The left arm is preferred since the balloon is located distal to the left subclavian artery. Upward displacement of the IABP catheter can readily be detected by damping of the left radial trace.
B. Connect pulmonary artery thermodilution catheter to pressure transducer and continuous flush system.	B. Accurate evaluation of left heart function and cardiac output is possible with this catheter.
C. Connect central IV line to a slow continuous infusion of 5% dextrose in water.	C. A central IV line must be kept available for the infusion of vasopressors. The right artial lumen of the PA catheter may be used in an emergency. However, if cardiac output measurements are to be made, vasopressors should not be infused in this lumen.
D. Connect peripheral angiocatheter to a slow continuous infusion of 5% dextrose in water.	D. A peripheral IV line should be kept available for the infusion of colloid, if necessary.
E. Connect transvenous pacing wire to pacemaker, on standby, unless otherwise indicated.	
F. Connect urinary catheter to drainage system.	F. Urinary output is a sensitive index of cardiac output.

ACTION	RATIONALE
10. Administer broad spectrum antibiotic, as prescribed by physician.	10. Adequate tissue levels of antibiotic should be established.
11. Shave and prep both groin sites.	11. In the event that balloon passage is impossible via one femoral artery, insertion in the other groin may be necessary.

ACTION	RATIONALE

12. Restrain the patient as necessary.

13. Ready standby medications.
 A. Attach vasopressor to central IV line via infusion pump.
 B. Place colloid and bolus medications near angiocatheter.

14. Connect dextran 40 to angiocatheter and adjust IV infusion rate to 10 to 20 ml./hour (optional).

14. This decreases platelet aggregation.

15. Mask, cap and gown all persons in immediate area.

16. Enclose "sterile" area and assist surgical team with preparation of the operative field.
 A. Drape patient, maintaining access to lines.
 B. Provide suction for operative field (surgical insertion only).
 C. Position overhead light.
 D. Provide requested equipment: antibiotic flush, heparin flush, local anesthetic, contrast material, balloon catheter.

 D. Contrast material may be injected through the central lumen of a double-lumen IABP catheter during insertion for visualization of vasculature.

17. Ready IABP console for start-up.
 A. Turn power on.
 B. Check gas tank or pressure gauge.
 C. Zero and calibrate pressure channels, as needed.
 D. Make preliminary timing adjustments, using appropriate controls. Select trigger logic, if necessary.
 E. Select 1:1 pumping ratio.

18. Note arterial systolic and diastolic pressures off IABP therapy, utilizing reference trace, if available.

19. Monitor ECG, pressures, and clinical status throughout procedure. Notify physician of significant change or pain.

19. Acute back pain, flank pain, or testicular pain may signify aortic dissection, warranting immediate notification of physician. Angina must be controlled to prevent infarction during insertion. Vasovagal responses secondary to aortic stimulation during catheter passage may require atropine.

ACTION	RATIONALE

20. Administer bolus of heparin approximately 3 minutes prior to arteriotomy or arterial puncture.

21. Evacuate and purge gas lines.
   A. If safety chamber present:
   (1) Extend and attach securely to balloon.
   (2) Evacuate air from safety chamber and balloon with syringe.
   (3) Fill safety chamber with gas.
   (4) Secure connections.
   B. If safety chamber not utilized:
   (1) Evacuate air from balloon during insertion by aspirating with syringe attached to IABP balloon plug.
   (2) Connect balloon plug to IABP console once balloon is positioned in the aorta.
   (3) Purge gas lines and fill balloon, using appropriate controls.

22. Initiate balloon pumping at low volume.

23. Adjust IABP timing, using the appropriate controls, visualizing the arterial trace (Fig. 1–59).

20. Despite the fact that the balloon surface is antithrombogenic, anticoagulation may be desirable.

21. For percutaneous balloons, air is evacuated manually prior to wrapping and insertion. IABP catheter is then connected to safety chamber (as in step A) or console (as in step B) and filled accordingly.

   (1) Aspiration reduces the diameter of the balloon, facilitating passage through the femoral artery.

   (3) Purging removes air from balloon catheter, filling lines with gas.

22. In the event of aortic dissection, pumping at low volumes minimizes trauma.

23. Timing should be adjusted to achieve maximal diastolic augmentation and reduction of afterload. The end-diastolic pressure on the balloon should be equal to or 5 to 15 mm. less than diastolic pressure off balloon. The exact timing of balloon inflation relative to the dicrotic notch depends upon the site used for arterial pressure monitoring (Fig. 1–59).

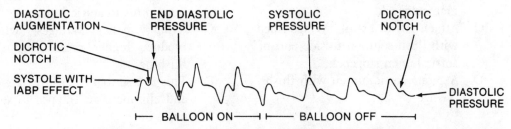

DIASTOLIC AUGMENTATION
DICROTIC NOTCH
SYSTOLE WITH IABP EFFECT
END DIASTOLIC PRESSURE
SYSTOLIC PRESSURE
DICROTIC NOTCH
DIASTOLIC PRESSURE
BALLOON ON
BALLOON OFF

Figure 1-59. Arterial trace with balloon on and off.

ACTION	RATIONALE

24. Evaluate balloon function by observing safety chamber or balloon pressure configuration.

25. Increase balloon volume to full capacity.

26. Recheck IABP timing and IABP pressure configuration.

27. Turn IABP console alarms on.

28. Assess peripheral pulses and record quality.

29. Apply sterile dressing, using sterile technique.

    29. Percutaneous balloon catheters should be anchored securely to the leg with adhesive tape to prevent displacement of balloon through the insertion sheath.

30. Arrange for a portable chest x-ray.

    30. A chest x-ray is essential to verify balloon position if fluoroscopic bed is not used during insertion. A chest x-ray should be obtained at least every other day with percutaneously inserted balloons to be certain that the balloon catheter has not changed position by displacement through the insertion sheath.

31. Connect the central aortic lumen to continuous flush system, if appropriate.
  A. Secure all connections of flush system and check flush for air bubbles before connection.

  B. Attach flush system to aortic lumen stopcock.
  C. Attach 10- to 12-ml. syringe filled with flush solution to side port of aortic lumen stopcock.
  D. Aspirate aortic lumen with flush syringe.

    A. Inadvertent disconnection may cause serious blood loss. Flush system may be air free because of lumen location in the central arterial vasculature.

    B. Aortic lumen stopcock should remain off to aortic lumen.
    C. Avoid smaller syringes, which produce higher pressures during flushing.
    D. This is essential to ensure patency and eliminate air trapped in stopcock.

ACTION	RATIONALE
E. *SLOWLY* flush line with syringe *after* aspiration.	E. Constantly observe for air or particulate matter while flushing. Eliminate by reaspiration if air or particulate matter noted.
F. *NEVER* flush line if clotted or if unable to aspirate.	F. Notify physician and shut off lumen stopcock.
G. Open aortic lumen stopcock to flush system. Cap side port of lumen stopcock with sterile Luer-Lok cap.	G. Continuous pressure monitoring with alarms is mandatory for detection of disconnection.
H. Turn on pressure module alarms.	
J. Inactivate fast-flush device of flush system.	J. Never fast-flush aortic lumen. Flush only with syringe after adequate aspiration.

Precautions

1. Protect balloon surface so that it does not come into contact with metal objects; perforation or damage to the antithrombogenic surface may result.
2. Avoid resterilizing or reusing balloons; the integrity and performance of balloons cannot be guaranteed under these circumstances.
3. Ensure that the IABP console senses the R-wave of the ECG to maintain accurate synchronization of balloon action.
4. Establish two potential routes of ECG input to the IABP console because of the ECG dependence: one via the direct patient cable and one indirectly via the bedside monitor.
5. Prepare emergency equipment and medications for the insertion.
6. Arrange for blood availability during insertion in the event of arterial trauma or hemorrhage.
7. Arrange for insertion of an arterial line prior to balloon insertion to ensure accurate balloon timing.
8. Adjust timing. Timing should be adjusted only by skilled personnel.
9. Avoid balloon deflation for more than 15 to 30 minutes. In the event of console malfunction, periodic quick manual inflation and deflation of the balloon with a 20-ml. syringe should prevent blood pooling and minimize potential clot formation.
10. Notify physician of recurrent angina during IABP therapy, since more aggressive therapy may be indicated.
11. Avoid inducing ECG artifact during chest physical therapy.
12. Monitor for contraindications. Aortic valve regurgitation and aortic aneurysm/dissection are absolute contraindications; severe peripheral vascular disease is a relative contraindication.

Related Care

1. Evaluate clinical and hemodynamic responses to IABP therapy every 15 to 60 minutes.
2. Assess quality of posterior tibial and dorsalis pedis pulses in both extremities hourly; note skin temperature and color. Doppler flow technique may be necessary to detect weak pulses.
3. Evaluate IABP timing hourly, and adjust as needed.
4. Maintain quality ECG signals for balloon activation.
5. Evaluate hematologic status to detect abnormalities: thrombocytopenia, fall in hematocrit (usually secondary to excessive blood loss during insertion or blood sampling), inadequate or excessive anticoagulation.
6. Perform routine respiratory care with minor modifications of position; head of the bed should not be elevated more than 45 degrees, nor should the involved leg be flexed.
7. Maintain strict aseptic technique during dressing changes. Dressing should be occlusive and should be changed every 48 hours. Change dressings on percutaneous balloon every 12 hours for the first 24 hours after insertion. Change more frequently as indicated. Outline any hematoma sites during dressing changes and record observations.
8. Continue antibiotic coverage for 24 to 48 hours after insertion.
9. Reduce the ratio of patient to IABP cycles (e.g., 1:1 to 1:8) during weaning, as prescribed by the physician; monitor patient's response closely.
10. Recreate the insertion environment during removal: organize equipment, reinstitute antibiotic coverage, turn IABP console off as ordered, aspirate or deflate balloon.
11. Evaluate peripheral pulses and patient tolerance after removal.
12. Assess incision for bleeding 15 minutes after surgical removal of balloon, then every 30 minutes times 2, then hourly for 8 hours. Bedrest is recommended for 24 hours after removal of surgical balloon; head of the bed should not be elevated more than 45 degrees.
13. Apply direct pressure either manually or with a mechanical clamp to the site of arterial puncture for at least 30 minutes after removal of the percutaneous balloon. Bedrest is recommended for 48 hours after removal of the percutaneous balloon; head of the bed should not be elevated more than 45 degrees.
14. Always connect the aortic lumen of double-lumen catheter to a continuous flush device to maintain patency and a pressure transducer/module for alarms. Otherwise the disconnected catheter will be undetected, and life-threatening arterial bleeding can occur.

Complications

Wound sepsis	Arterial trauma or dissection
Thrombocytopenia	Embolization of thrombi or
Thrombus formation on	plaque
balloon surface or catheter	Equipment malfunction

Suppliers

Datascope
Kontron

REFERENCES

Ford, P.J., and Buckley, M.J.: Circulatory assistance *In* AACN: Clinical Reference for Nurses. New York, McGraw-Hill, 1981.

Harvey, J.C., et al.: Complications of percutaneous intra-aortic balloon pumping (abstr.). Circulation, 62(Suppl. 3):41, 1980.

Leinbach, R.C., et al.: Percutaneous wire-guided balloon pumping. Am. J. Cardiol., 49:1707–1710, 1982.

Purrell, J.A., et al.: Intra-aortic balloon pump theory. AJN, 83:775–790, 1983.

Subramanian, V.A., et al.: Preliminary clinical experience with percutaneous intra-aortic balloon pumping. Circulation, 62(Suppl. 1):123–129, 1980.

EXTERNAL COUNTERPRESSURE WITH G-SUIT

Penny J. Ford, R.N., M.S.,
Rebecca A. Preston, R.N., B.S.N.
and
F. Michael Vislosky, Jr., R.N.

Overview

External counterpressure can also be exerted with application of the G-suit or antigravity suit. As opposed to the three-compartment MAST design, the G-suit is a single compartment garment enclosing the body from the xiphoid to approximately midcalf level. The G-suit can be used for (1) temporary preoperative control of subdiaphragmatic bleeding such as ruptured abdominal aortic aneurysms or massive trauma, until surgical correction can be undertaken; and (2) temporary postoperative control of intractable hemorrhage due to diffuse bleeding or coagulopathies, until clotting abnormalities are corrected. As with the MAST trousers, arterial pressure can be stabilized and bleeding sites compressed.

The G-suit consists of a double-layered polyvinyl suit with Velcro fasteners. The suit is connected to an external source of noncombustible gas by an extension tubing with an on-off flow valve. A separate tubing connected to a pressure gauge allows monitoring of suit pressure.

Objectives

1. To stabilize arterial pressure.
2. To redistribute intravascular volume proximally, maintaining perfusion of vital organs.
3. To act as a tamponade to stop bleeding.

Special Equipment

G-suit
Source of noncombustible gas, e.g., compressed air or nitrogen
Extension tubing and adapter for gas source
Lanolin
Bath blanket
Surgical pads, nonsterile
Gauze roll

Procedure

ACTION	RATIONALE
1. Apply lanolin to body surface.	1. Lanolin protects skin, minimizing irritation.
2. Spread G-suit on bed with arrow in center of mattress and Velcro down. Smooth bath blanket over surface of suit.	2. Blanket absorbs perspiration and minimizes blistering of skin.
3. Position patient so upper edge of G-suit lies beneath the xiphoid, with the arrow centered between the legs.	3. Compression of the thorax above the xiphoid will compromise ventilation. Suit must be centered with equal lengths of material on each side to facilitate closure.
4. Place surgical pads between knees and under coccyx; secure with gauze roll if necessary.	4. Padding minimizes pressure necrosis during compression.
5. Straighten all tubes and position them to ensure unimpeded flow.	
6. Wrap both ends of the blanket around the patient and smooth blanket.	6. Blanket should be as wrinkle-free as possible to prevent skin breakdown.
7. Wrap free edges of suit securely around patient and close with Velcro fasteners.	
8. Connect gas tubing to source of non-combustible gas.	8. Oxygen must *never* be used. The use of flammable gas is an unacceptable fire hazard.
9. Open flow valve between suit and gas source. Open gauge to suit for pressure monitoring.	
10. Closely monitoring arterial pressure, inflate G-suit with gas until (a) desired arterial pressure is achieved or (b) maximal recommended suit pressure of 20 to 30 mm. Hg is reached; 40 mm. Hg is not considered safe.	
11. Turn off gas flow and close valve once the desired pressure is reached.	11. Pressure gauge should remain open to suit for constant monitoring of pressure.

Precautions

1. Never use combustible gas because of fire hazard.
2. Avoid perforation of suit with sharp objects.
3. Pad all bony prominences and potential pressure points to minimize skin breakdown.
4. Never position G-suit above the level of the xiphoid to minimize interference with ventilation.
5. Avoid sudden deflation of the G-suit to prevent abrupt alteration in vascular volume and pressure.
6. Prevent kinking of the gas tubing to maintain designated pressure.
7. Minimize pressure and duration of inflation to prevent potential complications.

Related Care

1. Monitor arterial pressure closely.
2. Assess peripheral circulatory status at least hourly.
3. Check arterial blood gas levels within 15 to 30 minutes of application of the G-suit and as needed thereafter to detect signs of compromised ventilation.
4. If patient is ventilated, closely monitor ventilator function, especially inspiratory pressure and expired volume, to detect changes in lung compliance.
5. If patient is extubated, observe closely for signs of respiratory distress.
6. Check pressure gauge hourly or as needed to maintain designated pressure; replace gas as needed.
7. Use a portable tank of noncombustible gas during transport. Never use oxygen; never clamp. Pressure control must be precise.
8. Use a nasogastric tube if necessary during prolonged compression.
9. Monitor for indications for discontinuing the use of counterpressure: adequate volume replacement with control of bleeding or imminent surgical intervention.
10. Accomplish deflation by gradual release of pressure. Blood pressure should be monitored closely and volume replacement instituted immediately if pressure drops more than 5 mm. Hg. Subsequent release of pressure should proceed only after hemodynamic stabilization.
11. Administer sodium bicarbonate as ordered if metabolic acidosis is noted upon deflation.

Complications

Atelectasis	Skin necrosis and blistering
Pneumonia	Compartment syndrome
Pulmonary edema	Edema above the level of the suit

REFERENCES

Dove, A., et al.: Hemorrhage from pelvic fractures: Dangers and treatment. Injury, 13:375–381, 1982.

Hall, M., and Marshall, J.R.: The gravity suit: A major advance in management of gynecologic blood loss. Obstet. Gynecol., 53:247–249, 1979.

EXTERNAL COUNTERPRESSURE WITH MAST GARMENT

Penny J. Ford, R.N., M.S.,
and
F. Michael Vislosky, Jr., R.N.

Overview

External counterpressure or circumferential pneumatic compression is a noninvasive form of circulatory assistance of particular value in hemorrhagic shock or uncontrolled subdiaphragmatic bleeding.

The MAST (medical anti-shock trousers) garment is a one-piece, double-layered, polyvinyl suit with three separate pneumatic compartments enclosing both legs and the abdomen (Fig. 1–60). Velcro fasteners are used to secure the garment around the patient. The abdominal compartment extends from the lower margin of the rib cage to the pubis, maintaining access to the perineal region; the leg compartments extend to the ankles. Each compartment is connected to a separate tubing for gas flow/pressurization; compartment tubings are then interconnected and terminate in a single connection to a foot pump. Each gas flow tubing contains two valves: (1) an on/off flow valve allowing independent pressurization of compartments and (2) a pressure relief or pop-off valve so that inflation pressure cannot exceed 104 mm. Hg.

Application of the MAST trousers increases arterial pressure by two mechanisms. First, peripheral vascular resistance is increased by the reduction in blood vessel radius and blood flow under the garment. Second, com-

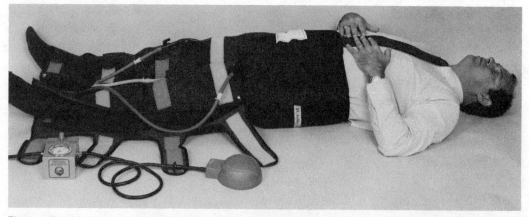

Figure 1-60.   Medical anti-shock trousers (MAST) garment. (Courtesy of St. Luke's Hospital, Cedar Rapids, Iowa.)

pression also redistributes blood flow from the periphery to the central circulation and vital organs. The magnitude of this volume displacement or autotransfusion remains controversial. In summary, arterial pressure is increased by alterations in afterload and preload. Tamponade of underlying bleeding sites is also achieved with external counterpressure. Finally the garment acts as a pneumatic splint, immobilizing fractures of the pelvis and lower extremities.

Objectives

1. To stabilize arterial pressure.
2. To redistribute flow from compressed regions to vital organs.
3. To act as a tamponade to stop bleeding.
4. To splint fractures of the pelvis and lower extremities.
5. To provide time for transport.

Special Equipment

MAST garment with foot pump
Equipment for in hospital only:
  Lanolin
  Bath blanket
  Surgical pads (nonsterile)
  Gauze roll
Optional equipment for in-hospital modification:
  Source of noncombustible gas (e.g.,
    compressed air or nitrogen)
  Extension tubing and adapter for gas source
  Pressure manometer
  Y connector
  Connecting tubing

Procedure

ACTION	RATIONALE
1. Apply blood pressure cuff and obtain baseline measurements.	
2. Open the garment with the Velcro fasteners down.	
3. Either slide garment underneath patient or move patient onto garment.	

ACTION	RATIONALE
4. Remove patient's clothing, apply lanolin, pad pressure points, and wrap in bath blanket (if time permits).	4. Lanolin protects the skin, minimizing irritation. Blanket absorbs perspiration and minimizes blistering of skin. Padding minimizes the potential for pressure necrosis.
5. Position upper border of garment at the lower margin of the rib cage.	5. Supradiaphragmatic compression interferes with thoracic movement.
6. Wrap garment around left leg; secure Velcro fasteners. Repeat with right leg, then abdomen.	
7. Position flow valves for sequential inflation of compartments. A. Open valve to left leg. B. Close valves to right leg and abdomen.	7. If single-step full inflation is preferred, all valves should be open. If two-step inflation is preferred, open valves to both legs only.
8. Attach foot pump or compressed air source.	
9. Closely monitoring arterial pressure for desired response, inflate left leg segment. Reposition flow valves and repeat with right leg, then abdomen.	
10. Continue inflation until: A. Desired arterial pressure is achieved. B. Maximal suit pressure is reached and pop-off valve is activated, approximately 104 mm. Hg.	10. The minimal pressure at which arterial pressure stabilization is achieved should be used to minimize potential complications. Slippage of Velcro straps may be noted at pressures less than the pop-off pressure for the relief valve, particularly in obese patients. Taping the straps in these situations may be required.
11. Close flow valve to abdominal compartment.	11. All flow valves should be closed at this time to maintain pressure.

Precautions

1. Avoid sudden deflation; blood pressure will fall precipitously. This includes opening the garment for examinations and procedures.
2. Never use combustible gas because of fire hazard.
3. Avoid perforation of suit with sharp objects.

4. Pad all bony prominences and potential pressure points to minimize skin breakdown, if time permits.
5. Never position MAST garment above the lower margin of the rib cage to avoid interference with ventilation.
6. Minimize pressure and duration of inflation to prevent potential complications, particularly in patients with lower extremity fracture.
7. Never utilize the abdominal compartment alone to avoid a tourniquet effect.
8. Do not inflate the abdominal portion in the latter stages of pregnancy.
9. Note that MAST application is contraindicated if the patient has pulmonary edema.

Related Care

1. Monitor arterial blood pressure closely.
2. Interpose a gauge between the pressure source and the compartment inflow tubing, if desired, for in-hospital monitoring and regulation of suit pressure.
3. Observe for early signs of compartment syndrome in the lower extremities: pain, swelling, redness, and tenderness. Loss of peripheral pulses is a late sign.
4. Insert a nasogastric tube if the abdominal compartment is to be used for a prolonged period.
5. Administer sedatives/analgesics as ordered for patient discomfort due to counterpressure.
6. Monitor respiration and oxygenation to ensure adequacy of ventilation. Mechanical assistance may be required.
7. Monitor for indications for discontinuation of counterpressure: adequate volume replacement with control of bleeding or imminent surgical intervention.
8. Accomplish deflation by gradual, sequential release of pressure in each compartment, beginning with the abdomen. Blood pressure should be monitored closely and volume replacement instituted immediately if pressure drops more than 5 mm. Hg. Subsequent release of pressure should proceed only after hemodymanic stabilization.
9. Administer sodium bicarbonate as ordered if metabolic acidosis is noted upon deflation.

Complications

Compartment syndrome
Skin breakdown or pressure necrosis
Edema above the level of
  MAST garment

Increased bleeding from
supradiaphragmatic sites
Respiratory compromise
Exacerbation of pulmonary
edema or congestive heart
failure

Suppliers

Armstrong (medical anti-shock trouser)
David Clark Company (MAST III-A)
Dyna Med (Anti-shock air pants)
Gladiator antishock pants

REFERENCES

Brotman, S., et al.: Management of severe bleeding in fractures of the pelvis. Surg. Gynecol. Obstet., *153*:823–826, 1981.

Brotman, S., et al.: MAST trousers improperly applied causing a compartment syndrome in lower-extremity trauma. Trauma, *22*:598–599, l982.

Gaffney, F.A., et al.: Hemodynamic effects of medical anti-shock trousers (MAST garment). Trauma, *21*:931–937, 1981.

Maull, K.I., et al.: Limb loss following military anti-shock trousers (MAST) application. Trauma, *21*:60–62, 1981.

McCabe, J.B.: Antishock trouser inflation and pulmonary vital capacity. An. Emerg. Med., *12*:290–293, 1983.

Reines, D., and Khoury, N.P.: Use of military antishock trousers in the hospital. Am. J. Surg., *139*:307–309, 1980.

Williams, T.M., et al.: Compartment syndrome after anti-shock trouser use without lower extremity trauma. Trauma, *22*:595–599, 1982.

TEMPORARY PACEMAKER MANAGEMENT

Betty W. Norris, R.N., M.S.N.

Overview

Pacemaker therapy improves cardiac output by restoring a more normal heart rate. The patient's need for temporary or permanent pacing is determined by the underlying condition. Indications may include: (1) atrioventricular blocks; (2) bifascicular or trifascicular blocks; (3) bradycardia — resulting in a low cardiac output, sinus bradycardia, junctional rhythm, sinoatrial block, carotid sinus sensitivity produced by drug therapy; (4) supraventricular rhythms unresponsive to medical therapy; (5) supraventricular rhythms with slow ventricular response; (6) sick sinus syndrome; (7) asystole; (8) ventricular dysrhythmias unresponsive to other therapy; (9) prophylactic measures during open heart surgery and following a myocardial infarction; (10) pacing-induced ischemia as a diagnostic test; and (11) pacing studies for sick sinus syndrome to determine sinoatrial recovery time. The critical

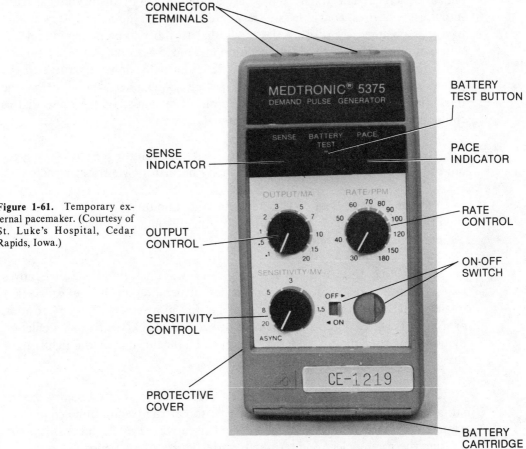

Figure 1-61. Temporary external pacemaker. (Courtesy of St. Luke's Hospital, Cedar Rapids, Iowa.)

CONNECTOR TERMINALS

BATTERY TEST BUTTON

SENSE INDICATOR

PACE INDICATOR

OUTPUT CONTROL

RATE CONTROL

ON-OFF SWITCH

SENSITIVITY CONTROL

PROTECTIVE COVER

BATTERY CARTRIDGE

care nurse contributes to multidimensional aspects of pacemaker therapy. The procedures presented in this section are offered to provide a greater perspective for pacemaker responsibilities.

Instrumentation

Regardless of the model, external temporary pacing units share basic components (Fig. 1–61).

Pulse Generator. This is the external battery-operated source that initiates electrical activity and controls the rate and intensity of each energy discharge. Its clear plastic cover enables the dials to be seen and protects the dial controls.

On-Off Lever. This controls the power component for activating the pulse generator. A safety lock protects against accidental termination of pacing. Two steps are required to turn off the pacemaker: (1) depress small button; (2) slide lever across top of the depressed button.

Mode Dial. Options include modalities for fixed rate pacing or demand pacing. The fixed rate, or asynchronous, mode disregards electrical impulses and fires continuously at a predetermined discharge. Fixed rate pacing is obtained by turning the mode dial to the maximum counterclockwise position. The demand, or synchronous, mode fires only after awaiting a signal through the exploring electrode. It is normally noncompetitive to the patient's electrical impulse. Demand pacing is obtained by adjusting the mode dial to the maximum clockwise position or adjusting the same dial as the sensitivity control for the R-wave signal.

Rate Dial. The rate dial regulates beats per minute. Atrial pacing requires higher rate options than those usually needed for ventricular pacing.

Ma. or Output Dial. This regulates the amount of energy delivered to the distal electrode. It is reported in milliamperes (ma.); it ranges from 0.1 to 20 ma.

Sense/Pace Indicator. Each time an R-wave is sensed the dial moves to the "sense" position or a light flashes, depending upon the pacemaker model. Each time the pacemaker fires the dial moves to the "pace" position or a light flashes. This component is utilized to check for battery depletion by observing the amount of deflection on the indicator dial or the light intensity.

Connector Terminals. The pacing electrodes to the temporary external pacemaker are usually connected at the top of the pacing unit; connector terminals are identified as positive (+) and negative (−). The mechanism for securing the pacing electrode terminals varies with different models.

Battery Cartridge. A small compartment on the lower portion of the pacing unit protects the battery. Newer models eliminate the need for tools in battery removal.

Temporary pacing systems are used for atrial or ventricular pacing, with provisions for variable rates of pacing and flexibility for continuous, synchronous, or demand modes. The pacing catheter is either bipolar or unipolar. The bipolar pacing catheter includes both positive and negative electrodes, positioned approximately 1 cm. apart. The unipolar electrode is the negative electrode and requires an indifferent, externally positioned electrode.

Temporary pacing catheters vary in design and are inserted by a physician using a transvenous pacing electrode procedure, a balloon-tipped pacing electrode procedure, or a transthoracic pacing electrode procedure. Epicardial pacing involves the placement of temporary epicardial pacing electrodes by a surgeon during cardiac surgery; these wires are secured and labeled externally for emergency pacing.

EMERGENCY INSERTION OF A TEMPORARY PACING ELECTRODE (ASSISTING WITH) _____

Objectives

1. To institute temporary pacing promptly when fluoroscopy is not immediately available.
2. To determine output threshold and sensitivity threshold, using an external temporary pacemaker.

Special Equipment

Select pacing electrode
External temporary pacemaker
Cable
Sterile towels
Masks
Sterile gown
Local anesthetic
Povidone-iodine prep solution
Suture with needle

ECG monitor and recorder
Defibrillator
Emergency cart and medications
For site care:
    Sterile gauze pads
    Povidone-iodine prep
      swabs
    Rubber glove
    Tape

Procedure

ACTION	RATIONALE
1. Connect patient to ECG monitor; monitor ECG recording continuously.	
2. Mask, gown, and glove all persons performing or assisting with the sterile procedure. All persons in the immediate area should be masked.	
3. Prep selected site with povidone-iodine solution; drape with sterile towels. A. Transvenous approach may include use of the jugular, subclavian, antecubital, or femoral veins. B. Transthoracic approach is through the chest wall to the heart.	B. This approach is often used during advanced life support therapy.
4. Anesthetize the area locally.	
5. Prepare external temporary pacemaker. A. Set the ma. on 6. B. Turn rate control to 10 beats/minute above patient's rate. C. Turn sensitivity dial fully clockwise.	B. The rate set above patient's rate will suppress the patient's natural pacemaking site.
6. Monitor patient while pacing electrode is inserted by a physician. A. Transvenous procedure: (1) A percutaneous puncture to the vein is performed. (a) The needle is removed and pacing electrode is passed through cannula. (b) Pacing electrode is positioned in right ventricle. (2) Connect pacing electrode to external temporary pacemaker, positive to positive and negative to negative. (3) Turn on external temporary pacemaker. (4) Adjust rate and ma. appropriately for effective capture.	

ACTION	RATIONALE
(a) Capture is indicated by a ventricular response after each pacemaker impulse.	
B. Balloon-tipped pacing electrode procedure:	
(1) Follow all preceding steps through 6(2).	
(2) Balloon inflation occurs when pacing electrode is in vena cava.	(2) The air-filled balloon allows blood flow to carry the catheter tip into desired position in right ventricle.
(3) Turn on external temporary pacemaker when pacing electrode is in the heart.	
(4) Observe ECG monitor.	(4) The ECG pattern is distinctive when the pacing electrode is in the vena cava, right atrium, and right ventricle.
(a) Assess ECG rhythm for small inverted P waves (Fig. 1–62).	(a) This depicts pacing electrode in vena cava.

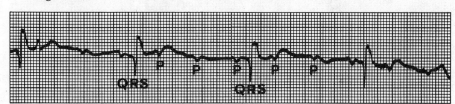

Figure 1-62. ECG rhythm: small inverted P-waves when pacing electrode is in vena cava. (Reproduced from Intensive Coronary Care, 4th Edition, by Lawrence E. Meltzer, Rose Pinneo, and J. Roderick Kitchell. Robert J. Brady Co., Bowie, MD, 1983.)

| (b) Assess ECG rhythm for tall biphasic P-waves (Fig. 1–63). | (b) This depicts pacing electrode in right atrium. |

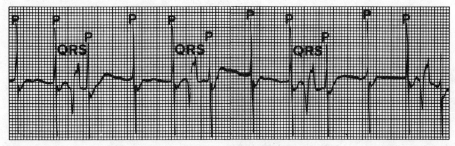

Figure 1-63. ECG rhythm: tall biphasic P waves when pacing electrode is in right atrium. (Reproduced from Intensive Coronary Care, 4th Edition, by Lawrence E. Meltzer, Rose Pinneo, and J. Roderick Kitchell. Robert J. Brady Co., Bowie, MD, 1983.)

ACTION	RATIONALE
(c) Assess ECG rhythm for large QRS complexes and progressively smaller P waves (Fig. 1–64).	(c) This depicts pacing electrode in right ventricle.

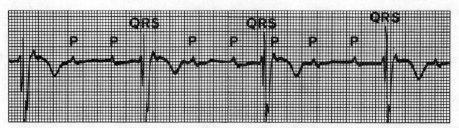

Figure 1-64. ECG Rhythm: large QRS complexes and progressively smaller P-waves when pacing electrode is in right ventricle. (Reproduced from Intensive Coronary Care, 4th Edition, by Lawrence E. Meltzer, Rose Pinneo, and J. Roderick Kitchell. Robert J. Brady Co., Bowie, MD, 1983.)

ACTION	RATIONALE
(d) Assess ECG rhythm for elevated ST segments (Fig. 1–65).	(d) This depicts pacing electrode wedged against endocardial wall of right ventricle.

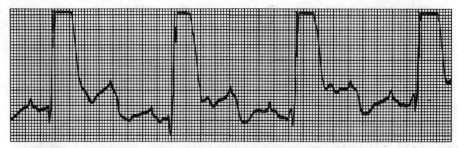

Figure 1-65. ECG rhythm: elevated ST segments when pacing electrode is wedged against the endocardial wall of the right ventricle. (Reproduced from Intensive Coronary Care, 4th Edition, by Lawrence E. Meltzer, Rose Pinneo, and J. Roderick Kitchell. Robert J. Brady Co., Bowie, MD, 1983.)

    (5) Capture is indicated by a ventricular response after each pacemaker impulse.
    (6) Deflate balloon.
  C. Transthoracic procedure:
    (1) A transthoracic puncture is made into the myocardium.
      (a) Needle and obturator are inserted transthoracically into ventricle through fourth intercostal space.

ACTION	RATIONALE
(b) Inner obturator is removed; pacing stylet is inserted through needle.	

(2) Secure stylet by taping or suturing.

(3) Attach stylet to external temporary pacemaker using connecting adapter.

   (a) Insert proximal end of stylet into adapter and tighten both locks.

   (b) Connect distal lead to negative pole of external temporary pacemaker and proximal lead to positive pole of external temporary pacemaker.

(4) Turn on external temporary pacemaker.

(5) Adjust rate and ma. appropriately for effective capture and pacing.

   (a) Capture is indicated by a ventricular response after each pacemaker impulse.

7. Determine stimulation threshold.

  A. Gradually decrease output until 1:1 capture is lost.

  B. Gradually increase output until 1:1 capture is regained; this is the stimulation threshold. Acceptable stimulation threshold is 1.0 ma. or less for most endocardial leads.

      B. If threshold exceeds these values, lead should be repositioned and procedure repeated.

8. Determine sensitivity threshold.

  A. Turn rate to 10 beats/minute less than patient's rate.

      A. The sense/pace indicator should deflect to sense zone as it senses R-waves.

  B. Turn the sensitivity control counterclockwise slowly (from the full clockwise position) until pacemaker begins to fire; this is the sensitivity threshold. Adequate threshold is in the 6 mV. range.

      B. The sense/pace indicator will deflect to the pace zone as it begins not to sense the R-waves. A low sensitivity threshold is indication for repositioning.

ACTION	RATIONALE
9. Set external temporary pacemaker at desired rate; set output at ma. of 3 to 5 increments above threshold.	9. P- or T-wave sensing may require sensitivity to be decreased.
10. Secure electrode wire at site of insertion by suturing or taping.	10. This prevents dislodgment of the electrode catheter.
11. Perform site care.	
A. Use sterile technique and cleanse pacing site with povidone-iodine prep swabs; apply sterile dry dressing.	A. A thoroughly dry dressing provides protective measure of safety insulation.
B. Label dressing: "pacing wire," "date," and "initials of one placing dressing."	

Precautions

1. Provide a defibrillator, emergency cart, and medications for immediate use. Pacemaker stimuli may inadvertently be delivered in vulnerable period during checking of threshold, causing lethal dysrhythmias. Passage of pacing electrode may irritate the ventricle, causing ventricular dysrhythmias.
2. Follow electrical safety guidelines for patients with pacemakers.
3. Observe monitor carefully during threshold checking. Do not be distracted.
4. Monitor ma. setting; insufficient ma. may result in loss of capture and dangerously slow rhythms; excessive ma. may result in irritability and lead to ventricular dysrhythmias.
5. Monitor sensitivity setting; excessive sensitivity may cause sensing of P- or T-wave, resulting in failure to pace at appropriate times; insufficient sensitivity will cause fixed rate pacing with the possibility of the pacing stimulus being delivered during the vulnerable period of the cardiac cycle, leading to lethal dysrhythmias.

Related Care

1. Facilitate physician's order for chest x-ray postinsertion to validate position of pacing electrode.
2. Perform site care daily; check external pacing electrode wire position, insulation, and security of catheter terminals within pacemaker connectors.
3. Assess pacemaker dressings for dryness; change immediately if damp or wet.

4. Check threshold profile daily; verify that pacemaker system is functioning properly.
5. Monitor patient's temperature every 4 hours.

Complications

Competitive dysrhythmias	Pneumothorax
Lethal ventricular dysrhythmias	Thrombophlebitis
Cardiac arrest	Infection
Cardiac perforation	Electromicroshock
Catheter electrode displacement or fracture	Equipment malfunction

Suppliers

Edwards Laboratory
Metronics

REFERENCES

Eldredge, T.: Protocol for nursing care of patients with temporary pacemakers. Crit. Care Nurse, 3:3, 47–50, (May/June), 1983.

Lang, R., et al.: The use of balloon-tipped floating catheter in temporary transvenous cardiac pacing, PACE, 4:491-496, 1981.

Luderitz, B.: Electrophysiology and indications for pacing in the 80's. PACE, 5:548-560, 1982.

INITIATING TEMPORARY EPICARDIAL PACING _____

Objectives

1. To facilitate emergency electrical stimulation of the heart, using an epicardial electrode that has been temporarily inserted into the atrial or ventricular myocardium, or both.
2. To control dysrhythmias.
3. To improve cardiac output.

Special Equipment

For site care:	ECG monitor and recorder
Sterile gauze pads	External temporary pacemaker
Povidone-iodine prep swabs	Steel needle or indifferent electrode
Rubber glove	Emergency cart and medications
Tape	

Patient cable
Rubber gloves
Defibrillator

Procedure

ACTION	RATIONALE
1. Obtain ECG recording.	1. This serves as baseline data.
2. Don rubber gloves.	
3. Expose pacing electrode.	
4. Select appropriate method.	
A. Bipolar ventricular pacing:	
(1) Connect ventricular pacing wire to negative pole of external temporary pacemaker.	(1) The electrode that is connected to the negative pole determines the type of pacing.
(2) Connect atrial wire to positive pole of external temporary pacemaker.	(2) In the bipolar system the current is between the electrodes.
B. Unipolar ventricular pacing:	
(1) Connect ventricular pacing wire to negative pole of external temporary pacemaker.	(1) The electrode that is connected to the negative pole determines the type of pacing.
(2) Insert a steel needle or indifferent electrode subcutaneously, usually in the upper abdomen.	(2) This serves as indifferent electrode.
(3) Connect needle or electrode to positive pole of external temporary pacemaker.	
C. Bipolar atrial pacing:	
(1) Connect the two atrial wires to positive and negative poles of external temporary pacemaker.	(1) Atrial pacing is fixed-rate pacing. The electrode that is connected to the negative pole determines the type of pacing.
D. Unipolar atrial pacing:	
(1) Connect an atrial wire to the negative pole of external temporary pacemaker.	(1) The electrode that is connected to the negative pole determines type of pacing.
(2) Connect a subcutaneously inserted indifferent electrode or steel needle to the positive	

ACTION	RATIONALE
pole of external temporary pacemaker.	
5. Set prescribed rate; set sensitivity mode and ma. at lowest settings.	5. It is dangerous to alter the rate in a fixed mode, since pacer spike may fall in the vulnerable period.
A. Use asynchronous (fixed) mode for atrial pacing.	A. Use of demand mode may result in failure to sense or capture.
B. Use asynchronous (fixed) or synchronous (demand) mode for ventricular pacing.	
6. Turn on the external temporary pacemaker; observe ECG monitor.	
7. Gradually increase ma. until complete capture is reached.	7. The myocardium requires time to adjust; turning the pacemaker on and off suddenly may be dangerous to cardiac electrodynamics.
A. Capture is indicated by a ventricular response after each pacemaker impulse.	
B. Increase ma. 3 to 5 increments above stimulation threshold.	
C. Note that atrial pacing requires a setting four to five times greater than that used for ventricular pacing.	
8. Secure ECG recording.	
9. Protect all exposed connections in rubber; secure with dressing.	

Precautions

1. Provide defibrillator, emergency cart, and medications for immediate use.
2. Protect connector sites from potential current leakage and moisture.
3. Wear rubber gloves when working with connective ends of pacing wires.
4. Follow electrical safety guidelines for patients with pacemakers.
5. Protect epicardial electrodes not in use.
6. Assess for pacemaker stimulation of the heart during the repolarization period (T-wave); this may cause lethal dysrhythmias.
7. Monitor ma. setting: insufficient ma. may cause failure to capture and bradycardia may continue; excessive ma. may cause irritability, leading to lethal dysrhythmias.
8. Monitor sensitivity setting: excessive sensitivity may cause sensing of P- or T-wave, resulting in failure to pace at appropriate times; insufficient

sensitivity will cause fixed rate pacing with the possibility of pacing stimulus being delivered during the vulnerable period of the cardiac cycle, leading to lethal dysrhythmias.

9. Facilitate epicardial electrode site identification at all times and availability of special equipment at the bedside for rapid emergency intervention.

Related Care

1. Ensure that pacing system is functioning properly; check that connections are secure and properly protected from potential sources of current leakage every 8 hours.
2. Perform pacing electrode site care daily or as needed if dressings become moist.
    A. Cleanse pacing electrode insertion site with povidone-iodine prep swabs, using sterile technique.
    B. Check insulation: exposed electrode wire should be insulated in a rubber glove.
    C. Maintain skin integrity by placing sterile gauze pads under rubber glove.
    D. Increase safety protection by placing gauze pads over rubber glove and sealing with tape.
3. Check ECG recording for appropriate pacing and sensing.
4. Assess threshold profile daily.

Complications

Lethal dysrhythmias
Competitive dysrhythmias
Cardiac arrest
Infection

Dislodgement of pacing wire
Electromicroshock
Equipment malfunction

Suppliers

Advanced Medical Systems, Inc.
Ethicon

REFERENCES

Underhill, S.L., et al.: Cardiac Nursing. Philadelphia: J.B. Lippincott, 1982, pp. 518–541.
Wulf, K.S.: Use of temporary epicardial electrodes for atrial pacing and monitoring. Cardiovasc. Nurs., *18*:1–5, 1982.

TEMPORARY A-V SEQUENTIAL DEMAND PACING _____

Objectives

1. To provide a variety of temporary modalities, i. e., asynchronous atrial or ventricular pacing, demand ventricular pacing, asynchronous or demand A-V sequential pacing.
2. To pace the atrium and ventricles in sequence, thereby allowing for more atrial contribution to ventricular filling and normal conduction to ventricles when A-V node is conducting normally.

Special Equipment

Atrial and ventricular pacing wires in place
A-V sequential temporary pulse generator (Fig. 1–66)

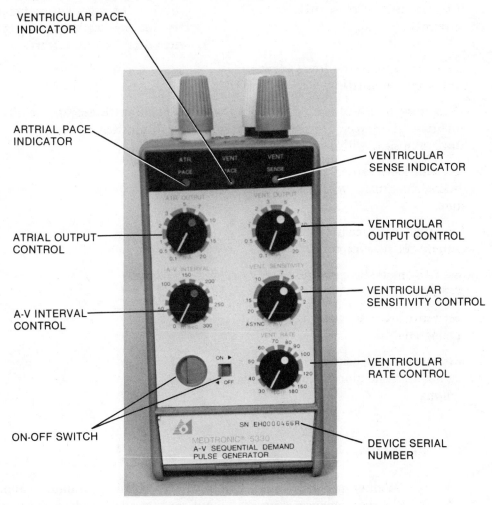

Figure 1-66.   Temporary A-V sequential demand pacemaker. (Courtesy of St. Luke's Hospital, Cedar Rapids, Iowa.)

ECG monitor with recorder
Defibrillator
Emergency cart and medication
For site care:
    Sterile gauze pads
    Povidone-iodine prep
       swabs
    Rubber gloves
    Tape

Procedure

ACTION	RATIONALE
1. Connect patient to ECG monitor.	
2. Connect atrial wires to atrial output terminals.	2. This may be used with pulmonary artery pacing catheter or epicardial wires, after cardiac surgery.
3. Connect ventricular wires to ventricular output terminals.	
4. Determine threshold (see "Emergency Insertion of Temporary Pacing Electrode (Assisting with").	4. Stimulation thresholds are 1.0 ma. or less to ventricular system.
5. Set ventricular output control at desired current for ventricular capture.	
6. Set atrial output control at desired current for atrial capture.	
7. Set A-V-interval control at desired A-V interval.	
8. Set ventricular rate control at desired pacing rate.	
9. Set ventricular sensitivity control at desired mV.value for adequate R-wave sensing.	

Precautions

1. Monitor patient's ECG rhythm closely when determining stimulation threshold changes, because stimuli may be delivered in the vulnerable

period of T-wave. Defibrillator and emergency equipment should be readily available.
2. Reduce gradually the pulse generator rate, using demand mode. Once a spontaneous rhythm is established, the pulse generator can be turned off.
3. Don rubber gloves when handling the pacing electrode tips.

Related Care

1. Perform site care daily; check insulation and security of pacing catheter terminals.
2. Check threshold profile daily; verify that system is functioning properly.
3. Monitor patient's temperature every 4 hours while external pacemaker is in use.

Complications

Asystole
Atrial fibrillation
Competitive dysrhythmias
Lethal ventricular dysrhythmias
Cardiac perforation

Catheter electrode displacement
  or fracture
Infection
Electromicroshock
Battery depletion

REFERENCES

Klein, L.: Temporary AV sequential pacing. Crit. Care Nurse, 3:36–41, (May/June), 1983.
Sutton, R. and Perrins, J.: Physiological cardiac pacing. PACE, 3:207–219, 1980.

CONVERSION FROM BIPOLAR TO UNIPOLAR SYSTEM WITH TEMPORARY PACING _____

Objective

To enhance the pacemaker's ability to sense electrical activity of the heart by increasing the distance between the electrodes, thereby increasing the electrical potential.

Special Equipment

ECG monitor and recorder
Small-gauge steel needle, or indifferent electrode, or
    ECG strap and metal plate
Patient extention cable with alligator-type clamps
Rubber gloves
Defibrillator
Povidone-iodine prep solution
Emergency cart and medications
For site care:
    Sterile gauze pads
    Povidone-iodine prep swabs
    Rubber glove
    Tape

Procedure

ACTION	RATIONALE
1. Obtain ECG recording.	1. This provides baseline data.
2. Turn off external temporary pacemaker.	
3. Prep select site on abdomen with povidone-iodine; insert steel needle subcutaneously and secure.	
4. Don rubber gloves.	4. These prevent the possibility of transmitting electrical current to myocardium.
5. Disconnect external temporary pacemaker from pacing electrode at terminals.	
6. Attach negative (black) alligator clip of patient cable to bipolar connector's pin for distal tip electrode.	
7. Convert to unipolar system (two options):	
A. Attach positive (red) alligator clip to steel needle or indifferent electrode placed subcutaneously in lower chest or abdominal area.	A. The needle becomes the indifferent electrode, thus increasing the distance between electrodes; it increases the electrical potential and makes it easier for the pacemaker to sense the heart's activity.

ACTION   RATIONALE

B. Attach metal plate, ECG strap,
    and bridging cable with alligator-
    type clamps. Cover exposed posi-
    tive tip with glove (Fig. 1–67).

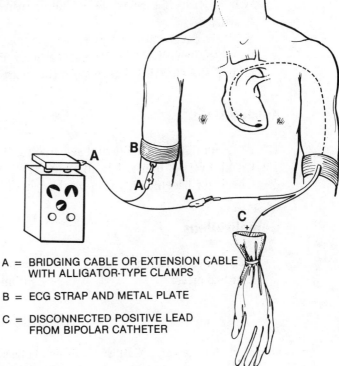

Figure 1-67. Conversion of a temporary transvenous bipolar electrode to a
unipolar electrode pacing system. Connect the positive terminal of the external
pulse generator via a bridging cable or
extension with alligator clips (A) to a
body surface electrode (B) instead of to
the positive catheter electrode (C). *All
exposed connections must be insulated
with a rubber glove or similar material.*
(Adapted from Preston, T.A., Yates
J.D: *Heart and Lung* 2(4):535, 1973.
Reprinted with permission.)

A = BRIDGING CABLE OR EXTENSION CABLE
    WITH ALLIGATOR-TYPE CLAMPS

B = ECG STRAP AND METAL PLATE

C = DISCONNECTED POSITIVE LEAD
    FROM BIPOLAR CATHETER

8. Connect patient cable to external
    temporary pacemaker, negative to
    negative and positive to positive.

9. Turn sensitivity dial fully clockwise;
    check that rate dial is set at desired
    rate and output is set at 6 to 10 ma.

10. Turn on external temporary pacemak-
    er; observe monitor.

11. Obtain ECG recording.

12. Secure alligator clips with dressing.

13. Protect all exposed connections in
    rubber; secure with dressing.

Precautions

1. Provide defibrillator, emergency cart, and medications for immediate use.
2. Wear rubber gloves when handling connector tips of pacing catheter
    electrode.

3. Follow electrical safety guidelines for patients with pacemakers.
4. Assess for lethal dysrhythmias, which may occur when the pacemaker fails to sense the patient's own heart beat. The pacemaker may stimulate the heart during the repolarization period (T-wave).
5. Decrease ma. if the muscle around the steel needle has a noticeable twitch with the paced beat, but continue to maintain capture of the heart.
6. Securely cover both of the exposed ends of the metal needle and the metal connector of the pacing catheter electrode with rubber glove to protect the electrical pathway to the heart.

Related Care

1. Note appropriate pacing and sensing on ECG monitor.
2. Check every 8 hours that all connections are secure.
3. Check for pacemaker firing by the patient.

Complications

Lethal dysrhythmias   Electromicroshock
Cardiac arrest   Equipment malfunction

REFERENCE

Underhill, S.L., et al.: Cardiac Nursing. Philadelphia: J.B. Lippincott, 1982, pp. 518–541.

ATRIAL ECG WITH TEMPORARY ATRIAL PACING ELECTRODE

Objective

To improve diagnostic accuracy of supraventricular dysrhythmias.

Special Equipment

12-Lead ECG recorder or modified bedside
  ECG monitoring equipment, selected cables,
  and bedside strip chart recorder
Rubber gloves
Defibrillator
Emergency cart and medications

For site care:
Sterile gauze pads
Povidone-iodine prep swab
Rubber gloves
Tape

Procedure

ACTION	RATIONALE

1. Don rubber gloves.

2. Expose atrial pacing electrode.

3. Select appropriate method.
   A. Bipolar system:
      (1) Connect one atrial electrode to RA connector and the other atrial electrode to LA connector on 12-lead recorder.
      (2) Place lower limb leads on ankles.
      (3) Turn lead selector to lead I (Fig. 1–68).

      (3) Left leg serves as indifferent electrode.

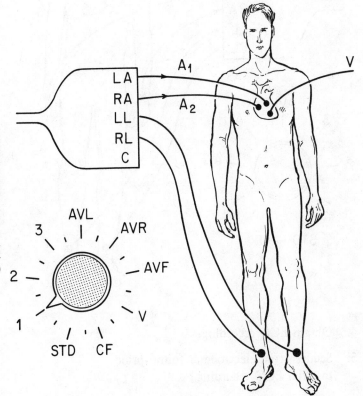

Figure 1-68. Connection for bipolar atrial lead. Attach two limb leads of ECG as usual. Using two alligator clip wires, attach each of the atrial pacing wires (A1 and A2) to the remaining limb leads. Run a rhythm strip in that limb lead position, i.e., lead I. (Adapted by permission of the American Heart Association, Inc., from Wulff, K.S: Use of Temporary Epicardial Electrodes for Atrial Pacing and Monitoring. *Cardiovascular Nursing* 18:1, 1982.)

ACTION   RATIONALE

B. Unipolar system:
  (1) Connect one atrial electrode to RA connector and the other atrial electrode to LA connector on 12-lead recorder.
  (2) Place lower limb leads on ankles.
  (3) Turn lead selector to lead II or III.
C. Alternative unipolar system:
  (1) Connect atrial wire to chest lead on 12-lead recorder.
  (2) Connect all limb leads.
  (3) Turn lead selector to V_1 (Fig. 1–69).

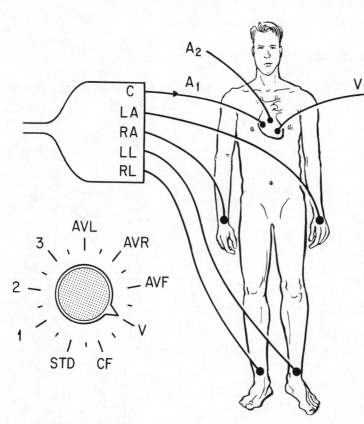

Figure 1-69. Connection of unipolar atrial lead. Attach four ECG limb leads. Use an alligator clip to connect the metal end of the atrial pacing wire (A_1) to the chest (C) lead cable of the ECG machine. Obtain rhythm strip with the dial in the V-lead position. (Adapted by permission of the American Heart Association, Inc., from Wulff, K.S: Use of Temporary Epicardial Electrodes for Atrial Pacing and Monitoring. *Cardiovascular Nursing* 18:1, 1982.)

4. Obtain ECG recording.

5. Secure atrial electrode as found prior to atrial ECG recording.

Precautions

1. Follow electrical safety guidelines for patients with temporary pacing electrodes.
2. Provide defibrillator, emergency cart, and medications for immediate use.
3. Observe for dysrhythmias.

Related Care

1. Perform site care after atrial ECG; protect all exposed connections.

Complications

Lethal dysrhythmias
Cardiac arrest

Electromicroshock
Equipment malfunction

REFERENCES

Mantle, J.A., et al.: A multipurpose catheter for electrophysiologic and hemo-dynamic monitoring plus atrial pacing. Chest, 72:285–290, 1977.
Wulff, K.S.: Use of temporary epicardial electrodes for atrial pacing and monitoring, Cardiovasc. Nurs., 18:1–5, 1982.

OVERDRIVE ATRIAL PACING ─────────────

Objective

To provide overdrive suppression of tachydysrhythmias.

Special Equipment

External atrial temporary pacemaker
ECG monitor or 12-lead ECG recorder
Defibrillator
Emergency cart and medications
For site care:
    Sterile gauze pads
    Povidone-iodine prep swabs
    Rubber gloves
    Tape

Procedure

ACTION	RATIONALE
1. Obtain initial ECG recording.	1. This provides baseline data.
2. Confirm that electrode is in right atrium by an atrial electrogram (AEG) tracing or fluoroscopy or both.	2. Accidental high rate stimulation of right ventricle could induce lethal dysrhythmias.

3. Prepare atrial external temporary pacemaker.
A. Connect lead connector tips to terminals.
  (1) Connect positive to positive, negative to negative.
  (2) An interconnecting cable is sometimes used between atrial pacemaker and electrode.
  (3) Adjust "rate" dial and "output" to desired setting on atrial pacemaker.	

4. Turn on external atrial temporary pacemaker, observing pacing activity on ECG monitor. A. Heart rate is increased. B. Observe for atrial pacing capture. C. Obtain ECG recording.	
5. Select prescribed method to achieve suppression of tachydysrhythmias. A. Terminate atrial pacing abruptly. B. Slow atrial pacing to an acceptable rate.	A. Abrupt cessation allows for SA node to assume pacemaking role.
6. Obtain ECG recording.	
7. Complete aftercare. A. Perform site care if pacing electrode is removed. B. Secure and insulate pacing electrode, perform site care, and check for dry dressing when: (1) Pacing electrode is left in place and pacemaker unit is disconnected. Tips of the pacing electrode should be	

ACTION	RATIONALE
placed in separate rubber gloves.	
(2) Pacing unit is turned off but remains connected.	

8. Monitor patient's response to therapy.

Precautions

1. Follow electrical safety guidelines for patients with pacemakers.
2. Provide defibrillator, emergency cart, and medications for immediate use.
3. Observe for dysrhythmias.

Related Care

1. Perform site care daily; check external pacing electrode wire position, insulation, and security of catheter terminals within pacemaker connectors.

Complications

Dysrhythmias	Altered skin integrity
Cardiac arrest	Equipment malfunction
Electromicroshock	

REFERENCES

Luderitz, B.: Electrophysiology and indications for pacing in the '80's. PACE, 5:548–560, 1982.
Wiener, I.: Pacing techniques in the treatment of tachycardiacs. Ann. Intern. Med. 93:326, 1981.

ASSESSING TEMPORARY PACEMAKER FUNCTION _____

Objective

To provide a systematic method of assessing temporary pacemaker function and to offer potential solutions.

Special Equipment

ECG recorder
Defibrillator
Emergency cart and medications

Procedure

ACTION	RATIONALE
1. Determine proper functioning of rate, current output, open circuit voltage pulse duration, and sensitivity. The function of a temporary or permanent pulse generator may be checked by using a specific pacing system's analyzer (see "Assessing Select Parameters of a Permanent Pacing System").	
2. Check pacemaker's performance using "sense/pace" indicator (Fig. 1–61).	
A. Note whether indicator needle is deflected to the right of center or pace light is flashing.	A. This indicates that a pacing stimulus has been delivered.
B. Note whether indicator needle is deflected to the left of center or sense light is flashing.	B. This indicates that an R-wave has been sensed, thus inhibiting the pacemaker output for one cycle.
C. Note if there is absence of deflection (or only slight deflection), or lights not flashing.	C. This indicates approaching battery depletion. This forewarning occurs before pacemaker output characteristics are significantly affected.
D. Note if there are erratic deflections (or quivering about center).	D. This indicates external interference strong enough to inhibit the pacemaker output temporarily.
3. Perform pacemaker battery assessment (Fig. 1–61).	
A. Turn on pacemaker and observe deflection on the "sense/pace" indicator or "sense/pace" lights.	A. No deflection (or only slight deflection) indicates that the battery is nearing depletion. This forewarning occurs before pacemaker output characteristics are significantly affected.
B. Facilitate battery replacement and enter in battery log record as required by hospital policy.	

ACTION	RATIONALE
C. Check battery for shelf life expiration date prior to inserting into pacemaker; label appropriately.	C. Close monitoring of battery shelf life expiration date is important for emergency life support equipment.

4. Check for failure to sense. This is illustrated by competitive pacing complexes (Fig. 1–70).

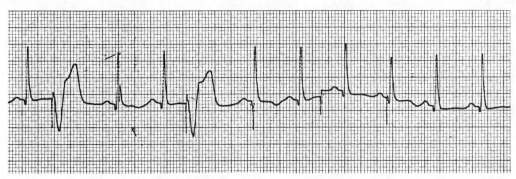

Figure 1-70. Example of failure to sense.

A. Check connection site.	A. Poor connection of positive or indifferent pole may result in failure to sense.
B. Check that "pace/sense" needle deflects to right, showing pacing, or pace light is flashing.	
C. Turn sensitivity dial to fully clockwise position and determine sensitivity threshold.	C. Sensitivity threshold can change with time.
D. Convert from bipolar to unipolar system (see "Conversion from Bipolar to Unipolar System with Temporary Pacing").	D. The unipolar system increases distance between the electrode and, in turn, increases ability to sense heart activity.
E. Provide defibrillator for immediate use.	E. Pacing spikes that occur in the vulnerable period can cause ventricular fibrillation.
F. Increase pacing rate above patient's heart rate to determine if pacemaker is operational when functioning in standby mode.	

ACTION	RATIONALE
5. Check for failure to pace. This is recognized by absence of pacing artifact on ECG recording at appropriate intervals (Figs. 1–71 and 1–72).	

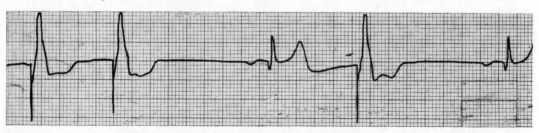

Figure 1-71.   Example of failure to pace.

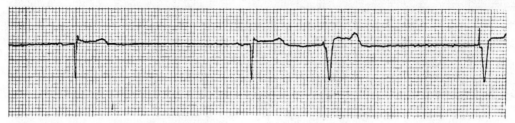

Figure 1-72.   Example of failure to pace.

ACTION	RATIONALE
A. Check lead connector sites.	A. Poor connections may cause loss of pacing.
B. Check for battery depletion; change battery if indicated or change external pacemaker unit.	B. Battery depletion signals vary with different brands.
C. Check for ungrounded equipment as potential interfering electrical field.	C. Electrical interference may cause demand mode to function improperly and result in erratic deflections or no deflection of "sense/pace" indicator.
6. Check for failure to capture. This is recognized by presence of pacing artifact without an accompanying QRS complex (Fig. 1–73).	

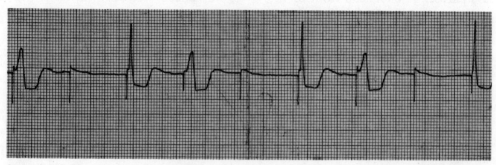

Figure 1-73.   Example of failure to capture.

ACTION	RATIONALE
A. Check security of connections.	A. Poor connection of negative pole may cause intermittent or continuous loss of capture.
B. Increase ma.; evaluate threshold for stimulation.	B. Fibrosis and drug-induced changes in myocardium can alter threshold with time.
C. If lead is dislodged: (1) Notify physician of possible lead dislodgment. Repositioning of pacing electrode is usually indicated. (2) Occasionally lifting or repositioning patient's arm or turning patient to left side may serve as temporary method of forcing lead back into position.	
D. Assess for pacing of diaphragm; this may be observed or palpated as muscle twitching in left lower chest with each paced beat.	D. With ventricular perforation, pacing may be unaffected, intermittent, or lost.

Precautions

1. Provide defibrillator, emergency cart, and medications for immediate use. Pacemaker stimuli may inadvertently be delivered in vulnerable period, causing lethal dysrhythmias.
2. Wear rubber gloves when handling connector tips of pacing catheter electrode.
3. Follow electrical safety guidelines for patient with pacemaker.
4. Observe monitor carefully during threshold checking. Do not be distracted.

Related Care

1. Monitor threshold profile daily. See   Emergency Insertion of Temporary Pacing Electrode (Assisting with) for determining stimulation and sensitivity thresholds.
2. Perform site care daily; check external pacing electrode wire position and insulation; check security of catheter terminals within pacemaker connectors.
3. Assess pacemaker dressings for dryness. Change immediately if damp or wet.

Complications

Competitive dysrthythmias   Infection

Lethal dysrhythmias   Electromicroshock

Cardiac arrest   Equipment malfunction

REFERENCES

Austin, J.L., et al.: Analysis of pacemaker malfunction and complications of temporary pacing in coronary care unit. Am. J. Cardiol., *49*:301–306, 1982.

Trusty, J.: Cardiac pacing postoperative considerations, Life Support Nurs., *5:3:18–27, (May–June), 1981.*

EMERGENCY APPLICATION OF TEMPORARY EXTERNAL CHEST PACING

Instrumentation

The external chest pacing system offers prompt noninvasive temporary pacing until fluoroscopy or permanent pacing therapy can be facilitated. Adhesive disposable pacing electrodes are applied directly to skin surface of the chest and connected to an external chest pacing unit. This unit can be battery operated with direct line current override (Fig. 1–74). The external chest pacing system operates as a fixed-rate pacemaker, and, also, inhibits initiation of pacing as long as the beat-to-beat interval is shorter than 750 milliseconds. At present, the transcutaneous pacing system is not a demand pacemaker. Other features include various ma. settings, and rate-limit circuitry to protect the patient form runaway pacing rates.

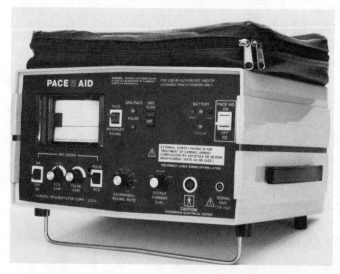

Figure 1-74. Temporary external chest pacing system. (Courtesy of Cardiac Resuscitator Corp.)

Special Equipment

External chest pacemaker
External pacing electrodes (adhesive and disposable)
ECG monitor defibrillator

Objective

To provide external chest pacing for treatment of cardiac arrest complicated by an asystole or severe bradycardia (rate less than 40/minute).

Procedure

ACTION	RATIONALE

1. Apply external pacing electrodes:
  A. Clean and dry skin sites.
  B. Connect electrode cable to external chest pacing unit.
  C. Apply adhesive, external pacing electrodes:
    (1) Anterior chest wall at V3 position (Fig 1–75).
	1. Electrode position is critical.
	
	    (1) Position anterior electrode with center over V3 ECG position for low pacing threshold.

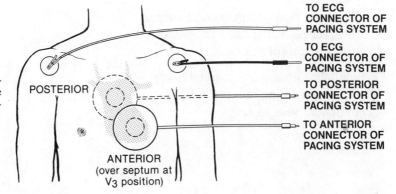

Figure 1-75. Temporary external chest pacing electrode placement. (Courtesy of Cardiac Resuscitator Corp.)

POSTERIOR

ANTERIOR
(over septum at V3 position)

TO ECG CONNECTOR OF PACING SYSTEM

TO ECG CONNECTOR OF PACING SYSTEM

TO POSTERIOR CONNECTOR OF PACING SYSTEM

TO ANTERIOR CONNECTOR OF PACING SYSTEM

(2) Posterior chest wall at midthoracic spine. (Fig. 1–75).	(2) Position posterior electrode to achieve effective pacer capture. In some patients, alteration of the posterior electrode position will be required to achieve capture. Sometimes, capture may be possible by locating the posterior electrode at the ECG V6 position.

ACTION	RATIONALE
2. Connect the external pacing electrodes to the external pacing cable per manufacturer's protocol.	
3. Connect the external pacing cable to the external chest pacing unit.	
4. Connect the monitoring ECG electrodes to the patient and external chest pacing unit per manufacturer's protocol.	4. Unless the monitoring ECG electrodes are connected to the external chest pacing unit, the QRS detector cannot control the initiation of pacing. (Lead II is recommended; however, another lead may be required.)
5. Check instrumentation to include ma. controls, recorder controls, battery-test controls per manufacturer's protocol. (See Fig. 1–74).	
6. Turn power switch on; observe for a 3 to 5 second QRS scan period, for the initiation of fixed rate pacing, and for a QRS/pace light trigger.	
7. Assess patient for mechanical cardiac action by palpation of femoral or carotid pulsations.	
8. Document pacing therapy and pacing effectiveness, using the ECG writer or pulse wave form writer.	
9. Facilitate for temporary invasive or permanent pacing therapy per physician's plan of care.	

Precautions

1. Provide a defibrillator, emergency cart, and medications for immediate use.
2. Disconnect the external chest pacing cable from the pacing unit during defibrillation. Delivery of defibrillation shocks directly into pacing leads may damage other protective circuits.
3. Follow electrical safety guidelines for patients with pacemakers.
4. Stay with the patient at all times and monitor effectiveness of pacing.

Related Care

1. Assess patient. Sedation may be appropriate for maintaining comfort level.
2. Monitor ma. setting. If pacing is not effective, increase the ma. output to "high." If pacing is effective, decrease output to "low." Continue pacing at the lowest level that ensures continuous capture.

Complications

Competitive dysrhythmias
Altered skin integrity
Equipment malfunction

Supplier

Pace-Aid—Cardiac Resuscitator Corporation

REFERENCES

Dalsey, W.C., Syverud, S.A., and Trott, A.: Transcutaneous cardiac pacing. *J. Emerg. Med.*, 1:201–205, 1984.

Dalsey, W.C., Syverud, S.A., et al: Transcutaneous cardiac pacing. *Ann. Emerg. Med.*, 13:410–411, 1984.

Syverud, S.A., Dalsey, W.C., Hedges, J.R., et al: Transcutaneous cardiac pacing: Determination of myocardial injury in a canine model. *Ann. Emerg. Med.*, 12:745–748, 1983.

PERMANENT PACEMAKER MANAGEMENT

Carolyn B. Chalkley, R.N., M.S.N.

Overview

An implanted cardiac pacing system is used in those patients who are at potential risk for lethal dysrhythmias or altered electrodynamics and subsequent altered hemodynamics (see the overview for "Temporary Pacemaker Management").

Components of a permanent pacing system include a pulse generator and one or more pacing catheter electrodes. The pulse generator contains the energy source; this can be a lithium iodide battery or nuclear battery (Fig. 1–76). Some pulse generators have batteries which are rechargeable by means of a transcutaneous technique and the use of an external power source. The pacing electrodes may be bipolar or unipolar. The pacing electrode(s) may be positioned by using an endocardial implant through a transvenous approach or an epicardial implant through a subcostal, subxiphoid, or median sternotomy approach during open heart surgery.

Permanent Pacemaker.

With the proliferation of pacemaker technology that has occurred in the past several years, a three-letter code was devised in 1974 by the Inter-Society Commission for Heart Disease to facilitate accurate communication between health care professionals and suppliers. The code was revised to a five-letter system in 1981 as follows:

First letter—Chamber paced
A = Atrium
V = Ventricle

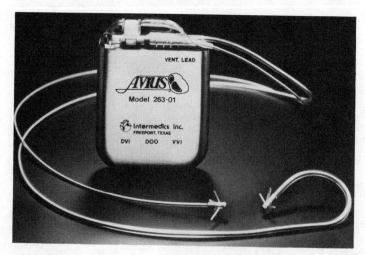

Figure 1-76. Permanent cardiac pacing system (pulse generator and pacing catheter electrode). (Courtesy of Intermedics, Inc.)

D = Double (dual) chamber
S = Single chamber

Second letter—Chamber sensed
A = Atrium
V = Ventricle
D = Double (dual) chamber
S = Single chamber
O = None

Third letter—Mode of response to sensed impulse
I = Inhibited
T = Triggered
D = Double
O = None
R = Reverse

Fourth letter—Programmability
P = Programmable rate or output
M = Multiprogrammability
O = None

Fifth letter—Tachyarrhythmia functions
B = Burst
N = Normal rate competition
S = Scanning
E = External
O = None

Examples of pacing systems now in common use:
AOO = Atrial asynchronous (fixed rate)
AAT = Atrial triggered ⎱ Atrial Demand
AAI = Atrial inhibited ⎰
VAT = A-V synchronous
VOO = Ventricular asynchronous (fixed rate)
VVT = Ventricular triggered ⎱ Ventricular Demand
VVI = Ventricular inhibited ⎰
VDD = Atrial synchronous (ventricular inhibited)
DOO = A-V sequential (fixed rate)
DVI = A-V sequential (ventricular inhibited)
DDD = Fully automatic dual chamber (A-V universal)

This section will focus on select procedures of permanent pacemaker management utilized within critical care units, the operating room or cardiac catheterization laboratory, intermediate care unit, and physician's office or clinic.

ASSESSING SELECT PARAMETERS OF
A PERMANENT PACING SYSTEM _____

      Basic Components of Analyzers. While pacemaker system analyzers (PSA's) differ among manufacturers, the basic components are as follows for the pacing and testing functions of the analyzer (Fig. 1–77).

1. Rate
    A. Allows adjustment of the PSA's pulse generator output to a wide range of pacing rates.
    B. Allows determination of the preset or programmed rate of the pulse generator being tested.
2. Output (volts, milliamps)
    A. Allows adjustment of the amplitude of the PSA's pulse generator to a wide range of current outputs to provide pacing for the patient before the permanent pulse generator is connected and during determination of pacing thresholds.
    B. Allows determination of the preset or programmed current output of the pulse generator being tested.
3. Pulse width (duration)

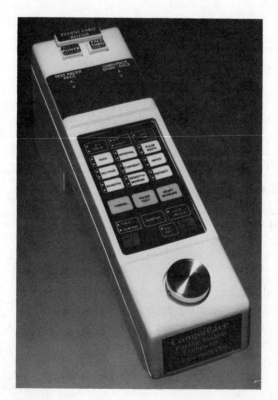

Figure 1-77. Pacing system analyzer. (Courtesy of Intermedics, Inc.)

    A. Allows adjustment of the duration of the impulse of the PSA's pulse generator.

    B. Allows determination of the preset or programmed pulse width (duration) of the pulse generator being tested.

4. Sensitivity

    A. Allows adjustment of the input sensitivity from asynchronous through an increasing range of sensitivity selections.

    B. Allows determination of the preset or programmed sensitivity of the generator being tested.

    C. Is used for determination of intracavitary R-wave and P-wave voltage.

5. A-V interval

    A. Allows adjustment of the time between the delivery of the atrial impulse and the delivery of the ventricular impulse.

    B. Allows determination of the preset or programmed time between the delivery of the atrial impulse and the delivery of the ventricular impulse by the pulse generator.

6. Slew rate

    A. Allows determination of the change in voltage (dv/dt) of intracavitary signals for proper sensing.

7. Lower rate

    A. Allows determination of the preset or programmed lower rate of the pulse generator being tested.

8. Upper rate

    A. Allows determination of the preset or programmed upper rate of the pulse generator being tested.

Objectives

1. To determine proper functioning of the following parameters on a pulse generator: rate, current output, open circuit voltage, pulse duration, upper and lower rates, A-V interval, refractory time, and sensitivity.

2. To determine the minimum intensity of a stimulus that causes depolarization of the heart via a permanently implanted pacing electrode.

3. To determine the adequacy of the intracavitary R-wave and P-wave signals to insure proper sensing by an implanted demand pulse generator.

4. To determine the integrity of the pacing electrode and its connection to viable myocardium.

5. To determine the proper function of a permanent or temporary pulse generator before patient use or in case of suspected malfunction.

Special Equipment

PSA	ECG monitor
Pacemaker test cable	Defibrillator
Pacemaker extension cable	Emergency cart and medications

Procedure

ACTION	RATIONALE

1. Establish continuous ECG monitoring.

2. Connect the pacemaker extension cable to the PSA. (The surgeon will connect the cable to the pacing electrode in the sterile field.)

3. Determine proper placement and function of the ventricular pacing electrode by testing the following parameters.

A. Stimulation threshold of the ventricle.

    (1) Follow manufacturer's instructions for operation of the PSA.

    (2) Establish 1:1 capture according to physician's directions or protocol.

    (3) Slowly decrease the output of the PSA until consistent capture is lost.

    (4) Increase the current output slowly until consistent capture is restored.

    (5) Compare the patient's ventricular stimulation threshold of the electrode and pulse generator to be implanted to the manufacturer's recommendations. The stimulation threshold may be measured in volts or milliamps.

B. Ventricular sensing threshold.

    (1) Follow manufacturer's instructions for operation of the PSA.

    (2) Compare the voltage reading of the patient's R-wave to the recommended ventricular sensing threshold of the pulse generator and electrode to be implanted.

A. This procedure determines the minimum intensity of a stimulus that causes depolarization of the ventricles via the permanently implanted pacing electrode.

(5) By comparison of the patient's ventricular stimulation threshold to the pacemaker manufacturer's recommendations, a margin of safety may be assured as the patient's ventricular stimulation threshold rises over a period after implant so that continued pacing is assured.

B. This determines the adequacy of the intracavitary R-wave signal to ensure proper sensing of the patient's intrinsic R-waves by the implanted pacemaker system.

ACTION	RATIONALE
(3) Note the voltage reading of any ectopic QRS complexes that may occur and compare to the recommended ventricular sensing threshold of the pulse generator to be implanted.	(3) Ectopic beats may have an R-wave vector or initial slew rate that is not sensed by the pulse generator, thus causing the pulse generator to fire during the vulnerable phase of ventricular repolarization and produce competitive rhythms, ventricular tachycardia, or ventricular fibrillation singly or in combination.

4. Determine proper placement and function of the atrial pacing electrode by testing the following parameters:

A. Stimulation threshold of the atrium.	A. This procedure determines the minimum intensity of a stimulus that causes depolarization of the atria via the permanently implanted pacing electrode.
(1) Follow manufacturer's instructions for operation of the PSA.	
(2) Compare the patient's atrial stimulation threshold to the recommended threshold of the electrode and pulse generator to be implanted. The stimulation threshold may be measured in volts or milliamps.	(2) By comparing the patient's atrial stimulation threshold to the pacemaker manufacturer's recommendation, a margin of safety may be assured as the patient's atrial stimulation threshold rises over time after implant so that continued pacing is assured.
B. Atrial sensing threshold.	B. This determines the adequacy of the intracavitary P-wave signal to ensure proper sensing of the patient's intrinsic P-waves by the implanted pacemaker system.
(1) Follow manufacturer's instructions for operation of the PSA.	
(2) Compare the voltage reading of the patient's P-wave to the recommended atrial sensing threshold of the pulse generator and electrode to be implanted.	

ACTION	RATIONALE
(3) Note the voltage of any ectopic P-waves that may occur and compare to the recommended atrial sensing threshold of the electrode and pulse generator to be implanted.	(3) Ectopic beats may have a P-wave vector or initial slew rate that is not sensed by the pulse generator, thus causing the pulse generator to fire during the vulnerable phase of atrial repolarization and produce atrial fibrillation.
5. Determine appropriate A-V interval for the patient by adjusting the A-V interval as directed by the physician or protocol.	5. This determines the optimum timing for delivery of the atrial and ventricular impulses to maximize cardiac output. Cardiac output may be reduced by loss of A-V synchrony.
6. Monitor blood pressure, pulse volume, patient's symptoms closely during this procedure.	
7. Determine lead impedance (resistance). A. Follow manufacturer's instructions for operation of the PSA. B. Compare the lead impedance to the lead manufacturer's recommendations for either a new or previously implanted lead. The lead impedance is measured in ohms.	7. This determines the integrity of the pacing electrode and its connection to viable myocardium. B. A higher than recommended lead impedance may indicate excessive fibrosis around a previously implanted lead. A lower than recommended lead impedance may indicate poor electrical integrity (Example: fractured lead). Erratic lead impedance readings may be due to a fractured lead that alternatively separates and approximates, loose connection between the lead and PSA, or unstable electrode position.
8. Determine proper functioning of a pulse generator (new or previously implanted). A. Follow manufacturer's instructions for operating the PSA to determine rate, pulse intervals, current voltage, pulse width (duration), sensitivity, lower rate, upper rate.	8. This determines the need for replacement of a previously implanted pulse generator, proper functioning of a new pulse generator to be implanted, and accuracy of newly programmed settings.

ACTION   RATIONALE

B. Compare readings to
    manufacturer's preset specifica-
    tions of the pulse generator to be
    implanted or the setting of the
    parameters at the time of the last
    programming of the pulse genera-
    tor.

Precautions

1. Provide defibrillator, emergency cart, and medications for immediate use.
2. Follow electrical safety guidelines for patients with pacemakers.

Related Care

1. Monitor patient's ECG and hemodynamic responses during select
    assessment/reprogramming of permanent pacemaker.
2. Record all measurements in permanent record.

Complications

Lethal dysrhythmias   Electromicroshock
Cardiac arrest   Equipment malfunction
Infection   Erosion of generator pocket

Suppliers

Biotronics   Intermedics
Coratomics   Medtronic, Inc.
Cordis Corporation   Pacesetter
C.P.I. ELA Medical   Siemens-Elema

REFERENCES

Intermedics: Compupace Pacemaker System Computer, Model 524-01. Freeport,
    TX, 1980.
Medtronic, Inc.: Medtronic 5311 A-V Pacing System Analyzer Operator's Guide.
    Minneapolis, MN, 1982.
Parsonnett, V., et al.: A revised code for pacemaker identification. PACE, 4:400,
    1981.

INHIBITION OF A PERMANENT PACEMAKER _____

Objective

To assess the patient's underlying cardiac rhythm by inhibiting permanent pacing temporarily through the use of an external temporary pacemaker.

Special Equipment

Temporary external pacemaker	ECG recorder
Pacemaker extension cable with alligator clips	Defibrillator
Two suction cup electrodes	Emergency cart and medications

Procedure

ACTION	RATIONALE
1. Locate the pulse generator by inspection or gentle palpation.	
2. Obtain initial ECG recording.	2. This serves as baseline data.
3. Determine model of pulse generator. This information may be found on patient's I.D. card, earlier charts, or by x-ray identification of pulse generator.	3. The effectiveness of this procedure will depend upon the model of pulse generator and the distance between skin surface and pacing system; therefore it cannot be used for all patients.
4. Apply suction cups to patient. A. If unipolar pacemaker is used, place one suction cup over pulse generator and another over tip of electrode. B. If bipolar pacemaker is used, place one suction cup over tip of electrode and other suction cup approximately 1 inch above and to the right (over the ring or proximal electrode).	
5. Connect suction cups to temporary external pacemaker, using extension cable (Fig. 1–78).	

ACTION   RATIONALE

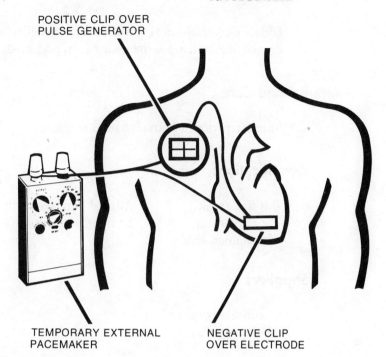

POSITIVE CLIP OVER
PULSE GENERATOR

Figure 1-78. Inhibition of permanent pacemaker using a temporary external pacemaker.

TEMPORARY EXTERNAL
PACEMAKER

NEGATIVE CLIP
OVER ELECTRODE

   A. Use positive clip connected to suction cup over pulse generator or proximal electrode.

   B. Use negative clip connected to suction cup over distal electrode.

6. Set sensitivity control of temporary external pacemaker on fixed rate.

7. Set rate of temporary external pacemaker at a value slightly higher than rate of the implanted unit; set amplitude at 4 ma. or higher, if necessary to inhibit permanent pacing.

8. Turn on temporary external pacemaker.

9. Record and assess ECG in usual fashion.

10. Disconnect the temporary external pacemaker.

11. Reprogramming to a lower rate may be done in place of this procedure if pacemaker is programmable.

8. The external pulses will inhibit the implanted pacemaker completely or partially, depending on its type.

9. Patient's own beats can be evaluated for change in the ECG that may not be evident during paced rhythm.

Precautions

1. Follow electrical safety guidelines for patients with pacemakers.
2. Provide defibrillator, emergency cart, and medications for immediate use.

Related Care

·1. Monitor patient's hemodynamic responses.

Complications

Cardiac arrest   Altered hemodynamics
Dysrhythmias   Equipment malfunction
Electromicroshock

Suppliers

Cordis Corporation
Medtronic, Inc.

REFERENCES

Medtronic, Inc.: Medtronic 5311 A-V Pacing System Analyzer Operator's Guide. Minneapolis, MN, 1982.
Intermedics: Compupace Pacemaker System Computer Model 524-01, Freeport, TX, 1980.

REPROGRAMMING A PERMANENT PACEMAKER _____

Instrumentation

The programmable parameters and programming procedures vary considerably among manufacturers and among different models produced by the same manufacturer (Fig. 1–79). Follow manufacturer's recommendations for operation of the programmer. *Programmers are not interchangeable.* The manufacturer and model of the pulse generator must be known, and the appropriate programmer must be used. This may be determined by x-ray if records are unavailable.

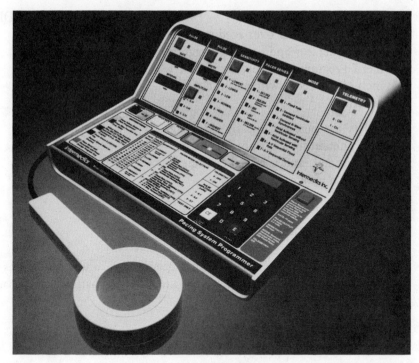

Figure 1-79. Pacing system programmer. (Courtesy of Intermedics, Inc.)

Objective

To change the rate, current output, sensitivity, A-V interval, refractory period, hysteresis, or pulse duration of a permanent pacemaker using a pacemaker programmer.

Special Equipment

Pacemaker programmer   Defibrillator
ECG recorder   Emergency cart and medications

Procedure

ACTION	RATIONALE
1. Adjust programmer to desired settings (see manufacturer's specification manual).	1. Parameters that may be programmed vary among manufacturers.
2. Locate pulse generator by inspection or gentle palpation.	

<table>
<tr><td align="center">ACTION</td><td align="center">RATIONALE</td></tr>
</table>

3. Place programmer over reed switch of pulse generator and activate programmer. Programmer must be within 1 inch of the reed switch of the pulse generator.

4. Verify the new settings by assessing ECG, obtaining a printout from the programmer, and pacemaker interrogation on applicable models.

Precautions

1. Provide defibrillator, emergency cart, and medications for immediate use.
2. Follow electrical safety guidelines for patients with pacemakers.

Related Care

1. Monitor patient's ECG and hemodynamic responses during select assessment/reprogramming of permanent pacemaker.
2. Record all settings in the permanent record.

Complications

Lethal dysrhythmias	Electromicroshock
Cardiac arrest	Equipment malfunction

Suppliers

Cardiac Pacemakers, Inc.	Intermedics
Cook	Medtronic, Inc.
Cordis Corporation	Telectronics
CPI	

REFERENCES

Cardiac Pacemakers, Inc.: Microlith-P Programmer Pacemaker System Physician's Manual. St. Paul, MN, 1980.

Cook Pacemaker Corporation: Physician's Technical Manual. Leechburg, PA, 1981.

Cordis Corporation Omnicor: Programmer Model 222B Instructions For Use. Miami, FL, 1979.

Intermedics: Physician's Manual Series 522 Cyber Lith Programmer. Freeport, TX, 1979.

Medtronic, Inc.: Censys Model 9701C Pacemaker Programmer Technical Manual. Minneapolis, MN, 1982.

Parsonnet, V., and Rodgers, T.: The present status of programmable pacemakers. Prog. Cardiovasc. Dis. 23:401, 1981.

Telectronics: Autima 2600 Programmer and 17 Series Charger Clinician's Information. Sydney, Australia, 1981.

USE OF A MAGNET

Objective

To temporarily convert a permanent demand pacemaker to fixed rate through the use of a magnet for such purposes as determining pacing rate, appropriate capture, or overriding dysrhythmias. (*Note*: Not all pulse generators respond to a magnet.)

Special Equipment

Appropriate pacemaker magnet, supplied
   by same manufacturer as pacemaker
ECG recorder
Defibrillator
Emergency cart and medications

Procedure

ACTION	RATIONALE
1. Initiate continuous ECG recording.	1. This provides baseline data.
2. Remove "keeper" from magnet (Fig. 1–80).	2. Keeper protects magnet until external application.

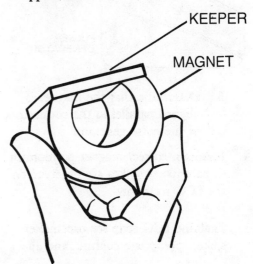

KEEPER

MAGNET

Figure 1-80. Keeper with magnet.

ACTION   RATIONALE

3. Apply magnet externally directly over
   the reed switch of the pulse generator
   (Fig. 1–81).

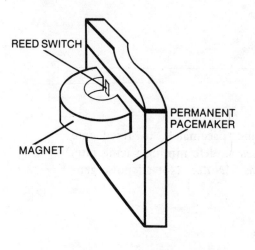

Figure 1-81. Positioning magnet over reed switch. (Position of reed switch varies among manufacturers.)

A. Place the magnet within 1 inch of   A. This activates the reed switch.
   the pulse generator (Fig. 1–82).

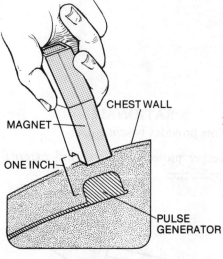

Figure 1-82. Placement of magnet within one inch of pulse generator.

B. Determine that the magnet is   B. This activates the reed switch.
   aligned parallel to the connectors
   of the pulse generator.

4. Maintain correct magnet position until pacemaker spikes are observed on
   the ECG recording.

5. Examine ECG strip for pacemaker   5. Each pacemaker spike falling outside
   spike, appropriate capture, and ap-   the refractory period should be fol-

ACTION	RATIONALE
propriate rate response, as specified by manufacturer.	lowed immediately by a paced depolarization. The magnet rate may be less than or greater than the preset rate, depending on the model.

6. Remove magnet; apply keeper.

7. Assess patient's ECG rhythm after magnet application.

8. Turn off ECG recorder.

Precautions

1. Follow electrical safety guidelines for patients with pacemakers.
2. Provide defibrillator, emergency cart, and medications for immediate use.
3. Note that some pacemakers exhibit a 20% increase in rate when the magnet is applied.
4. Observe for competitive rhythms, ventricular tachycardia, or ventricular fibrillation caused by fixed-rate ventricular pacing.
5. Remove magnet immediately if competitive rhythms occur.
6. Protect against reed switch breakage by using only a magnet supplied by the pacemaker manufacturer.

Related Care

Monitor patient's hemodynamic responses.

Complications

Cardiac arrest	Altered hemodynamics
Dysrhythmias	Equipment malfunction
Electromicroshock	

REFERENCES

Cardiac Pacemakers, Inc.: Microlith-P Programmer Pacemaker System Physician's Manual. St. Paul, MN, 1980.
Cook Pacemaker Corporation: Physician's Technical Manual. Leechburg, PA, 1981.
Cordis Corporation Omnicor: Programmer Model 222B Instructions for Use. Miami, FL, 1979.
Intermedics: Physician's Manual Series 522 Cyber Lith Programmer. Freeport, TX, 1979.
Medtronic, Inc.: Censys Model 9701C Pacemaker Programmer Technical Manual. Minneapolis, MN, 1982.

Parsonnet, V., and Rodgers, T.: The present status of programmable pacemakers. Prog. Cardiovasc. Dis., 23:401, 1981.

Telectronics: Autima 2600 Programmer and 17 Series Charger Clinician's Information. Sydney, Australia, 1981.

TRANSTELEPHONIC PACEMAKER MONITORING _____

Instrumentation

Transtelephonic monitoring systems have two basic components:

1. The transmitter consists of ECG monitoring electrodes that are placed on the patient's chest, wrists, or fingers and connected to the portion of the transmitter that converts the ECG into an audible signal (Fig. 1–83). The audible signal is then transmitted over the telephone, which has been placed in contact with the transmitter. (The transmitter is owned, rented, leased, or borrowed by the patient and is used in conjunction with a standard telephone from any location.)

2. The receiver consists of components that convert the audible signal received over the clinic telephone into an ECG signal that is printed on an

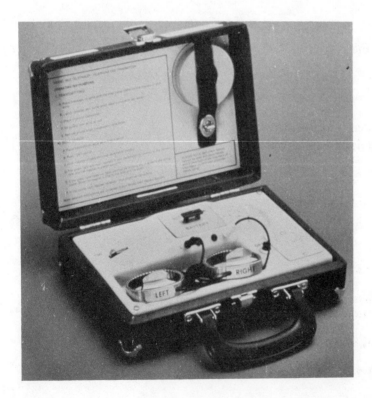

Figure 1-83. Transtelephonic *transmitter* for use by the patient. (Courtesy of Medtronic, Inc.)

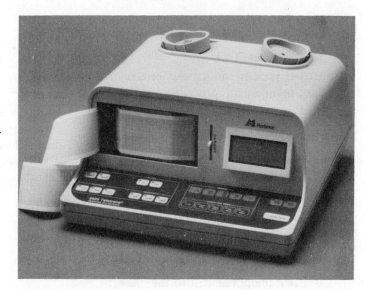

Figure 1-84. Transtelephonic *receiver* for use by the health-care professional. (Courtesy of Medtronic Inc.)

ECG recorder for analysis of pacemaker function and the patient's underlying cardiac rhythm (Fig. 1–84). Some receivers also have a digital display feature. The transtelephonic receiver is owned, rented, leased, or borrowed by the clinic, physician's office, or hospital.

Objectives

1. To determine proper function of a permanently implanted pacemaker system.
2. To assess patient for dysrhythmias.
3. To assess patient for adequacy of drug therapy for dysrhythmias.
4. To maintain ongoing patient follow-up.
5. To reduce the cost, time, transportation, anxiety, and inconvenience associated with more frequent office visits than the patient's general condition warrants.

Special Equipment

Transtelephonic transmitter system
Patient's (or neighbor's) telephone
Transtelephonic receiver system,
    including recorder
Physician or clinic's telephone

Procedure

ACTION	RATIONALE
1. Instruct patient and at least one significant other in the procedure and the schedule for calls and follow-up visits (Fig. 1–83):	1. Anxiety, illness, discomfort, and medications may interfere with the patient's usual ability to learn and recall information and procedures taught during hospitalization.
A. Prep skin/electrode site per transtelephonic manufacturer's recommendations.	A. This establishes a satisfactory skin-electrode interface.
B. Connect electrodes to wrists, fingers, or chest of patient, depending on transtelephonic manufacturer.	
C. Place telephone call to pacemaker follow-up clinic (include the following information: name, physician, date of last pacemaker check).	
D. Place mouthpiece of telephone over patient's pacemaker transmitter for a specified period (usually 1 minute).	D. The transmitter converts the ECG into an audible signal that is transmitted over the phone.
E. Await further instructions from pacemaker follow-up clinic.	
2. Facilitate pacemaker transtelephonic patient information by a health care professional (Fig. 1–84):	
A. Place the clinic's telephone into the transmitter receiver; turn on the strip-chart recorder.	A. The receiver converts the audible tones into an ECG recording that is viewed on a strip chart.
B. Examine digital readings and ECG rhythm strip for completeness.	B. Patient movement or interference in the telephone line may interrupt the signal.
C. Instruct patient to place the pacemaker magnet over the pulse generator and repeat the transmission (optional, depending on protocol).	C. The magnet temporarily converts the pulse generator from demand to fixed rate. In some models the pacing rate is also changed during the period when the magnet is used.
D. Record readings and ECG rhythm strip in patient's record for physician review.	

ACTION	RATIONALE
3. Elicit verbal information regarding the patient's condition, medication profile, health care treatments, or change in health instructions since previous pacemaker follow-up, and so on; provide patient instructions as appropriate.	3. Symptoms of altered hemodynamics may indicate the need for pacemaker reprogramming or other medical intervention. Signs and symptoms of other complications may be determined and appropriate intervention advised.

Precautions

1. Monitor patient's response closely during *optional* magnet application; magnet application may cause competitive rhythms, ventricular tachycardia, or ventricular fibrillation.
2. Monitor patient compliance with follow-up instructions, especially when health status indicates high risk situations.

Related Care

1. Verify patient's understanding of date for next transtelephonic pacemaker analysis.
2. Monitor patient's compliance with transtelephonic pacemaker analysis follow-up checks.

Complications

Lethal dysrhythmias
Skin irritation

Suppliers

Biotronics	Instromedix
Cardiac Monitoring, Inc.	Intermedics
Cardio Pace	Medtronic
Cook	Pacesetter
Coratomic	Seimens-Elema
Cordis	Survival Technology
C.P.I.	Telectronics
Ela Medical	United Medical Corporation

REFERENCES

Intermedics, Inc.: Housecalls. Freeport, TX, 1981.
Instromedix. A Pulse V transmitter. Beaverton, OR, 1981.
Medtronic, Inc.: Model 9408A Tele Trace Transmitter. Minneapolis, MN, 1981.

NONINVASIVE PERIPHERAL VASCULAR BLOOD FLOW MEASUREMENT

Karen L. Wheelock, R.N., B.S.N., M.A.

Overview

Monitoring changes in blood flow of the peripheral vascular system can often be accomplished through inspection, palpation, and auscultatory assessment. In persons with altered hemodynamics or acute onset of circulatory impairment due to thrombus, embolus, or spasms, the development of noninvasive peripheral vascular blood flow devices has enhanced the quality of obtaining data for rapid diagnosis of the patency or status of arteriovenous systems. There are two basic methods of noninvasive peripheral vascular blood flow measurement. These are ultrasonic velocity detection, which senses blood flow from the frequency shift of sound as reflected from blood cells flowing through vessels, and plethysmography techniques, which record dimensional changes in a portion of the body in response to either heartbeats or temporary occlusion of venous return. Plethysmography techniques differ according to the type of transducer used, and they include water, strain gauge, photoelectric, air, and impedance methods. Included in this section are procedures for use of the ultrasonic blood flow detector, and two of the easier to use plethysmography methods: strain gauge and a type of air recorder (pulse volume recorder).

ULTRASOUND BLOOD FLOW DETECTOR

Objectives

1. To detect blood flow in arterial and venous sytems of the periphery.
2. To obtain blood pressure readings when conventional auscultation is not reliable.
3. To aid in diagnosis and assessment of peripheral vascular problems.
4. To evaluate treatment of peripheral vascular problems.

Special Equipment

Ultrasound probe with stethoscope or automatic speaker amplifier (Fig. 1–85).
Ultrasound transmission gel

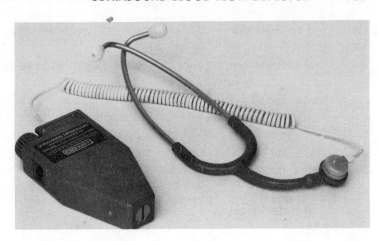

Figure 1-85. Ultrasound probe with stethoscope. (Courtesy of Medsonics, Inc. Mountain View, CA.)

Procedure

ACTION	RATIONALE
1. Apply ultrasound transmission gel to faceplate of probe.	
2. Position probe on skin surface over the vessel; tilt probe slightly toward the axis of blood flow.	2. Tilting (approximately 60-degree angle) the probe produces a better signal.
3. Auscultate for arterial sound. A. Normal arterial sound is a loud, high pitched systolic sound with one or more softer, lower pitched diastolic sounds. These sounds are repeated with each cardiac cycle. B. Normal venous sound is cyclic with respirations, higher pitched on expiration, and resembles a windstorm.	A. The rapid forward blood flow in systole, a lesser reverse flow in early diastole, and slight forward flow late in diastole produce this auscultatory sound.
4. Obtain blood pressure, using an ultrasound blood flow detector, if desired. A. Use conventional method, substituting prelubricated ultrasound probe for regular stethoscope. B. Adjust volume as necessary. C. Inflate cuff until arterial sound disappears, or pressure is 20 mm. Hg above brachial pressure; release cuff pressure slowly while checking for systolic and diastolic pressures.	

Precautions

1. Avoid using probe in the vicinity of the eye because of risk of damaging delicate nerve tissue.
2. Avoid compressing vessel with excessive probe pressure. Diastolic pressure is difficult to detect in critically ill patients.
3. Clean ultrasound probe as directed by manufacturer to prevent faceplate surface scratching; do not autoclave.
4. Avoid using alcohol as a transmission gel or to clean faceplate of probe.

Related Care

1. Integrate data with other information from circulatory assessment.
2. Turn off instrument following each use to preserve battery life.
3. Check volume control or battery or both if no auscultatory signal is elicited. Replace battery a minimum of every 6 months.

Complications

Nerve tissue damage (with high intensity ultrasound)
Altered skin integrity
Equipment malfunction

Suppliers

Corbin-Farnsworth
Medsonics Laboratories
Parks Electronics

REFERENCES

Barnes, R.W., and Hume, D.: Noninvasive Diagnostic Techniques in Peripheral Vascular Disease. Richmond Medical College of Virginia, Virginia Commonwealth University, 1980, pp. 5-14.

Durbin, N.: The application of Doppler techniques in critical care. Focus Crit. Care, *10*:45–46, (June) 1983.

PULSE VOLUME RECORDER

Objectives

1. To detect blood volume change in the extremities.
2. To obtain systolic pressure readings in the extremities.

3. To aid in diagnosis and assessment of peripheral vascular problems, both arterial and venous.

Special Equipment

Pulse volume recorder (PVR), portable or cart model (Fig. 1–86).
Blood pressure cuffs:
    Thigh cuffs for above the knee
    Regular adult cuffs for upper arm, forearm, calf, and ankle
    Pediatric cuff for foot measurements

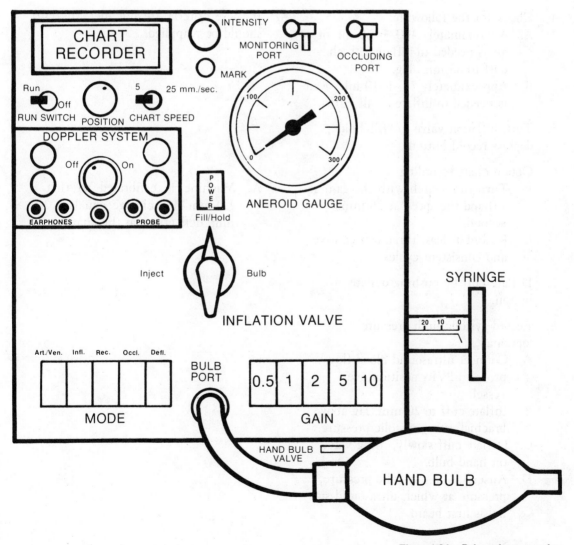

Figure 1-86.   Pulse volume recorder.

Procedure

ACTION	RATIONALE
1. Select appropriate cuff for site and place on extremity.	
2. Connect cuff to monitor port.	

3. Select inflation mode. Turn inflation valve to "bulb"; inflate cuff to arbitrary pressure.
  A. Use valve to inflate large cuffs; usually about 65 mm. Hg is required.
  B. Use syringe to inflate smaller cuffs.
	3. Using an arbitrary pressure setting provides for constant cuff volume around the extremity from reading to reading.

4. Check for the following.
  A. Approximately 400 $\pm$ 50 ml. of air is needed to inflate a thigh cuff to 65 mm. Hg.
  B. Approximately 75 $\pm$ 10 ml. of air is needed to inflate a calf cuff.
	4. If these criteria are not met, the cuff should be reapplied.

5. Turn inflation valve to "fill/hold"; depress record button.	

6. Obtain chart recording.
  A. Turn run switch with the gain at 1.0 and the speed at 25 mm./second.
  B. Record at least three consecutive and consistent cycles.
	A. Machine is calibrated so that a 1.0-mm. Hg change equals a 20-mm. deflection on the chart.

7. Deflate cuff by pushing deflate button.	

8. Record systolic limb pressure (optional).
  A. Connect ultrasound blood flow probe to PVR; position over vessel.
  B. Inflate cuff to 20 mm. Hg above brachial artery systolic pressure.
  C. Deflate cuff slowly, using valve on hand bulb.
  D. Auscultate for systolic pressure, pressure at which ultrasound signal is first heard.	

ACTION

RATIONALE

9. Measure systolic and diastolic pressures with PVR (optional).
   A. Place an occluding cuff proximal to the monitoring cuff.
   B. Read lower limb systolic pressure at site of occlusive cuff when its pressure obliterates recordings from monitoring cuff.
   C. Observe increase in amplitude of oscillation cuff. Pressure is slowly released from occlusion cuff.
   D. Read diastolic pressure at the point at which maximum excursions occur.

Precautions

1. Monitor for cuff error.
   A. At higher monitoring cuff pressures, distortion of recorded pulse wave form occurs.
   B. Ideally, monitoring cuff pressure should be below limb diastolic pressure.

Related Care

1. Assess circulation of extremity prior to and after the diagnostic test.
2. Integrate data with other information derived from circulation assessment.

Complications

Altered skin integrity
Equipment malfunction

Supplier

Life Sciences, Inc.

REFERENCES

Barnes, R.: Current status of noninvasive tests of venous disease. Surg. Clin. North Am. 62:489–499, 1982.

Bernstein, E. and Fronek, A.: Current status of noninvasive tests in the diagnosis of peripheral arterial disease. Surg. Clin. North Am. *62*:473–485, 1982.

Bernstein, E.: Diagnostic Techniques in Vascular Disease. St. Louis, C.V. Mosby, 1982.

Juergens, J.L., et al.: Peripheral Vascular Disease. Philadelphia, W.B. Saunders, 1980, pp. 139–219.

Waxham, R.: Doppler Ultrasound, Radiol. Today, (April-May), 1980, p. 1–7.

STRAIN GAUGE PLETHYSMOGRAPHY

Objectives

1. To detect volume flow in the extremities.
2. To aid in diagnosis and assessment of peripheral vascular disease.

Special Equipment

Strain gauges
Special blood pressure cuff
Plethysmograph recorder

Procedure

ACTION	RATIONALE
1. Place selected cuff at identified sites on larger extremity where a pressure reading will be taken: upper thigh, above knee, below knee, and ankle (Fig. 1–87).	

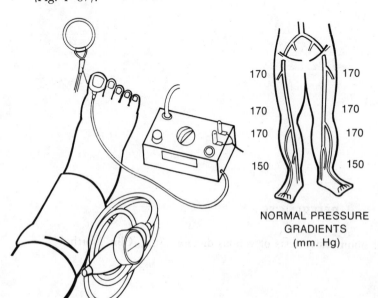

170   170
170   170
170   170
150   150

NORMAL PRESSURE
GRADIENTS
(mm. Hg)

Figure 1-87. Mercury strain gauge plethysmograph.

ACTION	RATIONALE
2. Place elastic strain gauge around digit.	
3. Turn on recorder; observe wave form.	3. This provides baseline data.
4. Inflate cuff until recorded pulses disappear. Gradually deflate cuff until small pulsations appear with each heartbeat.	4. At this point cuff pressure is equal to systolic pressure.
5. Turn off recorder.	
6. Complete systolic pressure measurements at four sites on each lower extremity: upper thigh, above knee, below knee, and ankle, following steps 1 through 5.	
7. Check for normal pressure gradients (Fig. 1–87). A. High thigh: 170 mm. Hg. B. Above knee: 170 mm. Hg. C. Below knee: 170 mm. Hg. D. Ankle: 150 mm. Hg.	7. Pressure differences of 30 mm. Hg or more indicate obstructive disease in the artery. Ankle pressure is normally within 15 mm. of brachial artery systolic pressure. Upper thigh pressure is normally 20 mm. or more above brachial artery systolic pressure.

Precaution

Check for cuff errors; an extreme pressure gradient exists across an obstruction.

Related Care

1. Determine the brachial artery and ankle pressures through a screening test.
2. Assess circulation of extremity prior to and after the diagnostic test.
3. Integrate with other information derived from circulation assessment.

Complications

Altered skin integrity
Equipment malfunction

Supplier

Parks Electronics

REFERENCES

Barnes, R.: Current status of noninvasive tests of venous disease. Surg. Clinc. North Am. *62*:489–499, 1982.

Bernstein, E. and Fronek, A.: Current status of noninvasive tests in the diagnosis of peripheral arterial disease. Surg. Clin. North Am. *62*:473–485, 1982.

Bernstein, E.: Diagnostic Techniques in Vascular Disease. St. Louis: C.V. Mosby, 1982.

Juergens, J.L., et al.: Peripheral Vascular Disease. Philadelphia, W.B. Saunders, 1980, pp. 139–219.

Waxham, R.: Doppler ultrasound. Radiol. Today. (April-May), 1980, pp. 1–7.

ROTATING TOURNIQUETS

Karen L. Wheelock, R.N., B.S.N., M.A.

Overview

Rotating tourniquet therapy is one of many therapeutic interventions frequently prescribed in the medical emergency of pulmonary edema. By rotating tourniquets on extremities systematically, venous return to the heart is decreased. Automatic devices for sequential rotation are available, or the therapy may be performed manually. Application, monitoring, and assessment of clinical response during therapy, as well as the proper discontinuation of therapy and assessment of the effects of altered hemodynamics, are major components of the procedure.

Objectives

1. To decrease circulating volume in such instances as acute pulmonary edema or severe congestive heart failure.
2. To provide temporary support therapy until additional definitive treatment is initiated.

Special Equipment

Automatic rotating tourniquet equipment, *or*
Four wide, soft rubber tourniquets
Four soft pads

Procedure

ACTION	RATIONALE
1. Place patient in semi-Fowler's position.	
2. Obtain baseline blood pressure reading.	
3. Select mode for rotating tourniquet therapy. A. Automatic rotating tourniquets: (1) Place cuffs high on appropriate extremity. (2) Secure air tubes to valves located on portable automatic rotating tourniquet equipment.	

ACTION	RATIONALE
(3) Close all outlet valves.	
(4) Adjust cuff release timer to the prescribed cycle length; multiply time selected by 3 to determine total time each cuff is to be inflated.	(4) Length of inflation is individualized and prescribed by physician.
(5) Set pressure to be maintained in the cuffs just above patient's diastolic pressure, using pressure control knob.	(5) This ensures impedance to venous return without interfering with arterial supply to the extremity.
(6) Activate alarm system.	(6) This permits an audible signal and a red alarm light to go on if machine fails to rotate cuffs or if there is an air leak.
(7) Open valves, one at a time, observing effect on patient.	(7) Machine will automatically inflate and deflate cuffs in rotation.
(8) Monitor blood pressure frequently.	(8) Use of rotating tourniquets may precipitate hypotension in some patients.
(a) Close valve to one of arm cuffs when deflated.	
(b) Disconnect air tube from valve.	
(c) Connect an aneroid sphygmomanometer to cuff.	
(d) Obtain blood pressure.	
(e) Reconnect to air tubing; open valve.	
(9) Facilitate safe transport and therapy, when necessary.	
(a) Close all four valves.	(a) This maintains pressure in three of the four cuffs.
(b) Leave cuffs connected and in place.	
(c) Turn off power.	(c) Never leave cuffs inflated longer than 45 minutes.
(d) Transfer patient to cart.	
(e) Turn on power; open valves.	
(f) Check and adjust pressure as needed.	

ACTION

(10) Discontinue therapy when prescribed. Close valve and disconnect air hose from cuff as each cuff deflates in a rotating fashion.

B. Manual rotating tourniquets:

(1) Place pads and tourniquets high on three extremities; position fourth pad and tourniquet next to, but not on, the fourth extremity.

(2) Palpate arterial pulses in three extremities while tourniquets are in place.

(3) Rotate tourniquets in a clockwise manner every 15 minutes (Fig. 1–88).

RATIONALE

(10) This permits gradual return of trapped blood into systemic circulation.

(2) Tourniquets should not obliterate arterial pulses.

(3) Tourniquets should not be left in place on any extremity for longer than 45 minutes.

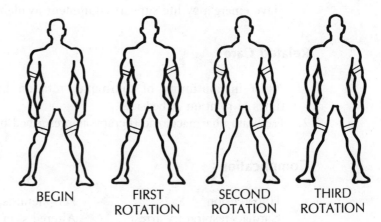

Figure 1-88. Pattern of 15-minute rotation of tourniquets.

BEGIN   FIRST   SECOND   THIRD
             ROTATION   ROTATION   ROTATION

(a) Remove first tourniquet and apply tourniquet to fourth extremity.

(b) Continue to rotate tourniquets in a clockwise manner every 15 minutes.

(4) Monitor blood pressure by placing cuff on arm that is tourniquet free.

(4) Use of rotating tourniquets may precipitate hypotension in some patients.

ACTION	RATIONALE
(5) Discontinue therapy when prescribed; remove tourniquets one at a time, at same time intervals, and in same clockwise rotation.	(5) This permits gradual return of trapped blood into systemic circulation.

4. Monitor patient status during and after therapy.

Precautions

1. Assess extremities frequently for the presence of an arterial pulse and skin integrity. It is anticipated that discoloration and temperature change will occur in the extremity while treatment is in progress.
2. Closely monitor the total time venous flow is impeded. Never leave cuffs inflated or tourniquets in place on an extremity for longer than 45 minutes.
3. Do not remove all tourniquets at once since this offers a high risk for circulatory overload, pulmonary edema or both.
4. Use of rotating tourniquets may precipitate hypotension in some patients.
5. Have emergency life support equipment available for use if needed.

Related Care

1. Assist in continuity of tourniquet rotation by keeping a diagram and times of rotation at bedside.
2. Facilitate pharmacologic therapy as prescribed by physician.

Complications

Hypotension   Peripheral ischemia
Cardiac/respiratory arrest   Altered skin integrity

Suppliers

Kidde Rotating Tourniquets
R.P. Scherer Rotating Tourniquets

REFERENCES

Luckmann, J, and Sorensen, K.C.: Medical-Surgical Nursing: A Psychophysiologic Approach, 2nd ed. Philadelphia, W.B. Saunders, 1980.
Phipps, W., Long, B., and Woods, N.: Medical-Surgical Nursing Concepts and Clinical Practice. St. Louis, C.V. Mosby, 1979, pp. 1009–1011.

THERAPEUTIC PHLEBOTOMY

Janice M. Casper, R.N., B.S.N.

Overview

The altered hemodynamic status of a critically ill patient can be purposefully improved by multidimensional and aggressive medical therapy. A therapeutic phlebotomy may be indicated (1) when it is necessary to remove blood from a patient to decrease the number of red blood cells in polycythemia, (2) to decrease intravascular volume in acute pulmonary edema, or (3) for potential autotransfusion. A phlebotomy is performed electively or as an emergency intervention within the critical care setting.

Objectives

1. To safely remove 250 to 500 ml. of blood in order to decrease central blood volume or red cell mass.
2. To ensure proper collection of blood for potential autotransfusion.

Special Equipment

500-ml. sterile blood bag containing anticoagulant solution
Blood collection tubing with 16–gauge, 18–gauge, or
   19–gauge needle
Tourniquet
Sterile gauze pads
Povidone-iodine prep swabs
Tape
Povidone-iodine ointment

Procedure

ACTION	RATIONALE

1. Prepare collection bag.
  A. Inspect bag for defects and clarity of solution. Discard defective bag.
  B. Close tubing clamp; insert needle-to-bag into inlet port, using sterile technique.	

2. Apply tourniquet and, using sterile technique, perform venipuncture.	

ACTION	RATIONALE
A. Select large vein and the largest needle possible.	A. A large needle lumen prevents clotting and decreases red cell lysis if autotransfusion is desired.
B. Prep with povidine-iodine swabs.	
C. Observe for flashback of blood; open tubing clamp.	
D. Prepare venipuncture site. (1) Secure needle to skin with tape. (2) Apply povidone-iodine ointment; cover with sterile gauze dressing.	(2) Povidone-iodine ointment provides a seal around needle at entry site and controls for infection.
3. Position bag low enough to allow gravity collection.	3. Bag may be upside down to aid mixing with anticoagulant solution.
4. Rotate the collection bag gently and at frequent intervals.	4. Rotation facilitates mixing of blood with the anticoagulant solution.
5. Assess patient continuously; closely monitor cardiopulmonary status during therapy.	5. Patients are high risks for altered hemodynamics.
6. Close tubing clamp when the prescribed amount of blood has been collected; remove needle from patient, preserving sterility of system.	
7. Apply a sterile gauze pressure dressing to venipuncture site.	
8. Rotate gently and invert collection bag post therapy.	8. Rotation facilitates mixing of blood with anticoagulant solution.
9. Send collection bag to blood bank immediately, when autotransfusion is anticipated.	9. Refrigeration and storage must be initiated promptly.

Precautions

1. Establish one IV route for potential emergency intervention prior to therapy.
2. Monitor patient's hemoglobin and hematocrit before and after therapy.
3. Do not remove more than 500 ml. blood at one time.

4. Bleed patient at a slower rate and provide a longer rest time after therapy when phlebotomy is prescribed electively.
5. Vacuum assist devices may increase risk of pulmonary emboli. If used, follow manufacturer's instructions.

Related Care

1. Monitor patient's vital signs, cardiac rhythm, and clinical symptoms prior to and during therapy, and every 15 minutes until stable following therapy.
2. Assess venipuncture site frequently for delayed hematoma formation.

Complications

Hypovolemia	Nausea, vomiting
Syncope	Hematoma
Convulsions	Vascular trauma
Cardiac or respiratory arrest	Infection

Suppliers

Cutter
McGaw
Travenol Laboratories (Fenwall Blood Pak)

REFERENCES

American Association of Blood Banks: Technical Methods and Procedures of the American Association of Blood Banks, 8th ed. Washington, D.C., American Association of Blood Banks, 1981.
Chwirut, D.J.: Danger of evacuated bottles for phlebotomy [letter]. N. Eng. J. Med., 306:302, 1982.
Metzer, Lawrence E. (ed.): Concepts and Practice of Intensive Care for Nurse Specialists. Bowie, Md., Charles Press Publishers, 1976, p. 132.

PERICARDIOCENTESIS
(ASSISTING WITH)

Karen L. Wheelock, R.N., B.S.N., M.A.

Overview

Pericardiocentesis is surgical aspiration into the pericardial space to relieve pressure on the heart or remove fluid for diagnostic testing or both. Fluid can be caused by pericardial effusion, myocardial perforation or rupture, and effusion from a tumor or chest trauma. In the life-threatening situation of cardiac tamponade, pericardiocentesis is performed as an emergency therapeutic intervention. Early assessment of altered hemodynamic parameters, facilitation of the emergency intervention, and follow-through monitoring of the patient for complications are vital contributions.

Objectives

1. To facilitate safe removal of fluid from the pericardial space by needle aspiration in such instances as pericarditis with effusion, post-trauma, acute rheumatic fever, other infections, tumors, or in the emergency intervention for cardiac tamponade.
2. To assess the patient's hemodynamic response to therapy.

Special Equipment

16- to 18-gauge short bevel
  needle
50-ml. syringe with three-way
  stopcock
Povidone-iodine prep solution
Local anesthetic
Sterile gloves
Ground wire
Sterile alligator clip or clamp for
  attachment of ECG lead to needle
ECG recorder
Defibrillator and resuscitation
  equipment

Procedure

ACTION	RATIONALE
1. Place patient in semirecumbent position, with head elevated approximately 30 to 60 degrees.	1. This position facilitates needle insertion.
2. Obtain baseline blood pressure.	
3. Attach limb leads of grounded ECG.	
4. Prepare resuscitation equipment and medications as appropriate.	4. Serious dysrhythmias can occur during the therapy
5. Attach lead V_5 of ECG to aspiration needle using sterile alligator clip or clamp (Fig. 1-89). Adequate threshold is in the 6 mV. range.	5. This enhances safe position since a sharp increase in QRS complex can be observed during needle penetration of the pericardial sac. Also, ST-segment elevation as needle advances suggests ventricular contact, and PR-segment elevation suggests atrial contact.

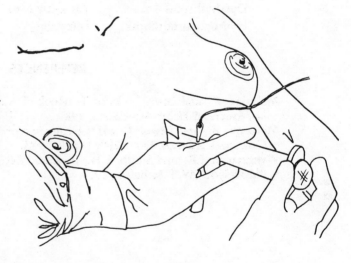

Figure 1-89. Pericardiocentesis using subxiphoid approach and Lead V_5 of ECG to aspiration needle. (From McIntyre, Kevin, and Lewis, James: Textbook of Advanced Cardiac Life Support. Dallas, American Heart Association, 1981.)

6. Prep skin site with povidone-iodine solution. The most common insertion site is subxiphoid, with the needle being inserted in the angle between the xiphoid and costal margin, directed toward the right shoulder.	
7. Monitor effect of therapy on patient during needle insertion and aspiration of fluid.	7. Aspiration fluid may be clear, cloudy, or bloody but should not clot.
8. Facilitate care and transport of specimen for appropriate laboratory analysis.	

Precautions

1. Observe presence of marked ST elevation, elevation of PR segment, or dysrhythmias, which indicate contact with epicardium or poor grounding.
2. Monitor blood pressure, pulse, and heart rhythm during entire procedure, and for 24 hours post-therapy.
3. Assess for signs and symptoms of cardiac tamponade.

Related Care

1. Facilitate obtaining written consent unless performed as an emergency intervention.
2. Assess skin integrity at site; provide site care post-therapy.

Complications

Cardiac tamponade	Laceration of coronary artery
Perforation of ventricle	Aspiration of blood from cardiac chambers
Cardiac arrest	
Dysrhythmias	Air embolism
Hydropneumothorax	Infection

REFERENCES

McIntyre, K., and Lewis, J., (eds): Textbook of Advanced Cardiac Life Support. Dallas, American Heart Association, 1981.
McIntyre, K., and Lewis, J. (eds.): Changing concepts of cardiac tamponade. Mod. Concepts Cardiovas. Dis: 52(4): (April), 1983.
Wyngaarden, J.B., and Smith, L.H., Jr. (eds.): Cecil Textbook of Medicine, 17th ed. Philadelphia, W.B. Saunders, 1984.

2

THE
PULMONARY
SYSTEM

AIRWAY MANAGEMENT

Jeannette McCann McHugh, R.N., M.S.N.

Overview

Situations can arise in which patients are unable to maintain a patent airway or adequate ventilation independently. In an acute situation, temporary measures may be taken until definitive airway management is possible. In certain cases, airway obstruction may be due to a flaccid tongue falling against the posterior pharyngeal wall. This may be relieved by hyperextension of the neck or forward displacement of the mandible or by the use of nasopharyngeal or oropharyngeal airways. Also used for rescue purposes is the esophageal obturator airway, which, when placed properly, blocks air flow into the stomach and allows ventilation through apertures located at the pharyngeal level.

When these measures are inadequate or when a respiratory crisis is not resolved quickly, the patient will most likely require endotracheal intubation. Endotracheal intubation may be performed on critically ill patients to facilitate bronchial hygiene, prevent aspiration, and provide mechanical ventilation or higher concentrations of oxygen, or both. Although intubation may be necessary for adequate respiratory care, the artificial airway interrupts the upper airway functions of humidification, filtration, and warming of inspired gases and also interferes with the cough and gag reflexes. Intubation also entails the potential hazard of tracheal injury. Once a patient is intubated, measures must be taken to compensate for the interrupted upper airway functions. Inspired gases must be humidified to prevent dryness of the respiratory mucous membrane, filtered to prevent deposition of foreign material in the lungs, and warmed to prevent loss of body heat.

Scrupulous attention to these details is essential, since the upper airway is the respiratory system's first line of defense against pathogenic organisms and sensitizing foreign particles. A breakdown in the respiratory mucous membrane, for example, may provide direct entry for pathogens into the cardiovascular network and thereby to the whole body. In addition, the intubated patient's inability to generate an effective cough necessitates the use of aseptic endotracheal suctioning to facilitate secretion removal. Additional techniques such as postural drainage, percussion, and vibration may be needed to move secretions from peripheral airways to a level within the tracheobronchial tree that is accessible to a suction catheter. (We cannot suggest that these techniques militate against evacuation of air from lung segments; so many factors promote suction-induced atelectasis.)

For the patient unable to maintain effective ventilation and oxygenation, a mechanical ventilator may be provided to assist or control repiratory rates, inspiratory/expiratory ratios, inspiratory volumes, and varying flow patterns.

Pressures of different levels and types above atmospheric pressure can be supplied to improve oxygen transport across the respiratory membrane.

For prolonged respiratory support, a tracheostomy is performed to improve access to the tracheobronchial tree and prevent upper airway trauma resulting from endotracheal tube pressure on the mouth, uvula, and larynx, as well as to alleviate patient discomfort and increased salivation. Indications for an emergency tracheostomy include severe facial or neck trauma and upper airway obstructions (e.g. tumors). When the respiratory crisis approaches resolution, consideration is given to termination of ventilatory support as well as eventual extubation. This weaning process may occur quickly or may be prolonged and requires additional innovative measures and devices that allow the patient to increase respiratory strength and decrease dependence on supportive measures. The prospect of a ventilator-dependent patient rightfully encourages the implementation of this process as early as possible.

Instrumentation

An emergency artificial airway is usually provided first by insertion of a plastic oropharyngeal device that generally conforms to the mouth from the lips to the base of the tongue. It is designed to hold the tongue of an unconscious patient forward, preventing obstruction of the posterior pharynx.

The esophageal obturator airway is a transparent device similar in appearance to an endotracheal tube. However, as a temporary airway it is quite different in several ways; the major differences are that the tube is inserted into the esophagus instead of the trachea, and its distal end is blocked. When it is inserted, an esophageal cuff is inflated, a mask is applied firmly to seal the nose and mouth, and air is forced into the trachea through tube perforations in the pharyngeal area. It is inserted blindly and can be placed quickly and easily. Those patients requiring further airway management will have an endotracheal tube inserted prior to removal of the esophageal obturator airway.

Both endotracheal and tracheostomy tubes are composed of polyvinyl chloride, silicone, or nylon, or combinations thereof, and disposable, although some silicone and nylon tubes can be steam- or gas-sterilized for reuse. These products are lightweight, soft, nontoxic, and have a longer shelf life than rubber. Standard size fittings (15 mm. male) provide easy connection to respiratory equipment. In addition, cuffs are bonded to the tube, resulting in less opportunity for cuffs to slip and herniate over the tip. Tubes should be selected with large volume (Fig. 2–1), low pressure cuffs that create a seal with less than 25 cm. H_2O (approximately 20 mm. Hg) pressure measured during expiration. Continuous in-line pressure gauges are available to assist in monitoring cuff pressures. Self-inflating foam cuffs are also available; these do not require monitoring, but it has been reported that they sometimes lose their elasticity within 48 hours.

The endotracheal tube is generally the airway of choice in an emergen-

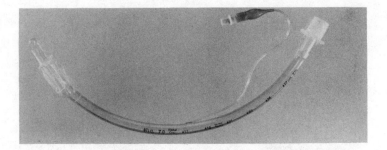

Figure 2-1. Endotracheal tube with large volume, low pressure cuff.

cy. The tube may be inserted via the oral or nasal route in about 1 to 5 minutes, while a tracheostomy takes approximately 15 minutes. Endotracheal tubes are radiopaque or have radiopaque markings to permit verification of tip position by x-ray. Although endotracheal tubes with large volume, low pressure cuffed tubes are preferred, red rubber low volume, high pressure cuffed tubes have been commonly used for short-term airway management during surgical procedures. However, the benefits of large diameter, thin-walled cuffed tubes and the known hazards of small volume cuffed tubes are obviating even this limited use. Methods are described in the literature for softening and stretching rigid cuffs to make them into high volume, low pressure cuffs. In addition, some endotracheal tubes are being developed that are more anatomically shaped to conform to the airway. In this way, pressure necrosis at the posterior subglottic area and tube tip site is thought to be minimized (Fig. 2–2).

When an artificial airway must remain in place for prolonged airway management, a tracheotomy is performed and a tracheostomy tube inserted.

Figure 2-2. The anatomically designed orotracheal tube (the Lindholm tube) conforms well to the structure of the airway. In the right upper corner a laryngotracheal specimen is shown with only minor injuries after three days of intubation. The specimen is incised along the anterior midline. Only some superficial abrasions and submucous bleeding are found bilaterally. (A) on the medial aspect of the arytenoid cartilage and (C) on the inner posterolateral aspect of the cricoid cartilage. (V) Vocal cord. (From Ledingham, I.McA.: Recent Advances in Intensive Therapy, No. 1. Edinburgh, Churchill Livingstone, 1977, p. 55. Reproduced by permission.)

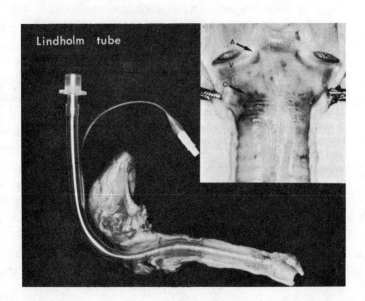

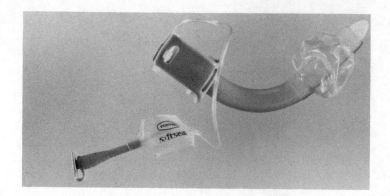

Figure 2-3. Single cannula tracheostomy tube.

Tracheostomy tubes are available in four styles: single-cannula, double-cannula, fenestrated, and "speaking" (Fig. 2–3). Double-cannula tubes are frequently used in the critical care unit for the patient requiring mechanical ventilation. The inner cannula is removable and allows cleaning of built-up secretions in the cannula. Fenestrated tubes, a type of double-cannula tube, have an opening above the cuff that permits air to flow through to the larynx. If mechanical ventilation is required, an inner cannula in some models occludes the fenestration. However, with the occluding inner cannula removed, the fenestration permits the patient to speak and, additionally, with the proximal end occluded, it is possible to evaluate the patient's ability to breathe spontaneously. Speaking tubes permit delivery of humidified air or oxygen through an accessory line to an outlet just above the cuff. The gas flows upward through the larynx, enabling the patient to speak.

Patients who are being weaned from tracheostomy tubes may be managed with the tracheostomy buttons that are used as interim airways. These devices consist of a cannula that extends from the skin surface into the trachea, a closure plug, and an adapter for intermittent positive pressure breathing or other respiratory treatments. When plugged, the button allows the patient to breathe and speak normally through the upper airways. The cannula, however, prevents stoma closure and facilitates tracheostomy tube insertion if needed.

Swivel connectors are available for lightweight, flexible connections to the ventilating system, providing improved patient comfort and positioning flexibility. They may be an integral part of the tracheostomy tube, or they may be added to either the tracheostomy or endotracheal tube. Two highly desirable features to look for in swivel adapters are (1) a suction port, to permit suctioning without disconnecting the mechanical ventilator; and (2) an effective antidisconnect method of securing the adapter to the ventilator tubing and add-on swivel adapter to the tracheostomy or endotracheal tubes.

Respiratory instrumentation continues to proliferate and become increasingly sophisticated. Careful, critical evaluation of these devices' positive and negative features regarding usefulness, efficiency, and safety must be undertaken; the devices will either hinder or improve airway management, depending upon how they are used.

ESOPHAGEAL OBTURATOR AIRWAY INSERTION

Objectives

1. To provide a route for rapid direct ventilation of the lungs.
2. To prevent insufflation of air into the patient's stomach, with consequent risk of vomiting and aspiration.

Special Equipment

Esophageal obturator airway (EOA) and attached mask
50-ml. syringe
Anesthesia bag/valve
Stethoscope

Procedure

ACTION	RATIONALE
1. Assess patient's respiratory and reflexic state.	1. The EOA is recommended for resuscitation of unconscious, areflexic, apneic, or near-apneic adults.
2. Administer mouth-to-mouth ventilations, or ventilate with bag/mask and supplemental oxygen. Ventilation is established while the EOA is obtained and prepared for use (mask attached, balloon fully deflated).	2. Mouth-to-mouth ventilation allows the rescuer to assess the patency of the upper airway.
3. Open the patient's mouth, using crossed-finger technique (Fig. 2–4).	

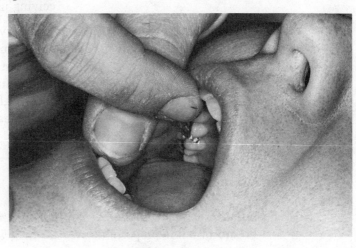

Figure 2-4. Crossed finger technique.

ACTION	RATIONALE
4. Grasp patient's tongue and mandible; pull jaw forward, flexing the patient's neck.	
5. Use other hand to hold EOA (connected to the mask); insert into patient's mouth at midline, and advance it along the natural curvature of the pharnyx.	
6. Apply steady, gentle pressure to advance tube until mask is securely seated on patient's face.	6. The balloon must be seated below the level of the tracheal bifurcation; positive pressure ventilation is not possible if the mask is not seated firmly upon the patient's face.
7. Hold mask firmly on patient's face and blow into tube or ventilate with bag/mask, checking tube position during ventilations. A. Observe chest excursion. B. Auscultate for breath sounds over the lateral lung fields.	7. If tracheal obturation has occurred the chest will not rise. The sound of air movement in the esophagus of improperly intubated patients may be transmitted to the anterior chest. Under these circumstances accurate assessment of breath sounds is more likely to be assured by auscultating the lateral chest at the midaxillary line
8. Inflate balloon with 30 ml. of air.	8. This seals off esophagus and directs inspiratory tidal volumes from pharynx into trachea and lungs. The balloon is *not* inflated before careful assessment of tube placement has been performed. Inflation and deflation of a malpositioned airway will consume time during which the patient is receiving no respiratory exchange.
9. Ventilate the patient with positive pressure and auscultate over the epigastrium.	9. This serves as a final determination of proper tube placement. If the trachea has been inadvertently intubated, the tidal volume will enter the esophagus and gurgling sounds will be heard over the stomach.

Precautions

1. Minimize risk of esophageal rupture by utilizing the EOA in patients who are of adult proportion (over 60 inches in height) and age (over 16

years). Avoid forcing the airway during insertion. If difficulties arise, discontinue the intubation and administer mouth-to-mouth ventilation.

2. Avoid the use of the EOA in conscious or semiconscious patients since the device may induce retching and vomiting.
3. Minimize esophageal trauma by avoiding the use of EOA's in patients with known or suspected esophageal disorders. This includes patients with esophageal varices or strictures and patients who have swallowed caustic substances.
4. Always deflate esophageal balloon before removing tube.
5. Reduce the risk of aspiration of vomitus during esophageal extubation by ensuring a protected trachea. This is usually achieved by tracheal intubation and cuff inflation prior to the removal of the EOA.
6. Minimize risk of esophageal rupture secondary to cardiopulmonary resuscitation over the high pressure esophageal balloon. Adhere strictly to American Heart Association standards for effective chest compressions and do not overdepress the sternum.

Related Care

1. Assess adequacy of ventilation frequently by auscultating both lung fields and observing for symmetric lung excursion continuously.
2. Insert nasogastric tube through aperture in esophageal airway and aspirate stomach contents prior to removal of airway.
3. Place the patient on his side, deflate the esophageal balloon, and remove the airway quickly when consciousness returns rapidly and gagging or retching begins.

Complications

Esophageal rupture/perforation
Tracheal intubation
Vomiting with aspiration during extubation
Gastric rupture

REFERENCES

American Heart Association: Textbook of Advanced Cardiac Life Support, 1981.
Crippin, D., Avey, S., and Graffis, R.: Gastric rupture: An esophageal obturator airway complication. Ann. Emerg. Med., 10:370, 1981.
Don Michael, T.A., and Gordon, A.S: The oesophageal obturator airway: A new device in emergency cardiopulmonary resuscitation. Br. Med. J., 281:1531, 1980.
Lindholm, C.E., and Grevnik, A.: Tracheal tube and cuff problems. Int. Anesthesiol. Clin. 20(3):103, 1982.
Long, J., and West, G.: The Olympic Trach-Button as an interim airway following tracheostomy tube removal. Respir. Care, 26:129, 1981.
Steve, J.F., and Brandstetter, R.D.: A new adult tracheostomy button in the management of a near drowning victim. Heart Lung, 11:299, 1982.
Perro, K.B., Goetze, C.M., and Monaghan, J.J.: Making every minute count with an esophageal gastric tube airway. Nursing 80, 10:61 (Aug.) 1980.

ENDOTRACHEAL INTUBATION

Overview

There are three routes by which an endotracheal tube may be placed.

Tracheotomy.   An endotracheal tube may be inserted through a tracheostomy when the upper airway is obstructed (e.g., tumor, severe facial trauma) or when the physical characteristics of the neck make nasal or oral placement impossible.

Nasotracheal Intubation.   A nasotracheal tube is often more comfortable for conscious patients than an oral tracheal tube. However, a nasotracheal tube is generally more time consuming to insert, and its diameter is limited by upper airway anatomy.

Oral Tracheal Intubation.   Oral tracheal intubation is generally preferred as the quickest and least traumatic means of emergency airway placement. This procedure will present the technique for oral endotracheal intubation.

Objective

To establish a patent airway by correct placement of an oral endotracheal tube.

Special Equipment

Anesthesia bag and oxygen source
Topical anesthesia: 4% lidocaine or 4% cocaine
Suction source
Sterile suction catheter
Sterile glove
Sterile normal saline solution
Laryngoscope with curved and straight blades
Low pressure cuffed endotracheal tube (usually 36 Fr. for adult males and
   32 to 34 Fr. for adult females; however, a range of sizes should be
   available)
Water-soluble anesthetic lubricating jelly
Malleable plastic or metal stylet
Magill forceps
Bite block or oral pharyngeal airway
Adhesive tape, alcohol swabs, tincture of benzoin
Swivel adapter

Procedure

ACTION	RATIONALE
1. Remove headboard from the bed.	1. This permits easy access to the head of the patient.
2. Check tube cuff, laryngoscope batteries, and bulbs.	2. This ensures properly functioning equipment.
3. Insert stylet into but not completely through selected tube.	A stylet protruding through an endotracheal tube may perforate or otherwise damage the tracheal mucosa.
A. Shape to desired curve for insertion.	
B. Lubricate tip of tube.	B. This decreases mucosal trauma and makes insertion of tube easier.
4. Prepare patient.	
A. Place patient's head on 2 to 4 inches of firm padding. (Fig. 2–5).	A. This is the "sniffing position" in which the axes of the oral cavity, pharynx, and trachea are approximately aligned.

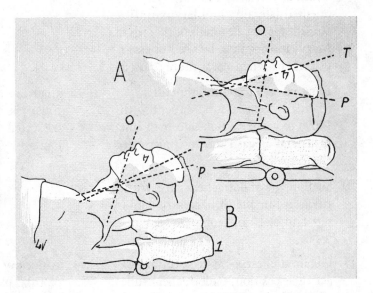

Figure 2-5. Position of the head for laryngoscopy and intubation of trachea. *A,* Ordinary position; *T,* axis of the trachea; *P,* axis of the pharynx; *O,* axis of the oral cavity. *B,* Modified position achieved with extra head rest. Flexion of cervical spine and extension at the atlanto-occipital joint bring the three axes more nearly into line. (From Dripps, R.D., Eckenhoff, J.E., and Vandam, L.D.: Introduction to Anesthesia, 6th ed. Philadelphia, W.B. Saunders, 1982, p. 186.)

B. Remove patient's dentures or partial plates and suction debris and secretions from mouth and airway, if necessary.	B. This prevents damage to dental prostheses and maintains a patent, visible insertion pathway.
C. Hyperventilate the patient with 100% oxygen.	C. This minimizes hemoglobin desaturation and hypoxia during the insertion process.

ACTION	RATIONALE
5. Open patient's jaw widely, using crossed-finger technique with right hand (see Fig. 2–4); spray pharynx with topical anesthetic.	5. This decreases gagging and discomfort.
6. Hold laryngoscope in left hand and introduce blade along right side of mouth. Advance blade and move centrally to displace tongue to left. A. Epiglottis is seen at base of tongue. B. Insert a straight blade beyond the epiglottis; a curved blade is positioned with its tip anterior to epiglottis.	B. Inserting blade too deeply causes entire larynx to be elevated, exposing the esophagus.
7. Hold wrist rigid; lift laryngoscope forward and upward at a 45-degree angle. At no time is leverage against the teeth used to effect exposure.	7. This elevates the mandible and exposes the larynx. Leverage on teeth may cause tooth loss or damage and possible airway obstruction.
8. Insert endotracheal tube (Fig. 2–6) with cuff deflated and concavity oriented laterally, into larynx until cuff disappears beyond vocal cords. Magill forceps may be used to assist placement when nasal route is used.	
9. Remove stylet and inflate cuff. Manually ventilate the patient with 100% oxygen. Auscultate both lung fields and epigastrium to confirm tracheal intubation.	9. Inadvertent esophageal intubation must be immediately detected and corrected to prevent hypoxic brain damage.
10. Suction the endotracheal tube with sterile technique, if necessary, and insert bite block or oropharyngeal airway.	
11. Obtain a chest x-ray to ascertain exact tube position; endotracheal tube tip should be at least 3 cm. above carina.	11. An x-ray provides visual observation of tube placement so that, if the tube has been inserted into the right main stem bronchus, it can be pulled back to proper position.

Text continued on page 218.

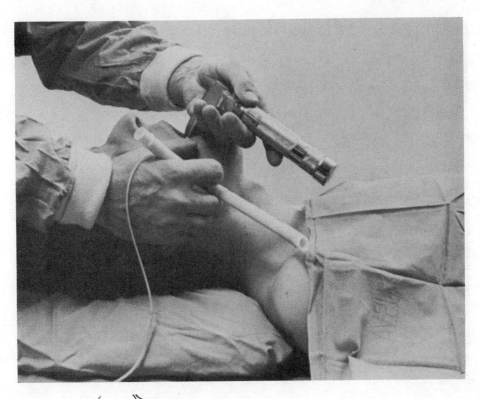

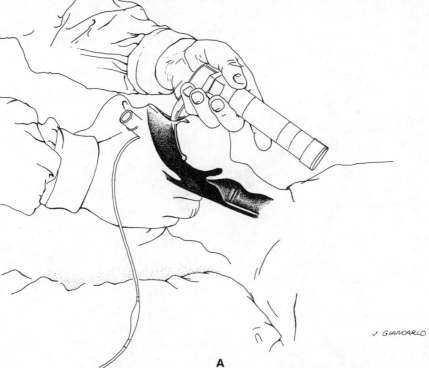

A

Figure 2-6.   Technique of orotracheal intubation. *A,* Laryngoscope blade is inserted into oral cavity from the right, pushing tongue to the left as it is introduced.

Figure 2-6 continues on following page.

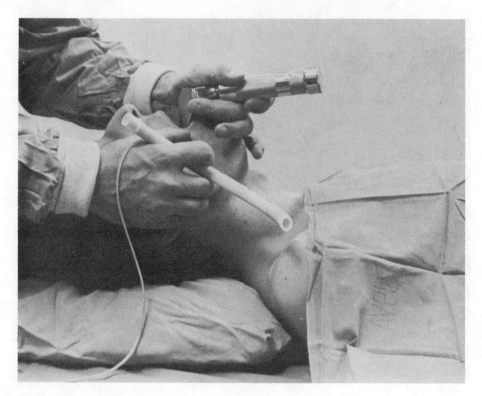

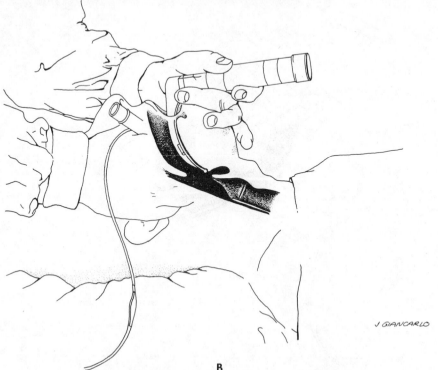

B

Figure 2-6. *Continued   B,* Blade is advanced into oropharynx and laryngoscope is lifted to expose the epiglottis.

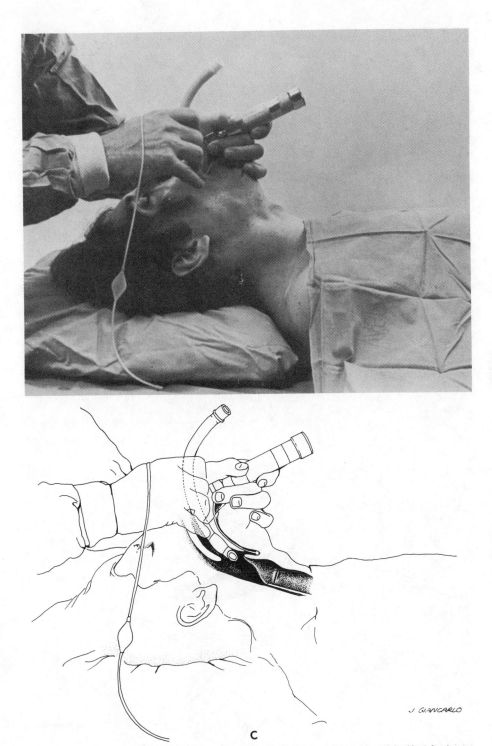

C

Figure 2-6. *Continued C,* Tip of blade is placed in vallecula, and laryngoscope is lifted further to expose glottis. The tube is inserted through the right side of the mouth.

Figure 2-6 continues on following pages.

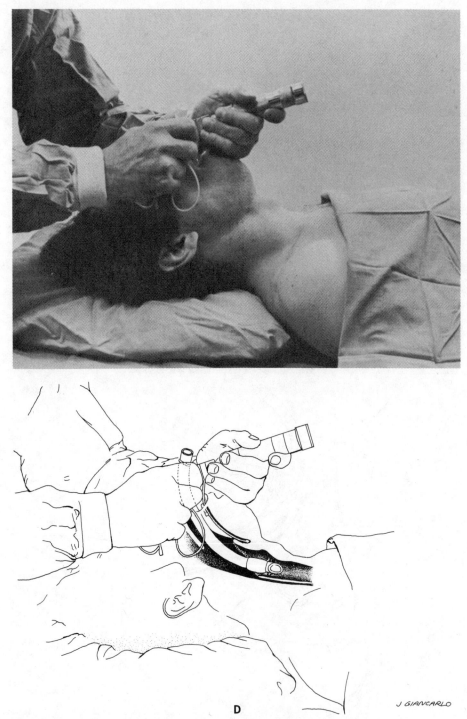

J GIANCARLO

D

Figure 2-6. *Continued*   *D,* Tube is advanced through vocal cords into trachea.

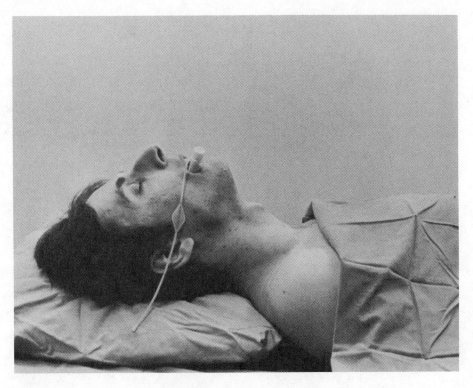

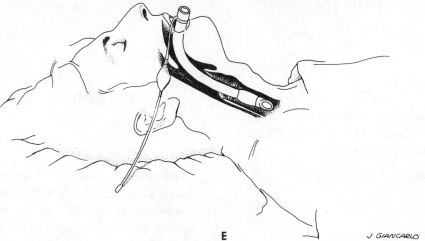

E   J GIANCARLO

Figure 2-6. *Continued*   *E,* Tube is positioned so that cuff is below vocal cords, and laryngoscope is removed.

Figure 2-6 continues on following page.

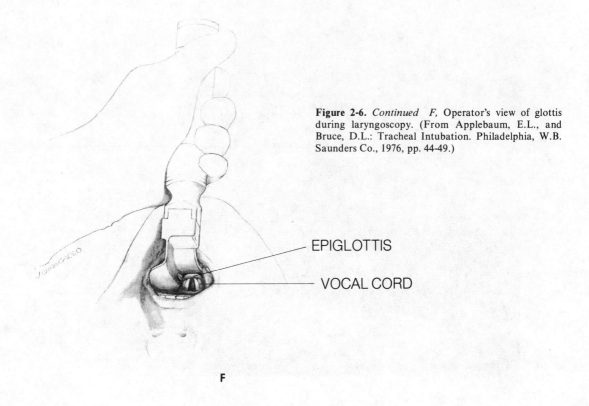

Figure 2-6. *Continued F,* Operator's view of glottis during laryngoscopy. (From Applebaum, E.L., and Bruce, D.L.: Tracheal Intubation. Philadelphia, W.B. Saunders Co., 1976, pp. 44-49.)

EPIGLOTTIS

VOCAL CORD

F

ACTION	RATIONALE
12. Cleanse patient's cheeks with alcohol, apply benzoin, and tape tube securely (see "Securing Airways").	
13. Mark tube at level of mouth.	13. This mark is checked at intervals to make sure that the tube has not been inadvertently pulled out or inserted deeper into the trachea.
14. Connect patient to humidified oxygen source or mechanical ventilator, using swivel adapter.	14. The swivel adapter reduces motion of the tube in the patient's mouth and trachea.
15. Recheck cuff volume to ascertain that minimum amount of air necessary to protect airway and permit ventilation is used.	15. Minimal occlusive volume for cuff inflation or intracuff pressure less than 25 cm. of water is an essential measure for preventing tracheal necrosis (see "Prevention of Tracheal Injuries").

Precautions

1. Avoid traumatizing mouth, pharynx, larynx, and esophagus; bruises, lacerations, and abrasions may occur during an emergency intubation. Trauma to lips may be avoided by spreading them away from laryngoscope blade and teeth; damage to teeth that are in poor repair may be unavoidable.
2. When the patient cannot be intubated within a reasonable period, prevent hypoxia by discontinuing the procedure and ventilating with 100% oxygen.
3. Observe for indications of esophageal intubation; these include abdominal distention and eructations with manual ventilation and absence of breath sounds across the lung fields. In such cases the tube must be removed and the patient reintubated.
4. Obtain information regarding possible cervical neck injury; extreme care must be taken in this case to prevent transection of the spinal cord.

Related Care

1. Insert a nasogastric tube to avoid gastric distention and aspiration. It may be connected to intermittent gastric suction, in the event of paralytic ileus, or it may be used for feedings or antacid administration or both.
2. Monitor patients undergoing intubation whenever possible. A wide variety of ectopy and conduction disturbances have been observed during intubation and have been ascribed to hypoxia and vasovagal reflexes. Careful preoxygenation and quick atraumatic intubation will minimize cardiovascular sequelae.

Complications

Bruises, lacerations, and abrasions
Tooth loss or damage
Hypoxemia
Cardiac dysrhythmias
Vomiting with aspiration
Laryngeal trauma
Intubation of right main stem bronchus
Tracheal rupture
Tracheoesophageal fistula

REFERENCES

Applebaum, E.L., and Bruce, D.L.: Tracheal Intubation. Philadelphia, W.B. Saunders, 1976, pp. 38–51.
Dripps, R.D., Eckenhoff, J.E., and Vandam, L.D.: Introduction to Anesthesia, 6th ed. Philadelphia, W.B. Saunders, 1982, pp. 180–195.

Orringer, M.B.: Endotracheal intubation and tracheostomy. Indications, techniques, and complications. Surg. Clin. North Am. *60*:1447, 1980.

Snow, J.C.: Manual of Anesthesia. Boston, Little, Brown, 1977.

ENDOTRACHEAL SUCTIONING _____

Overview

Endotracheal intubation is often necessary to maintain airway patency. Ironically, however, introduction of an endotracheal tube makes effective coughing difficult and reduces the patient's ability to raise tracheobronchial secretions. Under these circumstances, removal of accumulated secretions must be accomplished by endotracheal suctioning.

In addition, some disease states, pain, and surgical procedures will make effective coughing difficult and reduce the ability to raise tracheobronchial secretions. Endotracheal intubation may not be desirable, or the patient may have been recently extubated. In such cases removal of accumulated secretions may be accomplished by blind endotracheal suctioning.

Objectives

1. To remove tracheobronchial secretions, using sterile technique.
2. To mobilize tenacious secretions for removal, using sterile suctioning technique.

Special Equipment

Sterile gloves
Sterile catheter with intermittent suction control port
Sterile normal saline solution
Suction source
Anesthesia bag connected to 100% oxygen

Procedure

ACTION	RATIONALE
1. Assess patient's need for endotracheal suctioning; indications include: A. Coarse adventitious sounds. B. Coughing. C. Increasing inspiratory pressures for patients receiving mechanical ventilation.	1. Since endotracheal suctioning can be hazardous and cause discomfort, it is not recommended in the absence of apparent need.

ACTION	RATIONALE

2. Pour saline solution into sterile cup.

3. Open catheter packaging, maintaining catheter sterility. A 14 Fr. catheter is commonly used in adult patients; however, catheter should not exceed one-third the inner diameter of the airway.

3. Catheters exceeding one-third the airway diameter increase the possiblity of suction-induced hypoxia and atelectasis.

4. Preoxygenate patients with 100% oxygen.
   A. Use anesthesia bag, or
   B. Change oxygen setting on mechanical ventilator to 100%. Remember that ventilators cycle for variable times before oxygen delivery reaches 100%.

4. Preoxygenation may help minimize suction-induced hypoxia.

5. Glove and maintain sterility of dominant hand. Glove and maintain clean technique of nondominant hand.

5. This decreases the incidence of contamination and infection for the patient and the clinician and the possible transmission of microorganisms to others.

6. Using nondominant hand, remove ventilator or open suctioning port on swivel adapter. Ventilator tubing end may be:
   A. Placed on a sterile drape.
   B. Slipped inside a nonpowdered sterile glove.
   C. Held by a colleague. If contamination occurs, attachments should be replaced with sterile ones.

6. This prevents contamination of the ventilator tubing.

7. Using sterile gloved dominant hand, pick up catheter and connect to suction source; thumb of opposite "clean" gloved hand controls suction port.

8. Dampen catheter in sterile saline solution to lubricate.

8. Surgical lubricant is usually unnecessary and may accumulate on inner surface of the endotracheal tube.

9. Using sterile gloved hand, insert catheter fully into endotracheal tube. Do not force if an obstruction is encountered.

ACTION	RATIONALE
10. Apply intermittent suction by quickly opening and closing suction port; withdraw catheter, using a rotating motion. Entire suctioning pass should not exceed 10 seconds in duration.	10. Intermittent suction minimizes tissue damage from invagination of tracheal mucosa into the catheter tip; the rotating motion sweeps the catheter tip against all sides of the airway wall as the catheter is withdrawn.
11. Hyperinflate patient's lungs with 100% oxygen.	11. This re-expands sections of the lungs that may have been evacuated of air and collapsed and minimizes hypoxemia due to suction-induced atelectasis.
12. Reconnect patient to ventilator or close the suction port of the swivel adapter.	
13. Assess effectiveness of suctioning pass. If adventitious sounds, ventilatory difficulty, or patient discomfort persist, repeat steps 7 through 12.	
14. If secretions are tenacious, introduce no more than 5 ml. of sterile saline solution into airway and follow with several ventilatory cycles.	14. Introduction of saline may help mobilize secretions and aid in their removal.

Precautions

1. Immediately prior to suctioning, preoxygenate patients with 100% oxygen to minimize suction-induced hypoxia by raising PaO_2.
2. When suctioning has been successfully completed, return FIO_2 to prescribed settings.
3. Minimize suction-induced atelectasis and hypoxemia.
   A. Avoid the use of catheters larger than one-third the diameter of the airway.
   B. Administer one or more postsuctioning hyperinflations, using either an anesthesia bag or the manual "sigh" of a mechanical ventilator.
4. Maintain rigorous sterile technique when suctioning the intubated patient. Impaired pulmonary defense systems and invasive instrumentation of the pulmonary tract predispose these patients to colonization and infection. Never use the same catheter to suction the nose or mouth and then the trachea.
5. Limit the frequency of suctioning and avoid, as much as possible, catheter impaction in the bronchial tree when the patient is anticoagulated or when hemorrhage from suction-induced trauma is evident.
6. Minimize the frequency and duration of suctioning when the patient is on positive end-expiratory pressure or continuous positive airway pres-

sure. Small suctioning-induced changes may have profound effects on these marginally oxygenated patients.

7. Maintain awareness of the limitations of endotracheal suctioning. Maneuvers and catheter design have been proposed to increase the likelihood of passage into the left bronchus; however, thses have been shown to be of limited success. because the left main stem bronchus emerges from the trachea at a 45-degree angle from the vertical, suction catheters are almost inevitably passed into the right bronchus.

8. Remove cap or needle from syringe when introducing saline into airway. These may be propelled into the endotracheal tube and become aspirated foreign bodies.

Related Care

1. Include strategies to move secretions through peripheral airways. These measures are appropriate hydration, adequate humidification of inspired gases, coughing and deep breathing, frequent position changes, chest physiotherapy, and bronchodilating agents.

2. Monitor the patient carefully during endotracheal suctioning for ectopic dysrhythmias aggravated by suction-induced hypoxemia and other dysrhythmias, particularly conduction disturbances, related to catheter irritation of vagal receptors within the respiratory tract.

Complications

Hypoxemia
Atelectasis
Dysrhythmias
Nosocomial pulmonary tract infection
Mucosal trauma with increased secretions

REFERENCES

Imle, P.C., and Klemic, N.: Methods of airway clearance: Coughing and suctioning. In MacKenzie, C.F. (ed.): Chest Physiotherapy in the Intensive Care Unit. Baltimore, Williams & Wilkins, 1981, pp. 91–107.

Massachusetts General Hospital, Department of Nursing: Massachusetts General Hospital Manual of Nursing Procedures, 2nd ed. Boston, Little, Brown, 1980, pp. 266–268.

Morrison, M.L. (ed.): Respiratory Intensive Care Nursing, 2nd ed. Boston, Little, Brown, 1979, pp. 31–??.

BLIND ENDOTRACHEAL SUCTIONING _____

Objectives

1. To remove accumulated tracheobronchial secretions, using sterile technique.
2. To mobilize pulmonary secretions by stimulation of cough reflexes.

Special Equipment

Sterile glove
Sterile catheter (14 to 16 Fr. for adult patients), with
    intermittent suctioning control port
Sterile normal saline solution
Suction source
Oxygen source and mask capable of delivering high concentrations of
    oxygen
Sterile water-soluble lubricant
Sterile gauze pad
Soft rubber nasopharyngeal airway
Tissues

Procedure

ACTION	RATIONALE
1. Assess patient's need for blind endotracheal suctioning.	1. The patient will not need suctioning if evidence of accumulating secretions is not present, or if the patient can be educated and encouraged to cough and deep breathe effectively.
2. Prepare patient. A. Raise head of patient's bed to high or semi-Fowler's position, as tolerated. B. Insert lubricated soft rubber nasopharyngeal airway, if appropriate or requested by the patient. C. Preoxygenate patient with high concentration of oxygen for 5 minutes or more.	C. Arterial oxygen tensions are increased in anticipation of suction-induced decreases in PAO_2 and PaO_2.

ACTION	RATIONALE

3. Turn on suction source.

4. Open sterile saline.

5. Squeeze adequate quantity of lubricant onto sterile gauze pad.

6. Don sterile glove on dominant hand. Glove and maintain clean technique of nondominant hand.

                                               6. This decreases the incidence of contamination and infection for the patient and the clinician, and possible transmission of microorganisms to others.

7. Using sterile gloved dominant hand, pick up catheter and roll tip generously in lubricant.

8. Insert catheter into patient's nasal passage and advance into pharynx, approximately 8 to 10 cm.

9. Ask patient to breathe slowly and deeply as catheter is advanced.
   A. Listen for airway sounds transmitted mitted through catheter.
   B. If absent, withdraw catheter into pharynx and repeat.

                                             B. The absence of airway sounds transmitted through the catheter suggests entry into the esophagus.

10. Continue to advance catheter as fully as possible into trachea, withdrawing 1 to 2 cm. if obstruction is met at level of carina.

11. Attach catheter to suction source; apply intermittent suction with clean gloved hand while rotating and withdrawing catheter.

12. Hyperoxygenate patient as described in step 2-C, and encourage maximal deep breaths.

                                             12. These measures are employed to reverse suction-induced hypoxia and atelectasis.

13. Clear tubing by aspirating sterile saline solution through catheter.

14. Assess effectiveness of suctioning, repeating steps 8 through 11, if necessary.

15. Discard gloves and catheter and turn off suction.

16. Return patient to comfortable position.

Precautions

1. Preoxygenate for 5 minutes or more prior to suctioning in anticipation of suctioning-induced reductions in alveolar and arterial oxygen tensions.
2. Maintain scrupulous sterility during the suction process to minimize the risk of respiratory tract infection. Recognize that patients with excessive poorly mobilized secretions frequently have compromised pulmonary and systemic defenses against infection.
3. Recognize that oral and nasotracheal suctioning, even when performed with rigorous sterile technique, risks inoculation of lower airways with nose and mouth flora. Minimize spread of bacteria within the airways by limiting the frequency of blind endotracheal suctioning as much as possible.
4. Limit or avoid the use of blind endotracheal suctioning when there is a predisposition to or evidence of hemorrhage from suction-induced trauma. Conditions that predispose to hemorrhage include any bleeding disorder, esophageal varices, and treatment with anticoagulants.
5. Limit suctioning and catheter-induced trauma by using the nasopharyngeal airway, when appropriate, and avoiding the use of large suction catheters or high suction pressures.
6. Minimize suction-induced asystole or ectopy by scrupulous preoxygenation. Avoid the use of blind endotracheal suctioning in patients with increased vagal sensitivity, unstable conduction disturbances, or acute myocardial ischemia. Patients at any risk of suction-induced dysrhythmias should be monitored during suctioning.
7. Minimize the risk of catheter-induced gagging and consequent aspiration of vomitus by seating the patient upright prior to suctioning. Avoid suctioning patients within an hour of feeding, and never suction patients who complain of nausea.
8. Avoid hyperoxygenation of patients with lung disorders characterized by chronic hypercapnia. Strategies other than nasotracheal suctioning may need to be used in aiding these patients to mobilize secretions.
9. Limit the use of blind endotracheal suctioning to those circumstances in which patients are absolutely unable to mobilize secretions that impose an immediate hazard to airway patency. Never utilize blind endotracheal suctioning as a routine bronchial hygiene measure.

Related Care

1. Encourage postsuctioning deep breathing to reverse suctioning-induced atelectasis. If the patient cannot deep breathe voluntarily, administer several hyperinflations with an anesthesia bag and mask.
2. Pursue measures aimed at mobilizing peripheral airway secretions in any program of pulmonary hygiene. These measures include adequate hydration, humidification of inspired gases, chest physiotherapy, bronchodilators, frequent position changes and, if possible, ambulation.

Complications

Hypoxemia	Mucosal trauma with increased secretions
Atelectasis	Nosocomial pulmonary tract infections
Vomiting and aspiration	Hemorrhage
Dysrhythmias	

REFERENCE

Massachusetts General Hospital, Department of Nursing: Massachusetts General Hospital Manual of Nursing Procedures, 2nd ed. Boston, Little, Brown, 1980, pp. 266–268.

TRACHEOSTOMY CARE _____

Overview

Tracheostomy care is performed at least every 8 hours, or more frequently if needed, to keep the airway patent and free of sources of infection, as well as to make the tracheostomy more esthetically acceptable to the patient and visitors.

Objectives

1. To provide aseptic wound care and dressing of the tracheostomy and to keep the double-walled tracheostomy tube aseptically clean.
2. To maintain ventilation of the patient.

Special Equipment

Two sterile bowls	Sterile gloves
Sterile gauze pads	Tracheostomy ties
Cotton swabs	Tracheostomy dressing
Forceps	Anesthesia bag connected
Sterile water and sterile	to 100% O_2
hydrogen peroxide	Equipment for endotracheal
Tracheostomy care adapter for	suctioning
outer cannula	
Tracheostomy brush or sterile	
pipe cleaners	

Procedure

ACTION	RATIONALE
1. Assist patient to position of comfort that exposes tracheostomy and surrounding skin.	
2. Remove soiled dressing, using forceps.	
3. Pour hydrogen peroxide and water into separate sterile bowls.	
4. Dampen sterile cotton swabs in hydrogen peroxide and remove secretions from area, swabbing away from the tracheostomy toward the surrounding tissues.	4. This decreases odor and medium for bacterial growth. It moves contaminants from the "clean" wound area to the "less clean" surrounding tissues.
5. Dampen sterile gauze pads with saline, maintaining sterility, and place on skin for several minutes if secretions are encrusted. Repeat step 4.	5. This moistens and softens dry secretions.
6. Perform the following steps if patient has a double-walled tracheostomy tube: A. Remove inner cannula and immerse in hydrogen peroxide. B. Preoxygenate the patient and suction outer cannula, if necessary (see "Endotracheal Suctioning"). C. Using tracheostomy care adapter, reconnect ventilation or oxygen source to outer cannula. D. Don sterile gloves and, using tracheostomy brush or bent pipe cleaners, clean secretions from inside inner cannula. E. Rinse inner cannula in bowl of sterile water. F. Reinsert inner cannula into tracheostomy, making certain that locking mechanism is engaged, and reconnect ventilator or oxygen source.	

ACTION	RATIONALE
7. Change tracheostomy ties, if soiled; apply and secure clean ties *before* removing old ones. Ties should fit snugly against the skin but should be loose enough to allow two fingers to be slipped beneath them.	7. A tracheostomy tube that is untied, no matter how briefly, is in danger of being coughed or pulled out. Ties that are too tight will cause patient discomfort; ties that are too loose allow the cannula to slide too freely within the trachea and may cause mucosal damage.
8. Apply new tracheostomy dressing (Fig. 2–7). A. Fold a sterile gauze pad to form a triangle. B. Place under the flange of the tracheostomy tube with the "hypotenuse" against the tracheostomy. C. Fold and place another gauze pad similarly under the opposite flange so that pads cross in front of the tracheostomy. D. Prepackaged tracheostomy care kits are available that contain fenestrated gauze pads for use as dressings.	8. Gauze pads should not be trimmed or cut for use as tracheostomy dressings, since cotton filling or fibers could be aspirated into the airway or embedded in the surgical wound. In addition, tracheostomy dressings should be sterile and should not be prepared with contaminated instruments (scissors). Such a practice would provide contaminating microorganisms direct access to a surgical wound and the sterile lower respiratory tract.

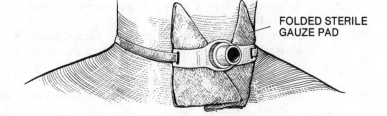

FOLDED STERILE GAUZE PAD

Figure 2-7. Triangular tracheostomy dressing.

Precautions

1. Observe for tracheal obstruction caused by accumulated secretions or cuff inflation.
   A. In such a case, a catheter is passed into the tracheostomy to ascertain the nature of the obstruction, and the cuff is deflated.
   B. If the obstruction is not relieved, the tracheostomy tube is removed, the stoma covered, and the patient ventilated with a bag/mask and supplemental oxygen until a new tracheostomy tube is inserted.
2. Prevent accidental decannulation by tying the tube securely in place and providing adequate slack in ventilator or oxygen connections. Restrain or sedate disoriented and agitated patients who are at risk of removing airways.
3. See also "Prevention of Tracheal Injuries."

4. Suction the oropharynx before deflating a cuff to prevent accumulated oral secretions from draining into the tracheobronchial tree.
5. Prevent obstruction secondary to accumulated secretions by providing adequate humidification of inspired gases, appropriate patient hydration, proper endotracheal suctioning, and chest physiotherapy.

Related Care

1. Obtain cultures of the wound site and sputum daily.
2. Change nebulizers and tubing connected to the tracheostomy tube daily, since they are potential sources of infection.
3. Use a large volume, low pressure cuff when using cuffed tracheostomy tubes to reduce tracheal complications.

Complications

Tracheal obstruction   Tracheobronchial tree infection
Accidental decannulation   Stomal stenosis
Tracheal mucosal damage   Tracheal stricture
Wound infection   Tracheoesophageal fistula

REFERENCES

Brown, I.: Trach care? Take care—infection is on the prowl. Nursing 82, 12:44(May), 1982.
Fuchs, P.L.: Providing tracheostomy care. Nursing 83, 13:139(April), 1983.
Massachusetts General Hospital, Department of Nursing: Massachusetts General Hospital Manual of Nursing Procedures, 2nd ed. Boston, Little, Brown, 1980, pp. 276–278.
Morrison, M.L. (ed.): Respiratory Intensive Care Nursing, 2nd ed. Boston, Little, Brown, 1979, pp. 100–104.

PREVENTION OF TRACHEAL INJURIES

Overview

Endotracheal intubation is often a necessary support for critically ill patients. However, cannulation of the trachea has been observed to cause a range of injuries, including tracheomalacia, tracheoesophageal fistula, tracheoinnominate artery fistula, and ulceration and scarring of the vocal cords.

Tissue changes, including necrosis of the posterior portions of the larynx, are common among patients treated with nasal and oral tracheal tubes. Although damage to larynx and vocal cords may be avoided by tracheostomy, the most common site of injury for all intubated patients is at the site of the endotracheal or tracheostomy tube cuff. For this reason, tracheal tube cuffs are inflated only when necessary to protect the airway from aspiration or to provide positive pressure ventilatory support. Various nursing measures may be undertaken to minimize these tracheal injuries.

Objectives

1. To minimize traction or torsion on the patient's endotracheal tube.
2. To inflate a tube cuff, permitting tracheal wall capillary perfusion.

Special Equipment

    10-ml. syringe
    Swivel adapter
    Intracuff pressure measuring gauge

Procedure

ACTION	RATIONALE
1. Suspend ventilator tubing above level of patient by adjustable support arms attached to ventilator. Tubing should be long enough to permit patient to turn from side to side.	1. Tubing that is too short or draped on bed or side rail will put traction on the patient's endotracheal/tracheostomy tube.
2. Connect relatively rigid ventilator tubing to patient's endotracheal/ tracheostomy tube with a fully flexible adapter (one type is the Morsh swivel adapter).	2. This allows freer movement of the patient's head, neck, and torso and prevents undue torsion on the endotracheal/tracheostomy tube.
3. Keep patient comfortable and at ease. Sedate or restrain confused or agitated patients, as appropriate, when a safe airway cannot otherwise be assured.	3. An agitated patient may dislodge or pull out a tracheal tube; thrashing and struggling may cause permanent vocal cord injury in patients with oral or nasal tracheal tubes.

ACTION	RATIONALE

4. Select technique for cuff inflation.

A. Inflate tube cuffs with minimal occlusive volume of air.

(1) Determine minimal occlusive volume while patient receives positive pressure ventilation. An anesthesia bag may be used for patients who do not require mechanical ventilation.

(2) Auscultate neck for inspiratory air leaks while air is injected slowly into inflation port of cuff.

(3) Continue to fill cuff with air until inspiratory air leak is obliterated.

(4) Withdraw a small amount of air until a slight leak is noted at peak inspiratory pressures.

A. Tracheal injury at the cuff site is due to distortion of tracheal anatomy and occlusion of tracheal capillaries. Necrosis is especially common with the use of low volume, high pressure cuffs. High volume, low pressure cuff designs conform more closely to tracheal contours and can achieve an airway seal at pressures that do not occlude mucosal blood flow. Overinflation of any cuff, however, can cause tracheal ischemia, distortion, and consequent injury.

B. Inflate a high volume, low pressure tube cuff with a minimal pressure between 15 and 25 cm. H_2O.

(1) Determine minimal occlusive volume as in step 4-A.

(2) Attach cuff pressure measuring gauge to cuff inflation tube.

(3) Auscultate neck for inspiratory air leaks while air is injected slowly into inflation port.

(5) Continue to fill cuff with air slowly until inspiratory air leak is obliterated.

B. Cuff pressure readings on small volume, high pressure cuffs have little or no relationship to cuff force applied to the tracheal wall. Greater-than-capillary pressure and consequent tracheal ischemia must be assumed whenever such an instrument is in use. Readings of less than 15 cm. H_2O pressure, measured on a high volume, low pressure cuff, indicates a risk of aspiration around the cuff. Pressure greater than 25 cm. H_2O increases risk of complications associated with diminished blood flow to tracheal wall capillaries; 27 cm. H_2O pressure is the approximate tracheal mucosal capillary blood pressure. When cuff pressure is maintained below this, capillary perfusion occurs.

ACTION	RATIONALE
(6) Leave cuff pressure measuring gauge connected to cuff. Pressure should be less than 25 cm. H_2O during the expiratory phase.	(6) This permits continuous in-line pressure monitoring.

Precautions

1. Suspect tracheomalacia at the cuff site when increasing amounts of injected air are required to achieve the minimal occlusive volume or maintain a given pressure.
2. Observe for stridor or respiratory distress following extubation; have emergency reintubation supplies immediately available.
3. Suction accumulated upper airway secretions from above the cuff before deflating and reinflating the cuff to prevent aspiration and possible infection.

Related Care

Deflate and inflate large volume, low pressure cuffs only when required to maintain the minimal occlusive volume or maintain the given low pressure. Routine periodic cuff deflations have been demonstrated to be of little or no value in preventing tracheal ischemia.

Complications

Tracheomalacia
Laryngeal edema
Tracheoesophageal fistula
Infection

REFERENCES

Massachusetts General Hospital, Department of Nursing: Massachusetts General Hospital Manual of Nursing Procedures, 2nd ed. Boston, Little, Brown, 1980, pp. 274–275.

Morrison, M.L. (ed.): Respiratory Intensive Care Nursing, 2nd ed. Boston, Little, Brown, 1979, pp. 87–111.

Powaser, M.M., et al.: The effectiveness of hourly cuff deflation in minimizing tracheal damage. Heart Lung, 5:734, 1976.

SECURING AIRWAYS _____

Objectives

1. To prevent inadvertent removal of the airway.
2. To minimize tracheal erosion by limiting sliding movements of the airway.

Special Equipment

Tracheostomy tube:
    Twill tape, single strand, 30 to 34 inches in length
    Hemostats or tweezers
    Scissors
Endotracheal tube:
    Twill tape, 30 to 34 inches
    Adhesive tape, ½-inch wide, 4 to 6 inches long
    Scissors

Procedure

ACTION	RATIONALE
TRACHEOSTOMY TUBE	
1. Obtain single length of twill tape prior to beginning tracheostomy care.	1. Mucus-encrusted tracheostomy ties should be changed as a part of routine tracheostomy care. Prepackaged kits may not include adequate lengths of twill tape.
2. Complete tracheostomy care regimen without removing old ties.	2. Untied tracheostomy cannulas are always at risk of being removed by sudden patient movements, even when handled by a second person.
3. Slip end of the clean twill tape under tracheostomy flange, and use hemostats or tweezers to pull tape through tie slot (Fig. 2-8, A).	
4. Thread this end of tape behind and around patient's neck (Fig. 2-8, B).	
5. Slip this same end of twill tape under second flange and, using hemostat or tweezers, through tie slots.	

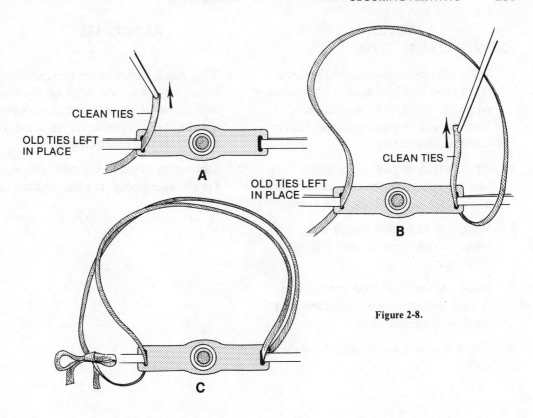

Figure 2-8.

ACTION	RATIONALE
6. Bring opposite end of clean twill tape behind and around patient's neck, but do not bring through tie slot (Fig. 2-8, C).	
7. Pull gently on two ends of twill tape until tie fits snugly around neck and tracheostomy flanges are flat against skin.	
8. Tie a firm knot at side of patient's neck.	8. The knot is less likely to become mucus-encrusted when tied some distance from the tracheostomy. The knot should not be over a cervical prominence where it can cause discomfort.
9. Carefully distinguish between old and new ties; snip and remove old ties.	
10. Recheck tracheostomy for snugness. Tape should allow one finger easily underneath against skin.	10. Loose-fitting ties may initially be obscured by close-fitting, soiled ties. Ties should be tight enough to prevent tracheostomy tube slippage but loose enough to prevent neck irritation and erosion.

ACTION	RATIONALE

ENDOTRACHEAL TUBE

1. With old ties removed, hold endotracheal tube and find mark that indicated proper point of tube emergence from mouth or nares (see also "Endotracheal Intubation").

2. Tie a length of twill tape tightly around tube, immediately below mark of emergence, and knot tape firmly.

3. Wrap a 4- to 6-inch length of adhesive tape around tube and over twill tape.

4. Bring ends of twill tape around and behind patient's neck; pull tape gently until snug against skin.

5. Tie in secure knot at side of patient's neck.

1. This mark indicates proper position of tube end below the level of the cords and above the tracheal bifurcation; if not marked, recheck the position and mark point of emergence.

2. Obscuring mark with tape will make future assessment of tube position difficult.

Precautions

1. Do not remove old ties in the tracheostomy tube prior to replacing with clean ones.
2. Use care not to extubate the patient inadvertently when replacing endotracheal tube ties.

Related Care

1. Ensure snug fit of airway ties. Ties should be close fitting and allow minimal in and out movements of endotracheal or tracheostomy tubes. They should be loose enough to allow two fingers to be slipped between the ties and the patient's neck.
2. Limit the movement of the tracheostomy and endotracheal tubes during tie changes. This minimizes stimulation of tracheolaryngeal reflexes and consequent patient discomfort.
3. Avoid buccal and lip membrane necrosis and erosion from oral tracheal tubes. Move tubes to the opposite side of the oral cavity at regular intervals.

Complication

Extubation

EXTUBATION

Objectives

1. To remove oral or nasotracheal tubes safely and atraumatically.
2. To observe for and minimize the hazards of laryngeal tissue reaction following extubation.

Special Equipment

Materials for endotracheal suctioning (see p. 220)
Anesthesia bag with universal adapter
Syringe
T tube
Face Mask
Humidifier (usually heated)
Supplemental oxygen source
Materials for endotracheal intubation (see p. 210)

Procedure

ACTION	RATIONALE

1. Assess patient's readiness for extubation. The patient should:
A. Be completely weaned from mechanical ventilation.
B. Be conscious and possess competent pharyngeal reflexes.
C. Be capable of generating an effective cough.
D. Have regained muscular control (e.g., be able to lift head and have adequate hand grasp).
E. Have acceptable respiratory parameters:
  (1) Minute volume (90 ml./kg.).
  (2) Inspiratory force (20 to 25 cm. H_2O).
  (3) Forced vital capacity (15 ml./kg.).
F. Have no serious cardiac dysrhythmias.
G. Have a stable pulse and blood pressure.	

ACTION	RATIONALE
2. Preoxygenate patient with 100% oxygen.	
3. Raise the head of the bed to semi-Fowler's or high-Fowler's position.	3. This position facilitates the patient's cough and minimizes the risk of vomiting and consequent aspiration.
4. Suction the endotracheal tube (see "Endotrachael Suctioning").	
5. Suction above endotracheal tube cuff and suction patient's mouth.	5. This removes pooled secretions above the cuff that may be aspirated into the lower airway when the cuff is deflated.
6. Change suction catheters.	6. Any further suctioning of the airway must be done with a sterile catheter.
7. Attach anesthesia bag to endotracheal tube and administer a maximal inflation with anesthesia bag as cuff is deflated.	7. This forces accumulated secretions away from lower airways as the cuff is deflated.
8. Attach patient to **T** tube and allow several breaths with cuff deflated.	8. The patient may need time to cough and stabilize respiratory pattern before proceeding.
9. Suction endotracheal tube, if necessary.	
10. Remove suction catheter from endotracheal tube and reoxygenate patient with 100% oxygen via **T** tube.	10. Catheter contact with vocal cords during extubation may precipitate trauma, spasm, or hemorrhage.
11. Ask patient to inspire maximally or inflate lungs maximally with anesthesia bag, and remove endotracheal tube at point of maximal inspiration.	11. This allows easier and less traumatic tube removal with expiration.
12. Suction pharynx, as necessary, and elevate head of bed if blood pressure is stable.	
13. Administer prescribed mixture of humidified oxygen via face mask.	13. Humidified inspired gases will aid in minimizing laryngeal edema.
14. Observe closely for increasing hoarseness or respiratory stridor.	14. Laryngeal edema or spasm may necessitate reintubation.

Precautions

1. Anticipate the presence of pooled oral secretions above the endotracheal tube cuff. Although suctioning above the cuff prior to extubation may be of some value, the removal of all secretions cannot be assured. Promote drainage of pooled secretions away from lower airways by placing patient in head-down position prior to cuff deflation and administering a postive pressure breath with the anesthesia bag simultaneously with deflation.
2. Observe for signs of respiratory stridor, gasping for air, increasing hoarseness or increased swallowing that may indicate development of laryngospasm or edema. Minimize laryngeal tissue reaction by providing warm humidification via face mask following extubation. Keep an endotracheal intubation tray at bedside in the event that laryngeal tissues begin to compromise airway patency.

Related Care

1. Provide constant calm reassurance and support to extubated patients. They may experience air hunger, thus heightening their anxiety level.
2. Encourage slow, deep breaths and, unless contraindicated, encourage patients with accumulating secretions to cough.
3. Provide heated humidified oxygen for most extubated patients to assist secretion mobilization. However, the patient who has had traumatic intubations or who otherwise exhibits signs of laryngeal edema may benefit from cold humidified oxygen.
4. Allow no oral intake for approximately 6 hours after extubation because the larynx is not usually competent for several hours. After this, only clear liquids should be permitted until the patient swallows with ease.
5. Assess arterial blood gas levels postextubation to determine minimal safe inspired oxygen level. Additional blood gas determinations should be performed as indicated.
6. Administer chest physiotherapy as necessary, usually four times a day.

Complications

Aspiration of pooled oral secretions into lower airways
Laryngospasm or laryngeal edema or both

REFERENCE

Morrison, M.L. (ed.): Respiratory Intensive Care Nursing, 2nd ed. Boston, Little, Brown, 1979, pp. 197–199.

VENTILATORY MANAGEMENT

Jeanette McCann McHugh, R.N., M.S.N.

Overview

Critical care nurses should be thoroughly acquainted with ventilator control settings, displays, and alarms. These features not only provide valuable data about the patient's pulmonary status but have a major impact upon

TABLE 2-1   Controls, Displays, Alarms, and Special Features of Several Mechanical Ventilators

	Servo	Bennett MA-1	Bennett MA-2
Flow Pattern	May be altered in several ways: (1) flow wave switch allows operator to select sine or square wave; (2) altering spring tension will increase or decrease driving pressure; (3) altering minute volume, inspiratory time , or rate controls will alter flow.	May be altered with peak flow control setting.	Same as MA-1.
Inspiratory Volume Control	Minute volume and rate are set by operator; tidal volume is determined by the ventilator. Imprudent unilateral changes in either minute volume or rate may therefore cause profound change in the tidal volume. On assist mode patient tidal volume remains constant. Patient may increase minute volume by increasing rate.	Tidal volume and rate determined by operator. Patient may increase minute volume by increasing rate.	Same as MA-1.
Inspiratory to Expiratory Ratio	A function of several settings: (1) rate; (2) minute volume; (3) inspiratory time ; (4) inspiratory hold .	Expiratory time determined by inspiratory plateau and expiratory retard settings. Inspiratory time determined by volume and flow settings. Alarm sounds if inspiratory to expiratory ration exceeds 1:1.	Same as MA-1.
Display/Monitoring Capabilities	Expiratory minute volume/inspiratory to expiratory ratio/tidal volume, and airway pressure/lung mechanics calculator/CO_2 analyzer calculates: end-volume CO_2 effective/ineffective tidal volume, CO_2 production.	Tidal volume spirometer/temperature inspiratory gases/inspiratory pressure gauge/assist light; indicates patient-initiated breath/sigh light/oxygen light; indicates oxygen enrichment.	Tidal volume spirometer/digital display of temperature of inspiratory gases/inspiratory pressure gauge/digital display of rate/digital display of FiO_2/oxygen light/assist breath/sigh light.
Alarms/Alerts	Alarm sounds if changes in controls effect a minute volume that is too high or too low. Upper limit pressure alarm/electric power failure.	Pressure limit alarm/oxygen failure alarm/adverse inspiratory:expiratory time ratio alarm/failure of spirometer to receive set volume within a set time initiates an alarm. Excessive inspiratory gas temperature alarm.	Pressure limit alarm/oxygen failure alarm/adverse inspiratory:expiratory time ratio alarm/failure of spirometer to receive set volume within a set time initiates an alarm. Excessive inspiratory gas temperature alarm/low pressure alarm/failure to cycle alarm.
Special Features	PEEP/CPAP/IMV/inspiratory hold.	PEEP (optional attachments)/negative expiratory pressure (optional attachments)/inspiratory hold/expiratory retard.	IMV/CPAP/PEEP/inspiratory hold.

it. Table 2–1 has been provided to help identify the controls of several types of ventilators in common use. Information for ventilators not listed may be obtained from the manufacturer's operating manuals, respiratory therapists, and several texts.

Pressure-preset ventilators are characterized by inspiratory cycles that terminate at preset peak pressures. Under these conditions, delivered tidal volumes may be decreased by increased airway resistance or by decreased lung-chest compliance. For this reason these ventilators are not preferred for prolonged mechanical ventilation.

TABLE 2-1 Controls, Displays, Alarms, and Special Features of Several Mechanical Ventilators (Continued)

	Bourns Bear-1	Ohio CCV-2	Emerson 3-PV (Post op)
Flow Pattern	Wave form alteration control allows operator to select sine or square wave.	Adjustable inspiratory flow control.	Provides inspiratory gases in a sine wave flow pattern.
Inspiratory Volume Control	Tidal volume and rate determined by operator. Patient may increase minute volume by increasing rate.	Tidal volume set by operator. Expiratory time control is titrated until desired rate is achieved.	Stroke volume adjustment knob is located in front of machine at approximately shin level. Rate is set by titrating inhalation and exhalation time controls (see below).
Inspiratory to Expiratory Ratio	Inspiratory to expiratory time will not exceed 1:1 when I:E switch is in "on" position.	A function of inspiratory volume flow and hold settings and expiratory time setting.	Inspiratory and expiratory times are set with two independent controls. When both controls are set similarly (both at 12' o'clock, for example) inspiratory and expiratory times are equal. Turning either control clockwise shortens the inspiratory or expiratory phase. Counterclockwise turns lengthen either phase. Turning *both* controls equal distance in similar directions will increase or decrease respiratory rate.
Display/Monitoring Capabilities	Airway pressure/digital display of expiratory volume/minute volume accumulate/inspiratory:expiratory ratio.	Tidal volume displayed by bellows spirometer. Digital display of rate/system pressure and patient pressure gauge/patient manifold thermometer.	A revolving needle spirometer is an available accessory. Zeroed during the inspiratory phase, the needle moves during expiration to a setting that will approximate tidal volume.
Alarms/Alerts	Low oxygen pressure alarm/low air pressure alarm/high inspiratory pressure alarm/adverse inspiratory to expiratory time ratio alarm/low CPAP alarm/low PEEP alarm/apnea alarm/ventilator failure alarm.	Oxygen failure alarm/power failure alarm/high inspiratory pressure alarm/failure to cycle alarm.	An alarm will sound to indicate power failure, massive lead, or disconnection of the patient. This alarm is an accessory and may not be present on all Emerson 3-PV ventilators.
Special Features	IMV/CPAP/PEEP/inspiratory hold.	PEEP/IMV/inspiratory hold.	PEEP is an available accessory. However, patient assist sensitivity cannot be adjusted to accommodate positive airway pressure. Patients must generate negative pressure to initiate an assisted cycle.

Volume preset ventilators are characterized by inspiratory cycles that terminate after a preset tidal volume has been delivered. Because of their greater precision and the availability of special features, these ventilators are preferred for complex respiratory care.

INSTITUTING MECHANICAL VENTILATION _____

Objectives

1. To institute respiratory support
2. To determine appropriate ventilator settings.

Special Equipment

Ventilator
Pressure-preset ventilator (Bird and Bennett series)
Volume-preset ventilator

Procedure

ACTION	RATIONALE
1. Prepare to institute mechanical ventilation in the presence of any one or more of the following laboratory and clinical criteria: A. Vital capacity less than 10 to 15 ml./kg. body weight B. Inspiratory force less than 15 to 20 cm. H_2O. C. $AaDO_2$ of 300 to 350 mm. Hg or more on 100% oxygen. D. Acute alveolar hypoventilation, causing pH of 7.25 or less. E. Dyspnea and increased labor of breathing in the presence of "normal" or rising $PaCO_2$. F. Hyperventilation with diminished or decreasing SaO_2 (85% or less). G. Impending physical and emotional exhaustion with the labor of breathing.	1. A total clinical picture must be considered before instituting mechanical ventilation. Laboratory and clinical findings aid the decision-making process.

ACTION	RATIONALE

2. Intubate the patient (see "Endotracheal Intubation").

3. Calculate or derive appropriate ventilator settings from nomograms.
   A. Tidal volume = 10 ml./kg. body weight.
   B. Rate = normal adult rate; approximately 15 breaths/minute.
   C. $$FIO_2 = \frac{AaDO_2 + 100 \text{ mm. Hg}}{\text{barometric pressure}}$$
   D. Determine appropriate airflow patterns.

3. These settings provide a minute volume approxiately twice normal. This is appropriate for most patients in respiratory failure since their disease is commonly associated with an increased physiologic dead space. When respiratory failure is secondary to a nonpulmonary disorder (barbiturate overdose, neuromuscular disease), minute volumes may be diminished by reducing the respiratory rate.

4. Be familiar with ventilator:
   A. Displays and data provided about the patient.
   B. Alarms, and their meanings.
   C. Current settings.

5. Repeat arterial blood gas determinations 30 minutes after the patient has stabilized on the ventilator (see "Arterial Puncture").

5. Blood gas results are used to verify that the ventilator settings are providing adequate ventilation and oxygenation.

Precautions

1. Observe carefully for signs and symptoms of reduced cardiac output, especially in those patients with hypovolemia or limited autonomic responses. Venous return and cardiac output may be reduced, particularly during prolonged inspiratory:expiratory ratio or during positive end-expiratory pressure (PEEP).
2. Prevent atelectasis with larger tidal volumes, thorough tracheobronchial hygiene, and regular position changes.
3. Detect a positive fluid balance and predict patient's fluid needs by maintaining accurate intake and output records and obtaining daily weights. A positive fluid balance may be due to complex physiologic changes induced by mechanical ventilation. In addition, properly humidified gases block insensible water loss from the respiratory tract in mechanically ventilated patients.
4. Employ every practical means of improving ventilation/perfusion relationships to make the need for high oxygen concentrations as temporary as possible. Alveolar damage occurs when high concentrations of inspired oxygen are delivered for prolonged periods.

5. When using larger tidal volumes and PEEP, the use of mechanically ventilated "sighing" or periodically cycled large volume breaths may not be necessary. In addition, sigh-breaths with PEEP have been associated with an increased incidence of pneumothorax.

6. Auscultate the chest carefully and frequently to detect early development of subcutaneous emphysema and pneumothorax. They are especially likely to occur following damage to airways or visceral pleura that allows air leaks during positive pressure inspiration. They are also more likely to occur among patients ventilated with PEEP or high inspiratory pressures. Chest tubes may be necessary to prevent total lung collapse.

7. Be prepared to relieve the building intrathoracic pressure of a tension pneumothorax rapidly. This may appear as sudden patient distress or ventilator malfunction or both, with the patient rapidly losing consciousness and the face appearing plethoric and cyanotic. The neck veins are distended and the trachea may be deviated away from the tension pneumothorax. A quick inspection of the chest shows one hemithorax becoming distended and tympanic to percussion. Insert one or more large-bore needles between the intercostal spaces and ventilate the patient manually until help is summoned and chest tubes are placed.

Related Care

1. Maintain strict asepsis in airway and bronchial hygiene measures and in the care of respiratory equipment. Respiratory disease or its treatment may impair nearly all host defenses.
    A. Change all ventilator hoses every 24 hours.
    B. Drain liquid condensed in the hoses in the same direction as the air flow. Never drain condensed liquid back into the humidifier.
    C. Wash hands thoroughly between patients as well as between "dirty" nursing tasks (such as Foley care) and "clean" tasks (such as endotracheal suctioning).

2. Use PEEP in circumstances in which diminished functional residual capacity (FRC) and shunt hypoxia are present. This treatment measure provides above-atmospheric pressure in patient airways throughout and between respiratory cycles. PEEP increases FRC and balances the distribution of inspired tidal volumes throughout the lungs, thereby reducing shunt hypoxemia. This frequently results in improved oxygenation at lower inspired oxygen concentrations and improved ventilation at lower peak inspiratory pressures. However, PEEP increases the risk of barotrauma and may be associated with decreased cardiac output.

3. Return arterial PCO_2 to normal in tachypneic patients who are overriding the ventilator respiratory rate settings and developing hypocapnia. When pharmacologic suppression of the patient's respiratory drive is not appropriate additional tubing may be added between the patient's airway and the inspiratory arm of the ventilating circuit. This increased mechanical dead space causes the patient to rebreathe a portion of the CO_2 expired and reverses respiratory alkalosis.

4. Suppress the respiratory drive of patients who are tachypneic and grossly overdriving a mechanical ventilator to prevent fatigue, decrease oxygen consumption, and improve blood gas levels. Patients who also because of fear, cerebral hypoxia, or dyspnea asynchronously "fight" the ventilator will require respiratory drive suppression. Respiratory drive may be suppressed by:
    A. Narcotics, such as morphine sulfate, given IV. These suppress central respiratory control centers and sedate the anxious patient.
    B. Neuromuscular blocking agents. These paralyze the respiratory muscles. These agents do not alleviate the patient's confusion, fear, or dyspnea but only block muscular responses to them. The nurse must be acutely aware of the patient's needs for constant reassurance and explanation regarding his temporary paralysis. The nurse should be aware of the pharmacology of drugs employed to suppress respiration, since they may be associated with reduced cardiac output, bronchospasm, or other remote effects.
5. Monitor stool or nasogastric aspirate daily, using guaiac test, as patients receiving prolonged mechanical ventilation are at increased risk of gastrointestinal bleeding. In addition, prophylactic antacid therapy or IV cimetidine titration may be prescribed to maintain gastric pH above 5. This will necessitate hourly testing of gastric pH.

Complications

Equipment malfunction	Gastrointestinal bleeding
Nosocomial infection	Subcutaneous emphysema
Instrumentation error	Tension pneumothorax
Microshock	Atelectasis
Positive fluid balance	Reduced cardiac output/venous return
Oxygen toxicity	Hyperthermia
Hypocapnia/hypercapnia	Cardiopulmonary arrest
Hypoxia/anoxia	

Suppliers

Bourns, Inc. (Bourns Bear-1)
J.H. Emerson, Inc. (Emerson 3-PV (Post op))
Ohio Medical Products (Ohio CCV-2)
Puritan-Bennett Corporation (MA-1, MA-2)
Siemens-Elema (Servo)

REFERENCES

Hunsinger, D.L., et al.: Respiratory Technology Procedure and Equipment Manual. Reston, VA, Reston Publishing, 1980, pp. 243–340.
McPherson, S.P.: Respiratory Therapy Equipment, 2nd ed. St. Louis, C.V. Mosby, 1981, pp. 216–248.
Rottenborg, C.C., and Via-Reque, E.: Clinical Use of Mechanical Ventilation. Chicago, Year Book Medical Publishers, 1981, pp. 175–179.

WEANING FROM MECHANICALLY ASSISTED VENTILATION

Objectives

1. To assess the readiness of the patient before weaning is attempted.
2. To wean a patient effectively.
3. To monitor qualitative (behavioral) and quantitative (ventilatory functions, vital signs) indications of blood gas derangements that may occur during weaning.

Special Equipment

Source of heated humidified oxygen of prescribed concentration
T piece adapter

Procedure

ACTION	RATIONALE
1. Determine that the original indication for mechanical ventilation has been corrected or adequately modified.	
2. Assess patient's readiness for weaning. A. $AaDO_2$ should be 350 mm. Hg or less on 100% oxygen. B. Dead space to tidal volume ratio (VD/VT) should not exceed 0.60. C. Patient should be able to generate an inspiratory force of −25 cm. H_2O or have a vital capacity of 10 ml./kg body weight. D. There should be absence of intercostal retraction, tracheal tug, or excessive use of accessory respiratory muscles during brief trial periods of spontaneous breathing.	
3. Suction patient, as necessary, and give sufficient time to recover from suction-induced dyspnea and hypoxia.	
4. Elevate head of patient's bed, if possible.	4. Proper positioning will reduce intraabdominal resistance to diaphragmatic excursion.
5. Remove patient from ventilator and connect to source of humidified oxygen, keeping ventilator connections sterile during weaning intervals. Oxygen concentrations are prescribed by	

ACTION	RATIONALE
the physician and are generally higher than those supplied while on the ventilator.	
6. Measure vital capacity, tidal volume, arterial blood gas concentrations, and vital signs before and after weaning periods. They may be measured during weaning periods as needed.	6. Weaning attempts are terminated if any symptoms of hypoxia or alveolar hypoventilation develop (see precautions, below).
7. At prescribed termination of weaning period: A. Remove **T** piece. B. Place the patient back on mechanical ventilation. C. Assist patient into a comfortable position.	
8. Reduce length of intervals between weaning periods gradually as weaning periods are lengthened.	

Precautions

Observe for signs of blood gas derangements during weaning, including rapid, shallow respirations with or without dyspnea. In addition, hypotension, cyanosis, ectopy or conduction disturbances or both, behavior changes, or decreased level of consciousness may also occur. In particular, agitation, fear, or air hunger during weaning should not be dismissed as a functional complaint but should be investigated in terms of alterations in vital signs, ventilatory parameters, and blood gas levels. Weaning should be terminated at any point that hypoxia or alveolar hypoventilation is suspected.

Related Care

1. Prepare patients for weaning from the beginning of mechanical ventilation. They should be reassured that the use of a ventilator is temporary. Patients are also told of any signs of improvement in their condition and are encouraged to look forward to trial periods off the ventilator.
2. Begin weaning patients from mechanical ventilation when they are able to tolerate as little as 10 minutes of spontaneous breathing without deterioration of clinical or laboratory findings.
3. Note that the need for PEEP to maintain FRC is not necessarily a contraindication for weaning. Continuous positive airway pressure (CPAP) can be easily maintained during weaning with intermittent mandatory ventilation (IMV). Similarly, CPAP devices can be adapted for weaning during periods of monitored discontinuation of mechanical ventilation.
4. Remain with the patient during weaning. Since he is unattached from the ventilator alarms and unable to summon help, a patient's deteriora-

tion may go unnoticed. In addition, patients are entitled to close support and encouragement during a procedure that they may perceive as threatening and frightening.

5. Do not attempt weaning at night until prolonged daytime periods of spontaneous ventilation are well established. Lack of staff for close supervision and patient fatigue at night results in suboptimal weaning.

6. Note that IMV is a more psychologic approach to weaning patients during mechanical ventilation. It permits the patient to remain attached to the ventilator while spontaneously breathing a humidified oxygen mixture. The ventilator is set to deliver a mandatory breath at specific intervals. These intervals are gradually lengthened until the patient breathes entirely independently of the ventilator.

Complications

Hypoxia   Hypotension
Dysrhythmias   Respiratory arrest

REFERENCES

Don, H.F.: Ventilatory management of the critically ill patient. *In* Berk, J.L., and Sampliner, J.E. (eds.): Handbook of Critical Care. Boston, Little, Brown, 1982, pp. 147–177.

Hastings, P.R., et al.: Cardiorespiratory dynamics during weaning with IMV versus spontaneous ventilation in good-risk cardiac surgery patients. Anesthesiology, 53:429, 1980.

Hunsinger, D.L., et al.: Respiratory Technology Procedure and Equipment Manual. Reston, VA, Reston Publishing, 1980, pp. 335–338.

McPherson, S.P.: Respiratory Therapy Equipment, 2nd ed., St. Louis, C.V. Mosby, 1981, p. 241.

MANUAL VENTILATION WITH POSITIVE END-EXPIRATORY PRESSURE (PEEP)

Objectives

1. To maintain increased FRC and minimize shunting in patients removed from mechanical ventilation with PEEP.

2. To provide optimal oxygenation and alveolar ventilation for patients who must be removed from mechanical ventilation with PEEP for transport, bronchial hygiene, or other purposes.

Special Equipment

Anesthesia bag with universal adapter
Oxygen source
Source of expiratory resistance (water column, PEEP valve, etc.)

Procedure

ACTION	RATIONALE

1. Begin flow of oxygen into anesthesia bag.

2. Attach source of expiratory resistance (Fig. 2–9).

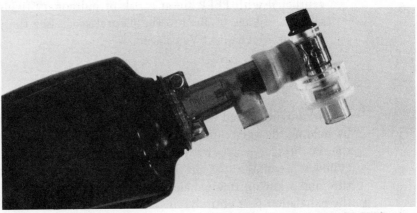

Figure 2-9.   Anesthesia bag with PEEP valve.

3. Remove ventilator hose from airway at end inspiration.

4. Attach anesthesia bag to airway during passive expiratory phase.

5. Observe patient's abdomen and chest for inspiratory efforts and supply breaths "on demand."

6. Encourage patient to breathe slowly and deeply.

7. Administer slow, full breaths at a rate of 10 to 12/minute to apneic or paralyzed patients.

8. Release inflation hold at end inspiration and allow patient to exhale against expiratory resistance.

9. Repeat respiratory cycles as described in steps 5 through 8 until patient can be returned to mechanical ventilation with PEEP.

5. Tidal volumes, and therefore alveolar ventilation, will be diminished if breaths are delivered against resistance or asynchronously with patient efforts.

Precautions

1. Minimize the risk of nosocomial pulmonary infections by employing aseptic technique in the management of all ventilatory equipment. Provide each patient with a sterilized anesthesia bag at least every 24 hours. Avoid using the same bag for more than one patient, thus reducing sources of cross infection. Replace any anesthesia bag that becomes contaminated.
2. Observe for sudden deterioration in ventilatory status that may indicate formation of a pneumothorax. Patients with poor compliance who are ventilated with PEEP are at a risk of pulmonary tissue rupture with consequent leakage of air into the pleural space (see the precautions for "Instituting Mechanical Ventilation").

Related Care

Maintain desired levels of PEEP when ventilating with Boehringer valves by holding the valve upright at all times. Expiratory resistance is provided by the Boehringer valve by means of weighted balls in a cylinder. If the cylinder becomes tilted the balls roll within the cylinder, opening the aperture and allowing free exhalation. Also, inverting the cylinders will occlude the exhalation port entirely.

Complications

Infection
Inadequate or excessive alveolar ventilation
Pneumothorax

REFERENCES

Manufacturer's literature
Massachusetts General Hospital, unpublished procedure.

CONTINUOUS POSITIVE AIRWAY PRESSURE (CPAP)

Objectives

1. To increase FRC and decrease the degree of pulmonary shunting.
2. To obviate the need for intubation and mechanical ventilation in acute, potentially reversible pulmonary disorder.

Special Equipment (Fig. 2–10)

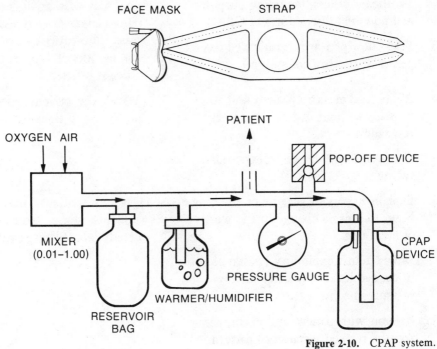

Figure 2-10.   CPAP system.

Oxygen source
Oxygen/air mixer
Reservoir bag
Source of warm humidification
Clear face mask of rigid material with soft, pliable seal
Straps for face mask
Inspiratory and expiratory tubing with one-way valves
CPAP device with safety pop-off feature
    PEEP valve
    Water column
    Spring-loaded membrane
    PEEP system of mechanical ventilator
Pressure gauge (cm. H_2O)
Skin Lotion

Procedure

ACTION	RATIONALE
1. Obtain baseline blood gas levels, vital signs and, if possible, central venous and pulmonary vascular pressures.	1. CPAP has profound respiratory and circulatory effects. The clinician must be able to detect early adverse as well as desirable reactions.

ACTION	RATIONALE
2. Explain procedure to patient and his significant others, including purpose and potential discomforts of CPAP.	2. Mask CPAP is a stressful experience that may last an indefinite time. Patient cooperation is essential for success. The patient in turn needs maximal emotional support of staff and significant others.
3. Begin flow of warm humidified oxygen mixture through system.	
4. Apply face mask to patient and strap in place without in-line expiratory resistance.	4. Allows the patient a few moments to adjust to the tight-fitting mask.
5. Connect CPAP device to expiratory tubing.	
6. Explain to patient that he or she may begin to sense a change in the work of breathing.	6. Dyspneic patients may panic if they suddenly sense interference in their already labored respirations.
7. Slowly adjust expiratory resistance until desired level of positive airway pressure is achieved.	
8. Remain with patient and encourage regular, relaxed respiratory pattern.	
9. Assess vital signs and central venous and pulmonary vascular pressures as soon as patient is stabilized. Determine blood gas levels as appropriate or prescribed.	9. These data provide a baseline from which the response to CPAP can be assessed.
10. Check the system frequently for air leaks, with particular attention to the face mask seal.	10. Air leaks will reduce the positive airway pressure.
11. Assess respiratory and circulatory parameters hourly, and more frequently as indicated.	11. CPAP imposes an increased workload on critically ill patients who are therefore at risk of slipping into respiratory failure.
12. Continue to provide close physical presence and emotional support.	
13. Discontinue CPAP for 10 minutes every 2 hours and provide warmed humidified oxygen via face tent.	13. The patient will need periods of rest from increased ventilatory workload as well as opportunity for verbalization, oral hygiene, and nourishment.
14. Assess skin around bony prominences of face and under any tubes (nasogastric tubes, etc.) that may protrude from under mask.	

ACTION

RATIONALE

15. Massage reddened areas with lotion.

16. Reassess non-CPAP respiratory and circulatory parameters as appropriate.

17. Reinstitute CPAP as described in steps 3 through 10.

18. Continue intermittent mask CPAP until pulmonary disorder resolves, or until more definitive respiratory support measures become necessary.

Precautions

1. Provide an expiratory tubing system that has an integral pop-off valve between the patient and the CPAP device. The valve should release to allow free exhalation if the system pressure exceeds desired levels of positive pressure; this could occur if the CPAP device malfunctions.
2. Ensure consistent levels of CPAP by checking the pressure gauge and observing the system for air leaks frequently. Air leaks around the face mask are particularly common.
3. Perform careful, periodic chest assessment to detect signs of pneumothorax. CPAP in patients with diseased, poorly compliant lungs may precipitate rupture, with the escape of air into the pleural space. The clinician should be particularly alert to this possiblity if high levels of CPAP are being attempted or if a sudden deterioration in ventilatory status occurs.
4. Observe respiratory efforts and chest excursion, as well as respiratory rate and depth frequently. Patients treated with CPAP are subjected to an increased respiratory workload on top of diseased, poorly compliant lungs. Fatigue and resultant hypercapnia may occur. An anesthesia bag with face mask, and in some cases an intubation tray, should be kept at the bedside.
5. Minimize the risk of infection by applying aseptic management of all CPAP equipment. Patients with pulmonary disease have compromised defense systems and are susceptible to infection. CPAP systems provide a warm, moist environment for bacterial growth and should be changed at least every 48 hours.
6. Avoid the use of opaque face masks, since they obscure patient vomiting and promote aspiration. Further minimize the risk of aspiration by checking the abdomen for distention frequently. Immediately attend to patient complaints of nausea by replacing the CPAP mask with the face tent and humidified oxygen.

Related Care

Provide the patient with an alternative means of communication while the CPAP mask is in place. If the patient must be left alone momentarily, provide a bell, buzzer, or other device for summoning help.

Complications

Ventilatory fatigue and failure   Excoriation of face
Pneumothorax   Infection
Diminished cardiac output

Suppliers

Boehringer Laboratories (Boehringer valve)
Puritan-Bennett Corporation (spring-loaded membrane
   obtained from MA-1 ventilator)

REFERENCES

Covelli, H.D., Weled, B.J., and Beckman, J.F.: Efficacy of continuous positive airway pressure administered by face mask. Chest, *81*:147, 1982.
Greenbaum, D.M., et al.: Continuous positive airway pressure without tracheal intubation in spontaneously breathing patients. Chest, *69*:615, 1976.
University of Wisconsin Hospitals Manual of Respiratory Therapy Procedures. Unpublished.

TRANSCUTANEOUS BLOOD GAS
——————— MONITORING ———————

Jeanette McCann McHugh, R.N., M.S.N.

Overview

Intermittent measurement of arterial blood gases is a common assessment of the condition and therapeutic responses of the critically ill patient. Samples of arterial blood are taken from indwelling catheters or by means of direct arterial puncture (see "Arterial Puncture"). Indwelling catheters and intermittent puncture impose many potential hazards upon the patient, not the least of which are embolism, infection, hematoma formation, nerve injury, and pain. For the critically ill neonate, frequent arterial sampling often requires umbilical artery catheterization with its consequent hazards.

Transcutaneous blood gas monitoring has become a practical reality in the care of critically ill infants and has demonstrated similar usefulness among adult patients. Instruments used for this purpose depend upon electrodes that are applied to the skin. Heating elements within these electrodes warm the skin to dilate and "arteriolize" the dermal capillaries. The partial pressures of O_2 and CO_2 as they diffuse transcutaneously ($PtcO_2$ and $PtcCO_2$) are measured by these electrodes, and these data are digitally or graphically displayed on the bedside unit.

$PtcO_2$, in particular, has been shown to be nearly identical to PaO_2 in normovolemic, normotensive neonates, and in spite of variable skin thicknesses $PtcO_2$ and $PtcCO_2$ correlated well with PaO_2 and $PaCO_2$ values in adult patients. Reduction in blood flow to the skin, however, is one of the earliest compensatory responses in developing shock states. Under these circumstances discrepancies will arise between PO_2 and PCO_2 measured arterially and transcutaneously. For this reason, when respiratory failure occurs in the normovolemic, normotensive patient, $PtcO_2$ and $PtcCO_2$ will accurately parallel PaO_2 and $PaCO_2$. But when circulatory systems fail, $PtcO_2$ and $PtcCO_2$ will reflect flow. Transcutaneous blood gas monitoring, then, serves as an accurate indicator of tissue oxygen delivery and provides an early clinical warning of low flow states.

Objectives

1. To obtain accurate measurements of $PtcO_2$ and $PtcCO_2$.
2. To make accurate inferences about the patient's ventilatory and circulatory status.

Special Equipment

Alcohol prep pad
Razor
Transcutaneous blood gas monitor and electrodes
Fixation rings
Electrolyte solution

Procedure

ACTION	RATIONALE
1. Calibrate the monitor as necessary (refer to operation manual).	1. Transcutaneous blood gas values will best correlate with arterial values when the electrode is positioned over sites of adequate dermal blood flow.
2. Replace electrode membranes as necessary (refer to operation manual).	
3. Set high and low alarms for PO_2/PCO_2 displays.	
4. Set electrode temperature.	4. Electrode temperature of 43° C. is recommended for newborns and 44° C. for adults.
5. Select an appropriate measuring site on the body. Take into consideration: A. The density of the capillaries. B. The adequacy of flow. C. Thickness of the horny skin layer. D. Deposits of subcutaneous fat. E. Right to left shunting. F. The presence of bony prominences.	 E. Electrodes placed on the lower trunk or extremities of infants with a patent ductus arteriosus will indicate $PtcO_2$ values that are much lower than true PaO_2.
6. Cleanse and prep the skin with alcohol pad. Shave site if necessary.	6. This removes oil and other substances through which gases must diffuse to contact the electrodes.
7. Apply two fixation rings for each electrode.	7. This provides for electrode site rotation.
8. Place prescribed electrolyte solution on the skin in the center of the fixation ring (refer to operation manual).	8. Manufacturers provide electrolyte solutions for specific instruments.
9. Attach electrode to the fixation ring.	

ACTION	RATIONALE
10. Allow 15 minutes or more for PO_2/PCO_2 readings to stabilize.	
11. Rotate electrode site every 2 to 4 hours.	11. Prolonged hyperthermia may result in skin burns.

Related Care

1. Recognize that transcutaneous blood gas values will rarely be identical to arterial values. In hemodynamically stable adults $PtcO_2$ may vary considerably from PaO_2, depending upon skin characteristics. Determine the difference in PO_2 (ΔPO_2) between arterial and transcutaneous data and utilize this factor to interpret monitor displays.
2. Recognize that $PtcO_2$ is always higher than $PaCO_2$ because of CO_2 production in the tissues at the electrode site. Determine PCO_2 between transcutaneous and arterial data and utilize this factor to interpret monitor displays.
3. Detect diminished $PtcO_2$ values and determine whether they reflect respiratory failure or impending circulatory collapse.
4. Inform parents that hyperemic spots caused by electrodes on infant skin will fade after 36 to 48 hours.

Precaution

Avoid skin burns by careful selection of electrode temperature and rotation of electrode sites.

Suppliers

Litton Medical Electronics   TCM20 TC carbon dioxide monitor
Radiometer/Copenhagen   TCM200 TC recorder
Servomed Oximonitor, SM 361   A7405 TC calibration unit
TCM2 TC oxygen monitor

REFERENCES

Beran, A.V., Tolle, C.D., and Huxtable, R.F.: Cutaneous blood flow and its relationship to cutaneous O_2/CO_2 measurements. Crit. Care Med., 9:736, 1981.
Dingle, R.E., et al.: Continuous transcutaneous O_2 monitoring in the neonate. Am. J. Nurs., 80:890, 1980.
Eberhard, P., Mindt, W., and Schafer, R.: Cutaneous blood gas monitoring in the adult. Crit. Care Med., 9:702, 1981.
Emrico, J.: Transcutaneous oxygen monitoring in neonates. Respir. Care, 24:(7), 1979.
Shoemaker, W.C., and Vidyasagar, D.: Physiological and clinical significance of $PtcO_2$ and $PtcCO_2$ measurements. Crit. Care Med., 9:689, 1981.
Tremper, K.K., and Shoemaker, W.C.: Transcutaneous oxygen monitoring of critically ill adults with and without low flow shock. Crit. Care Med., 9:706, 1981.
Tremper, K.K., et al.: Transcutaneous PCO_2 monitoring on adult patients in the ICU and operating room. Crit. Care Med., 9:752, 1981.

CHEST TUBE MANAGEMENT

Jeanette McCann McHugh, R.N., M.S.N.

Overview

The visceral and parietal pleura form a potential intrathoracic space that is filled with only 4 ml. of lubricating pleural fluid. Between these two membranes, which line the chest wall and cover the lungs, there is a fluctuating but always negative intrapleural pressure. Disease, chest trauma, or surgery may cause disruption of the lung, thorax, or pleura and enable air or fluid to flow into the pleural space. This interrupts full inspiratory excursion and may lead to complete lung collapse. Some injuries can result in a tension pneumothorax in which the lung collapses, mediastinal structures are displaced and the heart and great vessels are compressed, leading to sudden death.

Self-limiting but symptomatic pneumothorax may develop spontaneously or as the result of diagnostic or therapeutic measures such as subclavian vein catheterization or pulmonary biopsy. Under these circumstances, lung re-expansion may be enhanced by the use of a small, thin walled cannula connected to a flutter valve. The valve allows accumulated air to exit the pleural space during exhalation but prevents air from entering the chest with inspiration. This small flutter valve and cannula can be taped to the chest to allow the patient maximum mobility during resolution of the pneumothorax.

Patients requiring respiratory intensive care are subject to more severe pleural space disruptions secondary to thoracic surgery and ventilatory barotrauma as well as their own pulmonary disorders. Fluid in the pleural space such as blood or exudate or large volumes of air must be removed with conventional chest tube drainage systems. Once inserted into the pleural space the chest tubes may be connected to systems composed of one, two, or three parts, each of which provides a specific function. These functions can be described in terms of the classic three-bottle chest drainage system and provided by a bottle system or a disposable chest drainage unit.

CHEST TUBE PLACEMENT (ASSISTING WITH)

Objectives

1. To identify the signs of intrapleural air and fluid.
2. To assist the physician by anticipating needs during chest tube placement.

3. To attach the chest tubes to a drainage system and maintain chest tube patency.

Special Equipment

Antiseptic skin prep and swabs
Sterile drape(s)
Sterile gloves
Anesthetic with 2-ml. syringe and 5/8-inch 28-gauge and 21-gauge 1¼-inch needles
Scalpel blade and handle
Chest tubes with obturators in varying sizes
Suture material (3–0) needle and needle holder
Kelly clamps (2)
Hemostat
Forceps
Dressing materials:
    Sterile gauze pads/scissors/occlusive dressing (petroleum jelly gauze)/occlusive tape
Connecting tube and straight and **Y** connectors
Drainage/water seal/suction source

Procedure

ACTION	RATIONALE
1. Auscultate/percuss chest.	1. This identifies area of pleural space disruptions.
A. Pleural space disruptions may be manifested by decreased compliance and increased peak inspiratory pressures, decreased PaO_2, and increased $AaDO_2$.	
B. Intrapleural air may be manifested by distant breath sounds to absence of breath sounds, hyperresonance, or tympany to percussion.	
C. Intrapleural fluid may be manifested by distant breath sounds to absence of breath sounds, dullness, or flatness to percussion.	

ACTION	RATIONALE
2 Prepare drainage system "Three-Bottle Closed Chest Drainage System"). In an emergency, water seal may be provided by placing distal end of chest tube into bottle of sterile saline or water at a depth of about 2 cm.	2. If the tube is immersed under too much H_2O, accumulating pressure within the chest cannot escape.
3. Assist physician with chest tube insertion. Chest tubes are usually placed in the second intercostal space anteriorly to remove intrapleural air and in the eighth or ninth intercostal space posteriorly to remove fluid. If the pleural space contains both air and fluid, chest tubes may be placed at both sites.	
4. Connect tubing to drainage system. A. Tape connections securely. B. If two tubes are placed, a **Y** connector may be used to connect them to a single drainage system. C. Maintain drainage unit below level of the chest tube insertion site.	
5. Apply occlusive dressing (petroleum jelly gauze) to tube insertion site. Cover with dry, sterile gauze pads and tape in place with occlusive cloth tape.	
6. Turn on suction source, as appropriate.	
7. Place vertical strip of tape along collection bottle(s). Mark level of drainage and monitor every hour, or as circumstances indicate.	
8. Coil tubing and secure to bottom sheet in loose loop. Connecting tubing should be long enough for patient to turn 120 degrees and sit upright.	8. Fluid accumulating in lengths of dependent tubing interferes with flow of drainage into collecting system.
9. "Strip" or "milk" accumulated clots, fibrin, and drainage out of tubing.	

ACTION	RATIONALE

With the nondominant hand, firmly grasp the tubing proximal to the patient and prevent any traction from being applied to the chest tube during stripping. Pinch tubing with both hands, sliding fingers of dominant hand distally along tube. The entire length of each tube should be stripped hourly, or as indicated.

10. Make the following observations hourly.
    A. Water seal is maintained at 2 cm.
    B. Prescribed amount of suction is maintained.
    C. Continuous gentle bubbling is present in suction control bottle.
    D. Color and quantity of drainage are noted.

Precaution

Keep a bottle of sterile irrigating fluid at the bedside. If the chest tube becomes dislodged from its drainage connection, if a leak occurs, or if bottle no. 1 or no. 2 breaks, the chest tube should be immersed 2 cm. deep in sterile irrigating fluid and the physician notified. Once the problem has been resolved, cleanse the tubing ends with an iodine disinfectant, have the patient exhale, and reconnect the tubing. The patient should not be left unattended and should be observed for any signs of respiratory difficulty.

Related Care

1. Auscultate and percuss the chest to determine if a nonfluctuating water seal column is due to an obstructed chest tube or re-expansion of the lung. A patient breathing spontaneously should cause fluid in the water seal column to rise slightly with inspiration.
2. Observe for bubbling in the water seal bottle; this indicates an air leak into the pleural space from the lung or bronchus. Continuous slow bubbling should always be present in the suction control bottle, however. Lack of bubbling may indicate failure of the suction source or an "upstream" leak within the system or around the chest tube.

Complications

Infection	Hemothrorax
Hemorrhage	Equipment malfunction
Tension pneumothorax	

REFERENCES

Bricker, P.L.: Chest tubes, the crucial points you mustn't forget. RN, *43*(11) 21–26, 1980.

Connolly, J.E.: Thoracotomy and pleural resection. Surg. Clin. North Am., *60*:1489–1495, 1980.

Duncan., C., and Erickson, R.: Pressures associated with chest tube stripping. Heart Lung, *11*:166–179, 1982.

Erikson, R.: Chest tubes, they're not really that complicated. Nursing 81, *11*:34–43 (May), 1981.

Erickson, R.: Solving chest tube problems. Nursing 81,*11*: 62–68 (June),1981.

Harper, R.W.: A Guide to Respiratory Care. Philadelphia, J.B. Lippincott, 1981, pp. 289–310.

How to work with chest tubes. Am. J. Nurs., *80*:685–712, 1980.

Morrison, M.L. (ed.): Respiratory Intensive Care Nursing, 2nd ed., Boston, Little, Brown, 1979, pp. 343–358.

THREE-BOTTLE CLOSED CHEST DRAINAGE SYSTEM

Objectives

1. To re-expand the involved lung in a pneumothorax.
2. To observe and measure drainage via the chest tubes.

Special Equipment

Three sterile wide-mouthed gallon bottles

Three sterile caps or stoppers (two caps with two vents, third cap with three vents)

Two sterile glass pipets (longer than the depth of the bottles) and five small glass vents

Four lengths of sterile tubing

50-ml. irrigation syringe

Sterile water
1-inch adhesive tape and wire
Centimeter ruler
Sterile gloves
Needle holder
Kelly clamps (2)

Procedure

ACTION	RATIONALE
1. Open sterile packages of bottles and related equipment.	
2. Don sterile gloves	
3. Prepare water seal bottle (Fig. 2–11).	

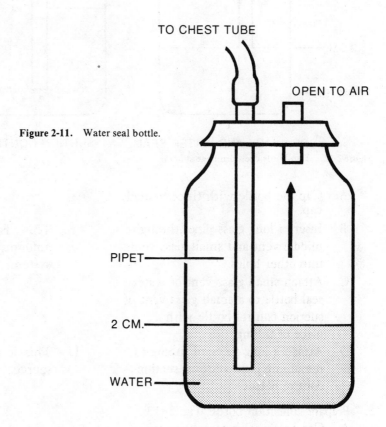

TO CHEST TUBE

OPEN TO AIR

Figure 2-11.   Water seal bottle.

PIPET—

2 CM.—

WATER—

A. Cap one bottle with a two vented cap.
B. Insert long glass pipet through one hole and a small glass vent in second hole.
C. Attach long tubing to long glass pipet.

ACTION	RATIONALE

4. Prepare the suction control bottle (Fig. 2–12).

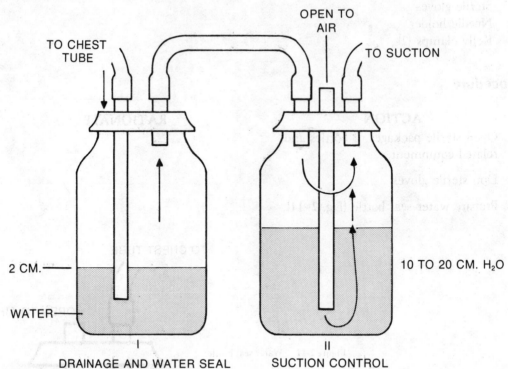

Figure 2-12. Two-bottle chest drainage system.

A. Cap the bottle with three-vented cap.

B. Insert a long glass pipet through middle vent and small glass vents into other holes.

    B. This is used to control the amount of suction applied by the system.

C. Attach small glass vent of water seal bottle to a small glass vent of suction control bottle with a piece of tubing.

D. Attach a long piece of tubing to remaining glass vent on suction control bottle.

    D. This is connected to the suction source.

5. Prepare collection bottle (Fig. 2–13).
   A. Cap bottle with remaining two-vented cap.
   B. Insert two small glass vents into holes.
   C. Attach long tubing from long glass pipet of the underwater seal bottle to small glass vent of collection bottle.

ACTION	RATIONALE

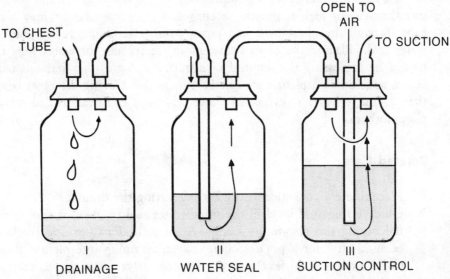

Figure 2-13. Three-bottle chest drainage system.

D. Attach a long tubing to remaining glass vent. Keep the end of this tube sterile.

E. Remove gloves.

F. Add sterile water to underwater seal bottle; position glass pipet tip 2 cm. under water level.

G. Add prescribed amount of sterile water to suction control bottle.

H. Tape all connections securely with occlusive cloth tape.

I. Secure bottles on floor at bedside. If possible, use wooden boxes built specifically to accommodate large drainage bottles. If these are not available, place bottles in wash basins. If absolutely necessary, tape bottles to the floor.

D. This connects the chest tubes to the collection bottle.

F. As the patient inspires, generating negative intrathoracic pressure, water rises in the pipet, but air is blocked from entering the pleural space.

G. The amount of suction delivered to the chest tube is determined by the length (cm.) of pipet beneath the water surface. Chest drainage systems are usually set to deliver 10 to 20 cm. H_2O negative pressure to the chest tube.

H. This provides extra protection against air leakage and separation.

I. This prevents accidental separation of tube connections or bottle caps in case the bottles are jarred or hit.

Precaution

Place the underwater seal pipet only 2 cm. under the water level. If an intrathoracic air leak is present, accumulating interpleural air may safely escape through the chest tube and pipet, causing bubbling at the point of the water seal. Placing the pipet below more than 2 cm. of water may cause a hazard by increasing the amount of intrathoracic pressure that must develop before accumulated pleural air can be blown off. Placing the pipet below less than 2 cm. of water risks loss of water seal from evaporation and subsequent pneumothorax.

Related Care

1. Precalibrate a collection bottle for measuring the drainage.
2. Observe the fluid level in the underwater seal column; it should rise and fall during the respiratory cycle. A single underwater seal bottle should be used only for a pneumothorax, since draining interpleural fluids will cause a rising fluid level and create progressive resistance to drainage. If underwater seal alone is used, the air vent is left open to air.
3. Provide suction when air enters the pleural cavity faster than it is forced out through the underwater seal.
4. Observe for bubbling in underwater seal. A small amount of bubbling may be normal.
   A. Absence of bubbling may indicate failure of suction source or reexpansion of the lung.
   B. Excessive bubbling may indicate a large pneumothorax or a leak in the system. Check by clamping each connection, starting at the chest tube insertion site, down to the collection chamber. When the bubbling stops the leak is distal to the clamp.

Complications

Pleural erosion and hemorrhage
Hematomas of lungs and chest wall

Failure of lung to re-expand
Tension pneumothorax
Infection

REFERENCES

Connolly, J.E.: Thoracotomy and pleural resection. Surg. Clin. North Am., 60:1489–1495, 1980.
Morrison, M.L. (ed.): Respiratory Intensive Care Nursing, 2nd ed. Boston, Little, Brown, 1979, pp. 343–358.

DISPOSABLE CHEST DRAINAGE UNIT _____

Objectives

1. To re-expand the involved lungs in pneumothorax.
2. To observe and measure drainage via the chest tubes.

Special Equipment

Chest drainage unit
50-ml. irrigation syringe
Sterile water

1-inch adhesive tape and wire
Needle holder
Two Kelly clamps

Procedure

ACTION	RATIONALE
1. Arrange tubings so they will not fall on floor. Make sure protective caps are securely attached to connectors.	1. This prevents contamination while equipment is being readied.
2. Attach sterile 50-ml. irrigation syringe, without barrel, to rubber tubing of water seal chamber.	
3. Fill water seal chamber up to 2-cm. line. If the patient will be on straight drainage, connector will be left off; otherwise, reapply.	
4. Remove cap from suction control chamber and, using same method as in step 3, fill to level necessary for desired amount of suction. Replace cap.	4. This will keep bubbling at minimum.
5. Fill the third chamber, found on some units, to a specified level in a similar manner.	
6. Hang unit from the bed or place in support device.	
7. Wire and tape the chest tube connection to the long tubing (see "Three-Bottle Closed Drainage System"	7. This prevents accidental disconnection and resulting pneumothorax.

Precautions

See precautions for the "Three-Bottle Closed Chest Drainage System."

Related Care

See related care for the "Three-Bottle Closed Chest Drainage System."

Complications

See complications for the "Three-Bottle Closed Chest Drainage System."

Suppliers

Argyle ("Double Seal" chest drainage unit)
Bard-Parker (Heimlich valve)
Cook Instrument Company (pneumothorax set)
Deknatel, division of Howmedica, Inc. (Pleur-evac)

REFERENCES

Connelly, J.E.: Thoracotomy and pulmonary resection, Surg. Clin. North Am., 60:1489–1495, 1980.

Massachusetts General Hospital Department of Nursing: Massachusetts General Hospital Manual of Nursing Procedures, 2nd ed. Boston, Little, Brown, 1980, pp. 258–288.

Morrison, M.D. (ed.): Respiratory Intensive Care Nursing, 2nd ed. Boston, Little, Brown, 1979, pp. 343–358.

CHEST PHYSIOTHERAPY

Jeannette McCann McHugh, R.N., M.S.N.

Overview

Airway obstruction is a common contributing factor in respiratory failure that causes ventilation/perfusion defects and frustrates the usefulness of ventilatory and oxygen therapy. Therefore measures are taken to alleviate bronchospasm and move secretions from peripheral to central airways from which they are more easily removed. In addition to the use of bronchodilating drugs, these measures include adequate hydration, deep breathing, and coughing exercises, postural drainage, and chest physiotherapy.

Postural drainage employs specific body positions to facilitate drainage of secretions from affected lung segments into the major airways. When several segments are involved, upper lobes are drained first, then middle, and finally lower lobes (Figures 2–14 through 2–22 illustrate the position employed for each segment of lung). Each position is maintained for 20 to 30 minutes if possible, although percussion and vibration should not exceed 20 minutes over each lung segment.

Objectives

1. To determine and place the patient in the appropriate drainage position.
2. To percuss and vibrate the chest effectively, loosening secretions and enhancing drainage.

Special Equipment

Towels
Several pillows

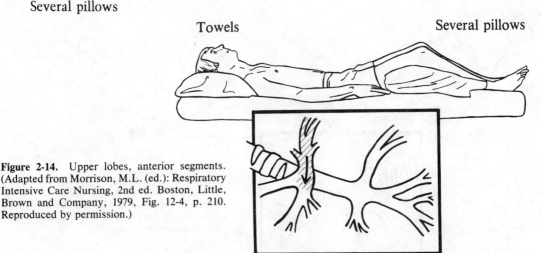

Figure 2-14. Upper lobes, anterior segments. (Adapted from Morrison, M.L. (ed.): Respiratory Intensive Care Nursing, 2nd ed. Boston, Little, Brown and Company, 1979, Fig. 12-4, p. 210. Reproduced by permission.)

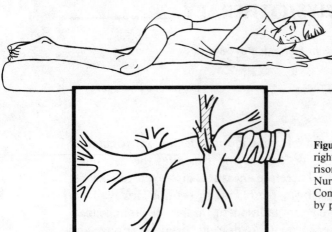

Figure 2-15. Upper lobe, posterior segment, right posterior bronchus. (Adapted from Morrison, M.L. (ed.): Respiratory Intensive Care Nursing, 2nd ed. Boston, Little, Brown and Company, 1979, Fig. 12-5, p. 210. Reproduced by permission.)

Procedure

ACTION	RATIONALE
1. Conduct an assessment using chest x-rays and auscultation to locate involved areas and estimate severity of obstruction.	1. The most severely obstructed airways permit less air movement and have *fewer* adventitious sounds. Diminished or bronchial breath sounds or absence of breath sounds may indicate a more severe disorder than loud rales and rhonchi.
2. Position patient appropriately and ensure that he is comfortably supported and relaxed (Fig. 2–16, Fig. 2–17).	

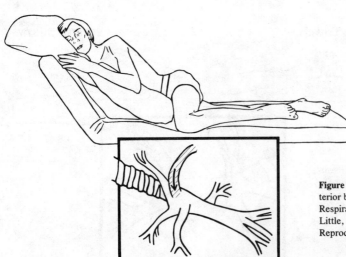

Figure 2-16. Upper lobe, posterior segment, left posterior bronchus. (Adapted from Morrison, M.L. (ed.): Respiratory Intensive Care Nursing, 2nd ed. Boston, Little, Brown, and Company, 1979, Fig. 12-6, p. 211. Reproduced by permission.)

ACTION   RATIONALE

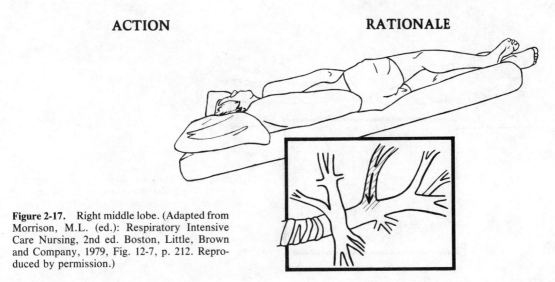

Figure 2-17. Right middle lobe. (Adapted from Morrison, M.L. (ed.): Respiratory Intensive Care Nursing, 2nd ed. Boston, Little, Brown and Company, 1979, Fig. 12-7, p. 212. Reproduced by permission.)

3. Provide tissues and receptacle for nonintubated patients or patients with deflated endotracheal tube cuffs.

4. Drape chest with towel.

5. Position yourself opposite site requiring therapy. Rhythmically clap chest wall. Hands should be held in cupped position; thumbs and fingers held together. Snap is applied only from the wrists. Elbows and shoulders are held loose and relaxed.

5. Air is caught under the cupped hand as it meets chest wall, causing an abrupt but cushioned blow. Percussion in the absence of chest trauma should not be strong enough to produce pain.

6. Stop periodically to encourage deep breathing and coughing.

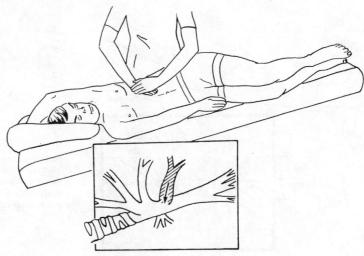

Figure 2-18. Left lingula. (Adapted from Morrison, M.L. (ed.): Respiratory Intensive Care Nursing, 2nd ed. Boston, Little, Brown and Company, 1979, Fig. 12-8, p. 212. Reproduced by permission.)

ACTION	RATIONALE

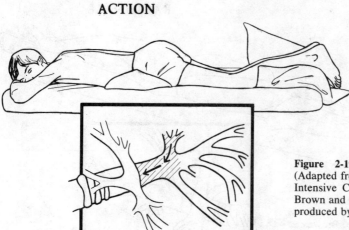

Figure 2-19. Lower lobes, apical segment. (Adapted from Morrison, M.L. (ed.): Respiratory Intensive Care Nursing, 2nd ed. Boston, Little, Brown and Company, 1979, Fig. 12-9, p. 213. Reproduced by permission.)

7. Vibrate chest wall.
   A. Place one hand over affected segment and second hand on top of first.
   B. Ask patient to inspire deeply and then exhale.
   C. Holding moderate pressure against chest wall, vibrate hands during expiration.
   D. If patient is being mechanically ventilated, synchronize vibration with passive expiratory phase.

8. Allow a few respiratory cycles for rest and coughing.

7. This assists the movement of secretions up and out of the tracheobronchial tree.

8. This avoids fatigue and hyperventilation.

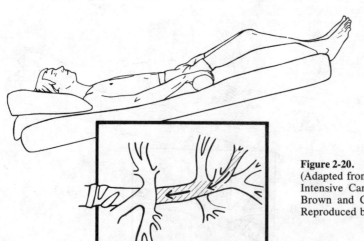

Figure 2-20. Lower lobes, anterior basal segment. (Adapted from Morrison, M.L. (ed.): Respiratory Intensive Care Nursing, 2nd ed. Boston, Little, Brown and Company, 1979, Fig. 12-10, p. 213. Reproduced by permission.)

ACTION   RATIONALE

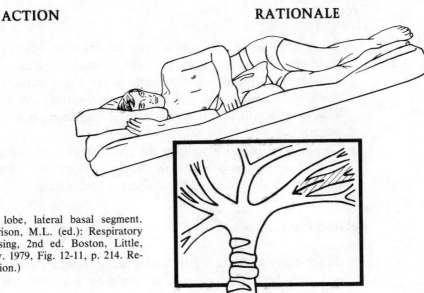

Figure 2-21. Lower lobe, lateral basal segment. (Adapted from Morrison, M.L. (ed.): Respiratory Intensive Care Nursing, 2nd ed. Boston, Little, Brown and Company. 1979, Fig. 12-11, p. 214. Reproduced by permission.)

9. Repeat. The amount of physiotherapy given to each segment is a clinical judgment based upon:
   A. Number of segments involved.
   B. Character and amount of secretions.
   C. Patient's ability to tolerate the total procedure.

10. Allow several minutes for drainage.

11. Advance to next involved segment, and repeat physiotherapy as indicated.

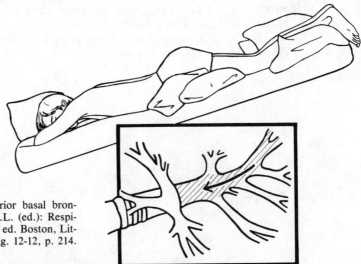

Figure 2-22. Lower lobes, posterior basal bronchus. (Adapted from Morrison, M.L. (ed.): Respiratory Intensive Care Nursing. 2nd ed. Boston, Little, Brown and Company, 1979, Fig. 12-12, p. 214. Reproduced by permission.)

Precautions

1. Avoid head-down and supine postural drainage after eating, since these positions may cause vomiting and aspiration. Head-down positioning may also be avoided in the presence of increased intracranial pressure.
2. Avoid postural drainage and physiotherapy during weaning intervals. Fatigue or abdominal pressure against the diaphragm may cause hyperventilation.
3. Do not percuss and vibrate in the presence of intrathoracic or intracranial bleeding, serious cardiac arrhythmias, or localized pulmonary infections that may be disseminated to unaffected lung tissue.

Related Care

Make every effort to see that pain medication, aerosolized bronchodilator therapy, and chest physiotherapy are given in a coordinated fashion and integrated into the patient's overall care plan.

Complications

Dysrhythmias   Disseminated pulmonary infections
Altered hemodynamics   Trauma
Hypoventilation/hyperventilation   Rib fractures
Fatigue

REFERENCES

Cielsa, N.: Postural drainage, positioning and breathing exercises. In McKenzie, C.F. (ed.): Chest Physiotherapy in the Intensive Care Unit. Baltimore, Williams & Wilkins, 1981, pp. 55–79.

Imle, P.C.: Percussion and vibration. In Chest Physiotherapy in the Intensive Care Unit. Baltimore, Williams & Wilkins, 1981, pp. 81–89.

Morrison, M.L. (ed.): Respiratory Intensive Care Nursing, 2nd ed. Boston, Little, Brown, 1979, pp. 205–209.

Rarey, K.P., and Youtsey, J.W.: Respiratory Patient Care. Englewood Cliffs, N.J., Prentice Hall, 1981, pp. 128–141.

___ THORACENTESIS (ASSISTING WITH) ___

Janice M. Casper, R.N., B.S.N.

Overview

Thoracentesis is performed to remove fluid or air from the pleural space or to instill sclerosing or antineoplastic agents between the two pleurae. This is accomplished by inserting a needle or trocar into the thoracic cavity at a selected site predetermined by x-ray findings and physical examination.

Thoracentesis using an anterior approach is usually performed as an emergency intervention for air removal and requires precise instrumentation and an understanding of thoracic anatomy. Thoracentesis using a posterior approach, however, is usually performed as a therapeutic intervention for fluid drainage or for obtaining a specimen for laboratory analysis. The critical care nurse shares responsibility in patient assessment before, during, and after this therapeutic intervention and must be cognizant of its potential effects.

Objectives

1. To remove fluid or air from the pleural space for the prompt relief of lung compressions or respiratory distress.
2. To obtain a fluid specimen for laboratory analysis.
3. To instill therapeutic agents into the pleural space.

Special Equipment

Thoracentesis tray
Sterile gloves
Sterile drapes
Local anesthetic
25-gauge, 20-gauge, and 18-gauge needles
Thoracentesis needles: 15-gauge, 17-gauge, 3-inch, short bevels
Two 10-ml. syringes
Two 50-ml. syringes
Three-way stopcock with 10 to 20 inches of tubing
Hemostat
Kelly clamp
Sterile fluid collection container
Scalpel blade (no. 11)
Laboratory specimen tubes
Sterile gauze pads
Povidone-iodine swabs
Povidone-iodine ointment
Tape

Procedure

ACTION	RATIONALE
1. Assess patient; obtain vital signs prior to therapy.	1. This information provides baseline data.
2. Position patient.	
A. Anterior thoracentesis approach:	A. An anterior-superior approach is used for air removal.
(1) Use supine position, with arm positioned under head.	
B. Posterior thoracentesis approach (options):	
(1) Have patient dangle at bedside with arms resting over a padded overbed table and feet resting on a footstool.	
(2) Use chair-straddle technique with arms resting on high back of chair or padded overbed table.	
2. Mask and gown all persons in immediate area and provide appropriately sized sterile gloves.	
3. Prepare skin site with povidone-iodine solution; drape area.	
4. Assess patient continuously while the thoracentesis is being performed.	
A. Support patient's position while skin zones are anesthetized; various gauges and lengths of needles are used for infiltration until parietal fluid is reached.	A. The patient may experience momentary pain on initial skin penetration and needle contact with the highly sensitive pleura prior to anesthesia infiltration.
B. Observe for pleural fluid return as needle is slowly advanced; as needle is withdrawn, note depth of penetration.	B. The depth of needle penetration to reach the pleural fluid is approximated and used as a guide during the advancement of the thoracentesis needle.
C. Instruct patient to breathe shallowly and to refrain from coughing as thoracentesis needle is advanced to pre-estimated depth and with constant aspiration; the thoracentesis needle is equipped with a preconnected 50-ml. syringe, three-way stopcock, and drainage tubing.	C. Shallow controlled breathing while the needle is in position minimizes risk of lung trauma. Also, the lung is re-expanded as fluid is removed; this brings the lung closer to the needle tip. Inform physician if patient experiences pain, nausea, dyspnea, cyanosis, or increased respiratory rate.

ACTION	RATIONALE
D. Support patient's position during immobilization period as thoracentesis needle is secured with Kelly clamp at skin puncture site and fluid is aspirated from pleural space (Fig. 2–23).	D. Securing the needle prevents inadvertent advancement during accidental movement.

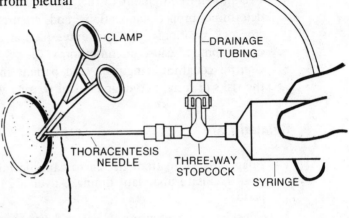

Figure 2-23. Thoracentesis.

E. Apply firm pressure to puncture site following removal of needle.

F. Assess puncture site; apply povidone-iodine ointment and secure sterile dressing.

5. Instruct patient to rest in bed after thoracentesis; monitor patient's vital signs and assess for pallor, cyanosis, dyspnea, tachycardia, hypotension, and bilateral breath sounds.

6. Note amount and appearance of fluid removed; facilitate prompt transport of specimen for prescribed laboratory analysis.

7. Assess post-thoracentesis chest films.	7. A chest x-ray provides data regarding the presence or absence of pneumothorax or residual pleural effusions.

Precautions

1. Assess health history for information regarding:
   A. Bleeding disorders and current medications, such as heparin or warfarin sodium (Coumadin), which could increase the risk of complications.
   B. Length of time of pleural effusion. Complete removal of a large pleural effusion present for longer than 3 months increases the risk of complications. Approximately 500 to 1000 ml. should be removed at one time in such cases.

2. Monitor the patient closely for perforation of the diaphragm or abdominal viscera if the puncture site is quite low in a posterior-inferior approach.
3. Monitor the patient for pain, nausea, cyanosis, dyspnea, and increased respiratory rate that might indicate pneumothorax.
4. Recommend equipment testing prior to thoracentesis needle insertion to determine proper connections and ensure familiarity with directional stopcock positions. Air can enter pleural space owing to faulty instrumentation and cause pneumothorax.
5. Control coughing, singultus, and patient movement; these will increase the risks of lung, nerve, and vessel trauma while needle is in position.

Related Care

1. Adapt procedure from needle to cannula insertion for therapeutic agents or to facilitate abundant drainage over a 24-hour, but less than 48-hour period.
2. Consider using vacuum collection bottles rather than a syringe-aspiration method for large volumes of pleural fluid. The vacuum method offers potential for lung tissue aspiration.
3. Assess puncture site for pain, erythema, edema, and warmth after 24 hours.

Complications

Pneumothorax

Mediastinal shift

Hemothorax; hemorrhage

Diaphragmatic injury

Penetration of abdominal viscera

Hypovolemic shock

Pleural shock

Infection

Protein depletion

Electrolyte imbalance

Suppliers

Kendall-Curity

American Pharmaseal

REFERENCES

Brunner, L.S., and Suddarth, D.S. (eds.): The Lippincott Manual of Nursing Practice, 3rd ed., Philadelphia, J.B. Lippincott, 1982, pp. 161–163.
Hamilton, H.K., & Rose, M.B. (eds.): Procedures, Nursing 83 Books. Springhouse, PA., Intermed Communciations, 1983, pp. 500–502.

3

THE
RENAL
SYSTEM

ACUTE HEMODIALYSIS

Anna J. Lavelle, R.N., B.S.N., M.N.,
Cheryl Tomich Wyman, R.N., B.S.N.

Overview

Hemodialysis can be defined as a method whereby desirable elements are retained on the blood side of a membrane, unwanted particles are passed through to a bath, and dangerous agents such as bacteria and viruses are prevented from entering the blood. The removal of these elements from the blood occurs by virtue of the differences in their diffusion rates through a semipermeable membrane.

There are a variety of clinical situations in which hemodialysis is therapeutically prescribed. Acute hemodialysis is used in cases of acute renal failure, congestive heart failure, hyperkalemia, and drug overdose. Long-term hemodialysis is used in cases of end-stage renal disease (ESRD). All of these clinical situations lead to some degree of renal impairment, resulting in fluid and electrolyte imbalances. The interpretation of blood chemistry findings, a diagnostic tool, is utilized to assess renal function, and this information can indicate the need for hemodialysis. It should be noted that some long-term hemodialysis patients do tolerate higher serum levels of electrolytes without manifesting clinical symptoms. To understand the basic principles of hemodialysis fully, the physiology of the processes of osmosis, diffusion, and ultrafiltration must be understood.

A patient's complete physiologic status must always be assessed before therapy is initiated. Such parameters may include:

1. Coagulation status or presence of fresh wounds, since heparinization is required to permit free flow of blood through the artificial kidney. Many patients in the critical care unit have undergone surgery or trauma or have bleeding problems. It is therefore important to administer heparin judiciously to avoid precipitating or increasing bleeding.

2. Cardiovascular status. Patients receiving digitalis therapy or patients with preexisting arrhythmias are already in a compromised condition. Sudden shifts in electrolytes, i.e., potassium, or intravascular volume loss, i.e., filling extracorporeal circuit, may result in further cardiac irritability or insufficiency.

3. Pharmacologic profile. Special attention must be given to antihypertensives, vasopressors, or antibiotics a patient may be receiving. Some medications are dialyzed from the blood, and additional doses may need to be given postdialysis. Blood levels of medications may need to be determined before and after dialysis.

Instrumentation

When hemodialysis therapy has been prescribed, a means of vascular access must be created. There are various ways to accomplish this.

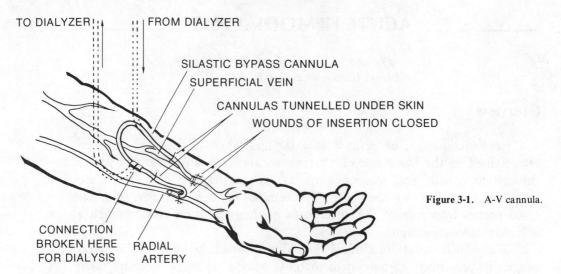

TO DIALYZER   FROM DIALYZER

SILASTIC BYPASS CANNULA
SUPERFICIAL VEIN
CANNULAS TUNNELLED UNDER SKIN
WOUNDS OF INSERTION CLOSED

CONNECTION
BROKEN HERE
FOR DIALYSIS   RADIAL
ARTERY

Figure 3-1. A-V cannula.

Shunt/Cannula.   These are artificial external shunts that create a connection between an artery and a vein (Fig. 3–1). Cannulas are commonly made of Silastic because of its flexibility, resistance to clot formation, and ability to withstand external mechanical trauma. The cannula can be inserted immediately during a crisis and can be left in place indefinitely, unless complications arise. A common insertion site is the distal portion of the arm or leg. One procedure presented will be directed to cannula access technique.

Arteriovenous (A-V) Fistula.   This is an alternative method of obtaining vascular access by which an internal connection is created between a patient's own artery and vein (Fig. 3–2). This type of access is not used in the critical care setting unless the patient has an already mature fistula. Access to the bloodstream is accomplished through venipuncture, using large-bore needles that are then connected to the blood tubing on the dialysis machine.

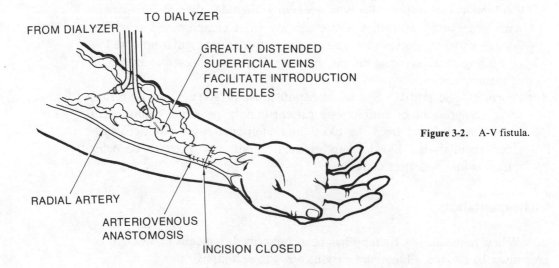

FROM DIALYZER   TO DIALYZER

GREATLY DISTENDED
SUPERFICIAL VEINS
FACILITATE INTRODUCTION
OF NEEDLES

RADIAL ARTERY

ARTERIOVENOUS
ANASTOMOSIS

INCISION CLOSED

Figure 3-2. A-V fistula.

Graft. Another means of obtaining vascular access is through surgical placement of a graft. A graft can be either a synthetic material, i.e., polytetrafluoroethylene or Dacron, or an inert vessel from cattle, i.e., bovine. The grafts are available in various sizes and have the advantage of being able to be used soon after insertion.

Femoral Vein Dialysis. This is sometimes used in the critical care setting when *immediate* access to the bloodstream is required. A catheter is inserted into the femoral vein and connected to the blood tubing on the machine, using a **Y** connector, and thus creating a venous and arterial access. A special accessory pump is used to facilitate blood flow through the dialyzer, thereby avoiding admixing of blood. Opinion varies as to how long this catheter should be left in place; however, as a rule, 72 hours is generally acceptable. The catheter must be kept patent between dialysis treatments by constant or intermittent infusion of a heparinized saline solution and kept secure by sterile protective dressings. The cannulated leg should be assessed frequently for circulatory compromise, hematoma formation, and catheter position. The patient is usually kept on bedrest.

Subclavian Catheters. Subclavian catheterization has been used for many years in medical therapy, e.g., fluid and medication administration, total parenteral nutrition, and invasive monitoring. With the advent of specially designed catheters, e.g., Shiley, Sorenson, access placement for short-term hemodialysis can be easily and safely accomplished via the subclavian route.

These catheters are available in either a single lumen or dual lumens. Depending on the type of catheter, a special accessory switching device may be needed. Further description of how this switching device functions can be found under related equipment in "Fluid Delivery Systems."

After the catheter is inserted per established protocol, the catheter itself should be secured either through the use of a special dressing, e.g., Op Site, or by skin sutures, and a chest film should be obtained *immediately* to confirm proper placement *prior to* initiation of dialysis. The catheter should be kept patent per physician's orders, e.g., IV fluid administration or heparinized saline administration by either constant or intermittent flush.

DIALYSERS/ARTIFICIAL KIDNEYS

There are three major types of artificial kidneys now in use (Fig. 3–3).

Parallel Plate. Sheets of cellophane membrane are placed in double layers like sandwiches and then placed between supporting plates. The plates are constructed so that the dialysate fluid can flow over the outside of the membrane, with the blood flowing between the cellophane layers. The parallel plate dialyzer operates on the principle of countercurrent flow—blood flows in one direction and dialysate flows in the opposite direction.

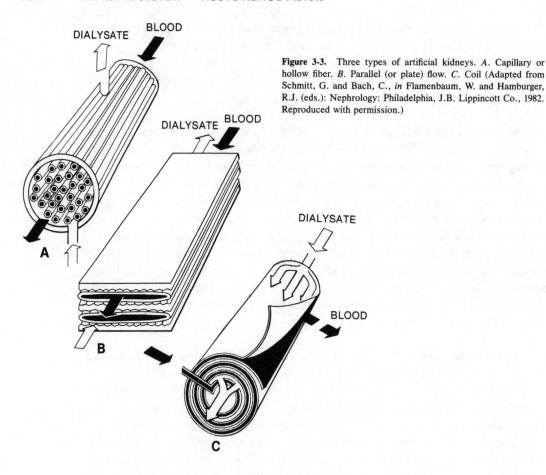

Figure 3-3. Three types of artificial kidneys. *A.* Capillary or hollow fiber. *B.* Parallel (or plate) flow. *C.* Coil (Adapted from Schmitt, G. and Bach, C., *in* Flamenbaum, W. and Hamburger, R.J. (eds.): Nephrology: Philadelphia, J.B. Lippincott Co., 1982. Reproduced with permission.)

Hollow Fiber.   This utilizes between 10,000 and 20,000 tiny hollow cellulose or Cuprophan fibers through which the blood flows, with the dialysate fluid surrounding the fibers. This type of dialyzer also utilizes countercurrent flow.

Coil.   This is composed of a long, flat envelope of cellulose tubing that is concentrically wound with a mesh supporting screen around a central core; bath fluid is pumped at a high flow rate through the support screen in a direction 90 degrees to that of the blood flow.

Hemoperfusion Biocompatible Cartridge.   This special cartridge, similar in appearance to a hollow fiber artificial kidney, is used on patients with drug overdose. The procedure is accomplished by dialysis personnel, using a dialysis machine. Many drugs have large, fat-soluble or protein-bound molecules that hemodialysis does not remove efficiently. Biocompatible hemoperfusion is often more effective.

Hemoperfusion is a process utilizing a special biocompatible cartridge *in place of* of an artificial kidney. It removes substances from the body, involving an extracorporeal blood pathway, but without dialysis solution. The cartridge contains an activated carbon adsorbent treated to preferentially adsorb toxins while allowing formed elements of the blood to pass through without hemodialysis. Heparinization and clotting time monitoring are necessary.

FLUID DELIVERY SYSTEMS

Essentially, all hemodialysis machines have similar basic components (Fig. 3-4). The purpose of the machine is to monitor and control the extracorporeal (blood pathway) circuit and the dialysate flow circuit. Various components may be integrated into the machine, e.g., blood flow pump or heparin pump, or they may be added equipment.

Each hemodialysis machine contains several monitoring systems (Fig. 3–5).

1. The extracorporeal circuit contains:
    A. Blood leak detector, which monitors outflowing dialysate for the presence of blood.
    B. Blood line pressure monitors, which measure the pressure in the extracorporeal circuit.
    C. Air leak detector, which monitors the presence of air or microbubbles in the extracorporeal circuit. This may be a photocell or an ultrasonic mechanism.

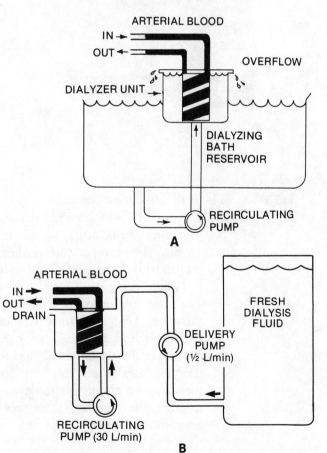

Figure 3-4. Fluid delivery system basic components. *A,* Total recirculating system used with coil dialyzer. *B,* Recirculating single-pass system with separate fluid supply. (Adapted from Gutch, C.F., and Stoner, M.H.: Review of Hemodialysis for Nurses and Dialysis Personnel, 4th ed. St. Louis, C.V. Mosby, 1984. Reproduced by permisssion.)

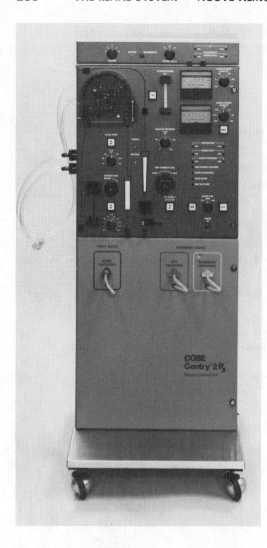

Figure 3-5. Dialysis control unit. (Courtesy of Cobe Laboratories, Inc.)

2. The dialysate circuit contains:
   A. Power "off," which monitors the failure of power to the machine.
   B. Dialysate temperature, which monitors the temperature of the dialysate. The temperature of the dialysate should be the normal body temperature; temperatures over 41°C (105°F.) may cause hemolysis and could be fatal.
   C. Dialysate conductivity, which monitors the ion concentration in the dialysate. Dialysis against hypotonic or hypertonic solutions produces hemolysis and cerebral and cardiac symptoms and may result in death. It should be noted that if either the temperature or conductivity violates preset limits, the machine will go into "bypass." This mode diverts the dialysate down the drain instead of having it flow through the dialyzer, thus preventing contact between blood and dangerous dialysate.

RELATED EQUIPMENT

Related equipment includes various types of mechanical equipment used for the hemodialysis treatment, such as:

Blood Pump. The blood must be circulated through the dialyzer at a given rate; without adequate blood flow, effective dialysis is not accomplished. Acceptable blood flow rates for adults average 150 to 250 ml./minute. The blood pump is usually placed on the arterial blood line side and is regulated by a variable speed control knob. All blood pumps should have a handle or some means by which manual circulation of the blood pump can be accomplished in the event of a power outage.

Heparin Infusion Pump. This device delivers heparin through the arterial side of the blood line at a constant fixed rate. Most of these pumps operate with a 30-ml. syringe and deliver heparin in milliliters (or fractions of) per hour.

Single-Access Machine/"Switcher." This device is used in addition to the blood pump when a single access (i.e., subclavian catheter) is used for hemodialysis. Single-access dialysis is characterized by a rhythmic, pulsatile blood flow through the dialyzer circuit. When the arterial clamp is opened (inflow of blood) the venous clamp (outflow of blood) closes, and vice versa. Single-access dialysis is controlled through settings of time, pressure, or combination of the two.

There are numerous single-access switchers available on the market. It will be necessary to refer to the manufacturer's recommendations for:
1. Proper use, setup procedure, and monitoring instructions.
2. Proper interfacing with the dialysis delivery system in use.
3. Need for single-access blood tubing.

Water Source. Concentrations of salts and minerals, e.g., sodium, calcium, and magnesium, vary geographically, and when these elements are present in high concentrations, water treatment may be necessary. State health departments conduct routine surveillance programs, and their analyses can be the basis for deciding what means are needed to treat the water and make it safe for dialysis. Some of these means are softening, filtration, distillation, deionization, and reverse osmosis. Periodic bacterialogical studies should also be obtained.

Electrical Power. Familiarity with the manufacturer's recommendations regarding the power source for the machine is of high priority. Correct voltage must be used to prevent overload to the circuitry as well as damage to the equipment. Also, it is necessary to ground the machine, especially when accessory equipment draws its power from the machine itself. When initiating hemodialysis, determine the closest emergency power outlet in case it becomes necessary to switch to emergency circuitry.

INITIATING HEMODIALYSIS: CANNULA COUPLING WITH BLOOD PUMP _____

Objectives

1. To obtain entrance to the patient's bloodstream by the established blood access.
2. To ensure safe, aseptic initiation of hemodialysis.

Special Equipment

Basin
Masks
Normal saline solution, 1000-ml. bag
1-inch paper and tape and ½-inch plastic tape
Sterile gauze pads
Sterile gloves
Linen saver
Cup with alcohol to soak blood tubing caps
Alcohol prep pads
Monitor lines (may be incorporated in manufacturer's blood tubing)
Cannula connector–Teflon connector
Cannula separators
Hemostats
"Bulldogs" or cannula clamps
IV administration set (macrodrip)

Procedure

ACTION	RATIONALE
1. Obtain and record patient's temperature, pulse, blood pressure, and weight.	1. This provides baseline information on the patient's condition.
2. Position patient comfortably in bed and make sure that blood lines are at same level as the bed.	2. This facilitates blood flow through machine and dialyzer, thereby not flowing against gravity.
3. Don mask and wash hands thoroughly.	3. This prevents infection of patient's cannula and prevents cross contamination between patients.
4. Don sterile gloves.	4. This protects one from blood contamination.

ACTION	RATIONALE
5. Place sterile gauze pads under cannula connection point and surrounding area of extremity.	5. This provides a sterile field when cannulas are disconnected.
6. Cleanse cannula connection with alcohol prep pad.	6. This decreases the possibility of contamination.
7. Clamp cannulas. A. Clamp arterial cannula with cannula clamp. B. Then clamp venous cannula with cannula clamp.	7. This prevents accidental separation due to arterial pressure, stops cannula blood flow, and prevents any blood loss.
8. Separate cannulas with cannula separator.	
9. Draw predialysis blood for analysis, as prescribed.	
10. Insert sterile Teflon connector into ends of both arterial and venous cannulas.	10. This accommodates the blood lines of the machine.
11. Cleanse end of arterial cannula with alcohol prep pad and connect to arterial blood line of machine.	
12. Place end of venous line into sterile basin.	12. This allows the saline solution in the dialyzer and lines to flow out of the venous line into the basin.
13. Remove all clamps. A. Begin with clamp at venous blood line. B. Then proceed to clamp on arterial line. C. Finally, remove clamp on arterial cannula.	13. This allows free flow of blood through the extracorporeal blood circuit.
14. Turn on blood pump, set at rate of 100 ml./minute.	14. A slow rate prevents symptoms of rapid fluid loss from the patient and also allows for assessment of the blood flow rate from the arterial cannula.
15. Instill heparin prime as blood enters the arterial chamber.	15. This prevents coagulation of the blood within the dialyzer.
16. Turn off blood pump and clamp venous blood line at basin when saline in venous drip bulb is light pink.	16. This prevents blood loss from the cannula and dialyzer.

ACTION	RATIONALE
17. Cleanse end of venous cannula with alcohol prep pad; attach end of venous blood line to venous cannula.	17. This completes the extracorporeal circuit.
18. Remove clamps: A. From venous blood line. B. From venous cannulas.	18. This allows free flow of blood through the circuit.
19. Turn on blood pump. Gradually increase rate to acceptable blood flow rate.	
20. Tape cannula connections securely and tape blood tubings to patient's extremity.	20. This prevents accidental separation of connections during dialysis.
21. Record initiation time of hemodialysis.	
22. Monitor patient's vital signs; assess effect of initial therapy on patient.	

Precautions

1. Ascertain patient's hepatitis status before dialysis is initiated and monthly thereafter while undergoing maintenance dialysis. If an HAA-positive patient is placed on the machine unknowingly, the virus may be transmitted to the internal workings of the machine and may then be passed on to another patient. In some institutions the machine is then considered to be contaminated and should be used only for the dialysis of HAA-positive patients. Minimize the possibility of hepatitis spread by proper hand washing between patients, wearing of clean gloves when in contact with blood, restricting eating or drinking within the unit, and by careful disposal of all needles and equipment.
2. Avoid inadvertent contamination when dialyzing a patient who is critically ill or immunosuppressed by utilizing sterile technique.
3. Observe for initial untoward effects that may be due to:
   A. Initial hypovolemia resulting from filling dialyzer (the amount of blood required to fill the dialyzer varies; it averages between 90 and 200 ml., depending upon the type of dialyzer used).
   B. Removal of metabloic waste products.
   C. Electrolyte shifts.

Related Care

1. Prior to heparinization, obtain a baseline clotting time to assess individual needs. Procedures for clotting times may differ from area to area. Generally speaking, a baseline clotting time should be obtained before dialysis. Thereafter, clotting times should be determined as often as neces-

sary to adjust heparin dosage to maintain safe coagulation status of the patient and prevent clotting of the dialyzer. Methods of obtaining clotting times are Lee-White clotting times (LWCT), activated clotting times (ACT) and whole blood partial thromboplastin times (WBPTT). The LWCT method is infrequently used in many dialysis units. Currently two methods are popular, the ACT and WBPTT, with the WBPTT gaining in popularity. With these two methods, a clotting time of 1 minute 30 seconds obtained is considered safe and acceptable for hemodialysis.

2. Methods for heparinization.

A. Constant: Most patients receive a "prime" or loading dose based on body weight and clotting status at the initiation of dialysis and may then receive 500 to 1000 units/hour by infusion.

B. Low dose: Usually 500 to 1000 units/hour is used, which is important in the patient with bleeding difficulties. In some cases, heparin is not used.

C. Regional: Protamine, a neutralizing agent for heparin, may be prescribed for infusion into the venous side of the blood tubing to decrease the patient's clotting time in the presence of a bleeding problem. This method may not be used as frequently as the low dose method.

3. Facilitate the removal of waste products, add selected substances, and prevent the removal of desired substances with the proper dialysate.

A. Two types of dialysate delivery systems are widely used.

(1) Proportioning system: This requires the use of a liquid concentrate that can be purchased commercially or mixed by personnel. Through the use of a proportioning pump operated by various devices, tap water and concentrate are constantly mixed at a specified dilution rate.

(2) Batch system: A given volume of dailyzing fluid is premixed at a certain concentration and stored in tanks from 100 to 300 liters or more in size.

B. A standard dialysate composition may be:

SUBSTANCE	CONCENTRATION (mEq./liter)
Total sodium	140.0
Sodium chloride	97.0
Sodium acetate	38.0
Calcium chloride	3.0
Magnesium chloride	1.0
Potassium chloride	Adjusted according to patient's own serum potassium level

Alterations to dialysate may include sodium bicarbonate substituted for sodium acetate for the acidotic patient who would profit from immediate buffering as soon as dialysis is initiated. Dextrose, as an additive, helps maintain the patient's serum glucose level, which is especially important in the diabetic patient. It also helps prevent the symptoms of rapid fluid removal, i.e., muscle cramps and nausea.

4. Assess the patency of the cannula by determining the blood flow rate. This procedure must be done when blood tubing is out of the blood pump and is to be done at the beginning and at the end of dialysis, or anytime in between if flow appears to be altered. An ideal blood flow rate is 150 to 250 ml./minute. This measurement is made by timing the progress of an air bubble through a 50-cm. length of tubing specifically marked on the blood line. An ideal bubble time is 2.0 to 3.0 seconds. The length of dialysis may need to be extended beyond the usual 2½ to 4 hours if inadequate blood flow rates are obtained. Factors affecting blood flow include condition of cannula, blood pressure, and cardiac output. Also consult manufacturer's information, since flow rates are dependent upon the lumen size of the blood tubing.

5. Understand the principle of ultrafiltration. Ultrafiltration is the removal of excess water from the patient's blood, using both positive and negative pressure exerted across the semipermeable membrane. Formulas are available to calculate fluid removal, thus predicting and providing control of fluid loss.

6. Use sequential ultrafiltration (SUF) to remove large amounts of water quickly without causing symptoms of rapid ultrafiltration, i.e., muscle cramps, nausea, vomiting, hypotension. SUF can be done alone or in tandem with dialysis. If necessary, dialysis follows SUF because clearance of electrolytes and uremic waste products does not happen while the fluid is being removed. After the extracorporeal circuit is filled with blood and the dialysate pathway is filled, dialysate is diverted away from the artificial kidney. Pressure is then exerted on the blood pathway in the artificial kidney to force fluid out of the blood and into the dailysate compartment. This process requires either additional equipment or a specially designed fluid delivery system. Accurate weights are important for these patients.

Complications

Altered integrity of vascular access
Emboli
Hepatitis
Infection
Disequilibrium syndrome
Mechanical complications
Hypovolemia
Heparin allergy

MONITORING HEMODIALYSIS _____

Objectives

1. To assess patient status during prescribed hemodialysis therapy to determine tolerance for procedure.
2. To ascertain equipment performance and take corrective action, as needed.

Special Equipment

Stopwatch
Gloves
Hemastix
Normal saline solution, 1000 ml
IV administration set (macrodrip)
Flow sheets

Syringes with needles
Needle discard receptacle
Alcohol prep pads
Equipment for testing
    clotting times

Procedure

ACTION	RATIONALE
1. Infuse heparin, as prescribed.	1. This maintains adequate blood flow through the dialyzer and prevents clotting.
2. Instill air into each drip chamber to displace blood approximately ½ inch below top of chamber.	2. This allows visualization of blood flow rate into drip chambers, maintains patency of monitor lines, and provides accurate pressure reading.
3. Connect monitor lines on both arterial and venous drip bulbs, as specified by manufacturer.	3. This establishes mechanism for reading pressures.
4. Set alarm parameters.	4. This detects pressure changes.
5. Set air bubble detector mechanism on venous drip chamber (may be photocell or ultrasonic device).	5. This provides a means to detect air in the system and prevent air embolus to the patient.
6. Hemastix the dialysate outflow.	6. This ensures operation of blood leak detector and detects blood leaks within the dialyzer.

ACTION	RATIONALE
7. Perform initial machine check and document on log sheet (includes checking of monitoring system).	7. This establishes baseline of machine functioning and assesses functioning of alarm system.
8. Assess patient; record vital signs on log sheet.	8 This establishes baseline tolerance level of patient to the initial volume depletion.
9. Obtain clotting times and record on clotting log.	
10. Gradually begin to increase negative pressure, if prescribed.	10. This prevents rupture in the membrane of artificial kidney, achieves ultrafiltration, and prevents sudden hypotension.
11. Place 1000 ml. of normal saline with macrodrip tubing on an IV pole and connect to saline input line.	11. This will treat hypotension immediately and may be used to discontinue dialysis quickly, if necessary.

Precautions

1. Keep cannula clamps (smooth surfaced and without teeth) on cannula dressing at all times. In case of accidental separation, these must be used on the Silastic cannulas, as opposed to hemostats, to avoid puncturing cannulas.
2. Keep two hemostats available at all times. In an emergency (e.g., air embolus, clots in blood line returning to patient, or failure of bypass mechanism) these must be used on the blood line tubing. Note: Keep scissors in separate place away from hemostats to avoid inadvertent use in an emergency.

Related Care

1. Check the machine and assess the patient (including clotting times) at least every hour (or more frequently, if warranted).
2. Monitor the patient's response to the hemodialysis therapy. The following are possible causes of hemodialysis intolerance:
   A. Rapid blood flow rate in a patient with known cardiac disease.
   B. Myocardial oxygen deprivation.
   C. Electrolyte shifts, especially sodium and potassium.
   D. Initial hypovolemia.
   E. Air infusion during fluid administration.
   F. Blood line separation or dialyzer leak or rupture.
   G. Excess ultrafiltration.
   H. Pyrogenic reaction.

    I.   Too rapid return of blood at termination of dialysis.

    J.   Disequilibrium syndrome.

    K. Improper heparinization.

    L.   Transfusion reaction if receiving blood.

    M. Muscle cramps.

    N. Nausea, vomiting.

3. Support blood pressure, as prescribed by physician. The following may be used to treat hypotension or support the blood pressure or both.:

    A. Normal saline.

    B. Plasmanate/albumin.

    C. Blood.

    D. Vasopressors.

    E. Mannitol.

    F. 50% Dextrose (for diabetics).

4. Administer medications, as prescribed, via the venous blood line or a designated blood port.

5. Identify equipment malfunction. When a monitoring system is violated, prompt intervention is necessary to insure patient safety.

6. Monitor the patient's response to heparin. There are special blood ports or rubber sleeves on the arterial and venous blood lines; these are used to draw blood from the machine. For regional dialysis, blood is drawn from the arterial sleeve for the patient's clotting time, while blood drawn from the venous sleeve (before protamine infusion) is considered to be for the machine's clotting time.

Complications

Angina	Hemolysis
Dysrhythmia	Fever/chills
Air embolus	Headache
Exsanguination	Convulsion
Hypotension	Pruritus
Shortness of breath	Clotting in dialyzer

TERMINATING HEMODIALYSIS: CANNULA UNCOUPLING USING SALINE/AIR RINSE _____

Objectives

1. To conclude hemodialysis safely and to return the blood within the extracorporeal system to the patient.

2. To reestablish blood flow through cannulas.
3. To assess patient's status after hemodialysis therapy.

Special Equipment

Masks
Normal saline solution,
    1000-ml. bag
1-inch paper tape and ½-inch plastic
    tape
Sterile gauze pads
Sterile gloves
Linen saver
Alcohol prep pads
Cannula connector–Teflon
    connector or cannula infusion **T** or both
Cannula separators
Hemostats
"Bulldogs" or cannula clamps
IV administration set (macrodrip)

Procedure

ACTION	RATIONALE
1. Reduce negative pressure to zero.	1. This minimizes blood volume in dialyzer.
2. Drape venous blood line on bed.	2. This allows visualization of all tubing as rinse progresses.
3. Don mask.	
4. Remove dressings and tape; expose cannula connection sites; preserve integrity of blood tubing system.	
5. Don gloves.	
6. Place sterile gauze pads under connection points of tubing.	6. This provides a sterile field for separated cannulas.
7. Cleanse arterial connection with alcohol prep pad.	
8. Turn off blood pump and clamp arterial cannula and arterial blood line tubing.	8. This prevents blood loss when cannulas are separated.
9. Use separating forceps to separate arterial tubing from cannula.	

ACTION	RATIONALE
10. Connect IV line of normal saline solution to arterial tubing. Open clamps on saline line and arterial tubing. *Note*: Arterial cannula stays clamped.	
11. Turn on blood pump at rate of 100 ml./minute until prescribed amount (approximately 150 to 200 ml.) of saline is infused.	11. This initiates saline rinse of blood tubing.
12. Turn off blood pump and clamp arterial blood tubing and saline line.	
13. Disconnect saline tubing from arterial blood tubing.	
14. Open clamp on arterial blood tubing and turn blood pump on at 100 ml./minute.	14. This initiates air rinse of blood tubing, which maximizes return of red blood cells to the patient.
15. Return blood to patient until air reaches air detector alarm in venous drip chamber.	
16. Turn off blood pump and clamp venous blood tubing and then venous cannula.	
17. Cleanse venous connection with alcohol prep pad; separate tubing.	
18. Insert Teflon connector or infusion-**T** halfway into venous cannula; attach arterial cannula over exposed area of connector and remove clamps from venous and then arterial cannulas.	
19. Tape connection securely.	
20. Perform cannula site care.	
21. Remove all needles, syringes, and traces of blood from machine and work area; dispose of in safe manner, as required by institution.	21. This prevents possible spread of hepatitis.
22. Obtain postdialysis weight, pulse, temperature, and blood pressure.	22. This determines the efficiency of dialysis in regard to weight loss and patient's tolerance of procedure.

Precaution

Avoid any interruptions or distractions during termination procedure.

Related Care

1. Assess cannula and site at frequent intervals after terminating hemodialysis.
2. Perform cannula and site care (see the next procedure, "Hemodialysis Cannula and Site Care").

Complications

Air embolus	Hemorrhage
Infection	Cannula displacement

Supplier

Cobe Laboratories, Inc.

HEMODIALYSIS CANNULA AND SITE CARE _____

Objectives

1. To promote integrity of cannula by monitoring and maintaining adequate blood flow through cannulas and protecting from trauma or accidental separation.
2. To assess and clean exit sites to prevent or detect infection.

Special Equipment

Masks	Sterile gauze pads
Soap and water	Povidone-iodine ointment
Hydrogen peroxide solution (3%)	Tape
Sterile cotton swabs	Sterile flexible gauze roll
Alcohol prep pads	Telfa pads, if necessary

Procedure

ACTION	RATIONALE

1. Mask all persons in immediate area.

2. Remove dressing; expose site.

ACTION	RATIONALE

3. Assess cannula site for:
  A. Secure connections.
  B. Proper alignment, no tension at sites.
  C. Absence of infection at sites.
  D. Absence of hematoma or clotting problems.
	
	D. Dark blood in cannula indicates first stage of clotting. Granular appearance of blood indicates second stage of clotting. Syneresis, an indication of the third stage of clotting, shows separation of blood with clot and clear plasma observed within the cannula.

4. Cleanse extremity with soap and water; rinse and dry well. Carefully lift cannulas to do this, but do not wash within immediate area of the exit sites.	4. This avoids contamination of exit sites with skin bacteria.

5. Cleanse each exit site with hydrogen peroxide and sterile cotton swabs.
  A. Start at exit site.
  B. Work outward to cover immediate area. Do not go over cleansed area with used applicator stick.
	5. This cleanses and gently removes crusts around exit sites.
	
	B. This prevents cross contamination from one exit site to another.

6. Dry exit site with cotton swabs, using same technique as in step 5.	6. Dampness predisposes the patient to infection.

7. Cleanse both arterial and venous cannula tubing with alcohol prep pad.
  A. Start at exit site.
  B. Work toward the connection.
	7.
	
	B. This prevents contamination of exit sites.

8. Apply povidone-iodine to exit sites, if prescribed.	8. This prevents infection and provides a seal at exit sites.
9. Place a sterile gauze pad over exit sites, touching only side that will be away from skin. (If there is any drainage or bleeding from exit sites, use Telfa on sites first.)	9. This protects exit sites.
10. Place second sterile gauze pad over cannulas, allowing only a small loop of cannula to be exposed.	10. This allows for ease in assessing cannula for signs of clotting.

ACTION	RATIONALE
11. Secure sterile gauze pads to skin with paper tape; do not encircle extremity with tape.	11. This avoids constriction, which may lead to clot formation.
12. Wrap area with soft, flexible gauze roll, in such a way that dressing is secure but not constrictive; tape end of roll in place.	12. This insures padding and protection of cannula.
13. Put cannula clamps on dressing.	13. This allows for immediate access at all times in case of accidental separation.

Precautions

1. Restrict blood pressure determinations on cannulated extremity.
2. Restrict blood drawings or vascular invasive procedures on cannulated extremity above cannulas.
3. Restrict use of constricting device on cannulated extremity over or above cannula.
4. Wash hands well before handling cannulas.

Related Care

1. Perform cannula care every 24 hours, or if dressing becomes soiled or wet, or if exit sites have been exposed (e.g., after dialysis, after inspection of cannulas).
2. Draw blood from the cannula and administer medications via a heparin infusion-**T** that can be inserted into the cannula. Connectors may, however, increase the chance of the cannula clotting, as a result of its small lumen.

Complications

Infection
Disconnection
Clotting

CANNULA DECLOTTING _____

Objectives

1. To reinstate integrity of cannula by removing the blood clot that is obstructing the blood flow through the cannula.
2. To assess the rate of blood flow after declotting.

Special Equipment

Masks
Sterile gloves
Sterile drapes
Sterile gauze pads
Linen protectors
Syringes
Cannula aspirators
Sterile Teflon pliers or hemostat
1-inch paper tape and ½-inch plastic tape
500 ml. normal saline
Heparin 1000 units/ml.
Povidone-iodine solution
Cannula clamps
Sterile cannula separators
Sterile flexible gauze roll
Cannula infusion-**T** or cannula connector
Sterile basin
Sterile pitcher

Procedure

ACTION	RATIONALE
1. Assess circulatory status of the cannulated extremity for presence of pulses, temperature, and color and presence or absence of pain. Notify physician of any compromise in circulation before the declotting procedure.	1. The assessment provides baseline data for evaluating effects of the declotting.
2. Assess patient's weight and postural vital signs.	2. These factors will help determine cause of cannula clotting.
3. Heat normal saline in a pan of hot water to body temperature.	3. Normal saline is warmed to body temperature to avoid venospasm from cool solution or hemolysis from hot solution.
4. Don mask.	4. Mask is worn to avoid contamination of the cannula exit sites.
5. Remove all cannula dressings, tape tabs, and bridge. Place linen protectors under extremity.	

ACTION	RATIONALE
6. Place sterile gauze pads in sterile basin and cover with povidone-iodine solution.	
7. Pour warm sterile saline into sterile pitcher and add heparin as ordered.	
8. Don sterile gloves.	8. This is to protect the nurse from blood contamination.
9. Prep cannulated extremity and cannula with povidone-iodine–soaked gauze pads for 5 minutes, including all surfaces of the extremity and hand or foot.	9. This disinfects all areas that may be exposed during procedure.
10. Place extremity on sterile drape when prepping is complete.	
11. Don a new set of sterile gloves and continue to place sterile drapes around extremity, including hand or foot. Leave only cannula bodies exposed.	11. This provides a sterile field for declotting, which is considered a sterile procedure.
12. Use cannula separator to gently separate cannulas. Use a sterile gauze pad to remove any clot extending from the cannulas. Use Teflon pliers or hemostat to remove cannula connector.	12. Gentle separation helps keep any clot intact for easier removal.
13. Fill syringe and cannula aspirator with warm heparinized saline solution. Attach aspirator to arterial cannula. Aspirate for clots. Repeated attempts may be necessary.	13. Attempts are made to declot the arterial cannula first because it is usually easier to declot. The venous cannula is more often the cause of clotting. Also, arterial pressure will assist with aspirating pressure to dislodge the clot into the aspirator and syringe.
14. Evaluate declotting of arterial cannula with aspirator. If cannula remains clotted, attach the polyethylene declotting tubing to a syringe and fill it with heparinized saline. Insert polyethylene tubing into the cannula and aspirate clots.	14. The polyethylene tubing fits inside the cannula and can get close to the clot for more secure attachment.
15. Evaluate blood flow from the arterial cannula; then irrigate cannula gently and slowly with heparinized saline; clamp cannula.	15. Unless the cannula is flushed completely with saline, it will reclot immediately.

ACTION	RATIONALE
16. Attach polyethylene tubing to a syringe and fill with heparinized saline. Insert polyethylene tubing into venous cannula and aspirate for clots. Repeated attempts may be necessary.	16. An attempt to declot the venous cannula by means of direct connected aspiration is avoided to prevent collapse of the vein by pulling it in a direction opposite to the blood flow.
17. Evaluate declotting of venous cannula. If the cannula appears free of clots, fill it with heparinized saline via polyethylene tubing.	17. A backflow from the declotted venous cannula is not necessarily obtained.
18. Attach aspirator and syringe filled with warmed heparinized saline to the venous cannula. Irrigate venous cannula several times. *Note*: Before irrigating the vein, be sure that all the clots are removed. Note that clots may be located in the cannula tip or vessel beyond the reach of the polyethylene tubing.	18. Warmed irrigation solution helps relax venous spasm. Evaluate ease of injection of solution to determine cannula patency.
19. Reattach cannulas, if both are patent, using heparin **T** or Teflon connector as ordered.	
20. Apply heparin lock to patent cannula if the opposite cannula is still clotted. Obtain orders for strength of heparin solution and frequency of injection.	20. A patent cannula needs to be flushed with heparin saline solution or it will immediately clot.
21. Apply empty sterile syringe to end of clotted cannula.	
22. Redress cannula.	
23. Reassess circulatory status of extremity.	
24. Record procedure in chart and notify physician of results of cannula declotting, resultant blood flow, vital signs, weight and any other factors that may have contributed to cannula clotting.	

Precautions

1. Avoid dislodging clots or introducing air into cannulated vessels during declotting.

2. Do not clamp clotted cannulas prior to separating them during declotting. This aids in easier removal of the clot in its entirety. However, the cannula must be observed carefully throughout the procedure for the need to clamp off blood flow.
3. Gently handle infected cannulas to prevent dislodgement and spread of infection.
4. Do not inject into the clotted arterial cannulas as the clot may be dislodged into the arterial circulation and result in blockage of circulation to the extremity distal to the cannula.
5. Do not irrigate either cannula if there is any uncertainty that all the clot has been removed.

Related Care

1. Observe hypotensive patient's cannulas hourly for signs of clotting, cool temperature and separation of blood and serum.
2. Notify the physician of patients undergoing dialysis whose blood flow is slow. A heparin **T** may need to be inserted into their cannulas after dialysis and systemic intermittent heparinization begun to maintain cannula patency, or a cannula revision may be indicated. In any event, their cannulas need to be observed frequently for signs of clotting.
3. Teach patients to not wear watches, bracelets, or tight sleeves on their cannula arms as these will restrict blood flow. They must not be allowed to lie lie on their cannulated arm or leg.
4. Perform daily cannula care to provide a time for observation and to prevent infection.

Complications

Hemorrhage	Air embolus
Exit site infection	Septicemia
Clot embolus	

INITIATING HEMODIALYSIS: SUBCLAVIAN CATHETER COUPLING

Overview

The single-lumen subclavian catheter is used to provide temporary vascular access for hemodialysis. The end of the catheter used to connect the catheter to the blood lines is in a **Y** configuration. This **Y** connection provides the means to hook up to the arterial and venous blood tubing to complete the extracorporeal circuit. A switcher device is then necessary to provide for the cyclic flow of blood through the dialyzer circuit.

Objective

To initiate hemodialysis therapy, using a single-lumen subclavian catheter as temporary vascular access.

Special Equipment

Sterile gauze pads
Povidone-iodine solution
Alcohol prep pads
10-ml. syringes (3)
Bulldog clamps (2)
Heparin prime (as ordered by physician)
Clean gloves (1 pair)
Masks (2)
Switcher*
Normal saline solution for IV administration, 1000-ml. bag; heparinized
    (heparin 1000 units/ml.; heparin, 4 ml./1000 ml.)
IV administration set

---

*Prior to the beginning of the couping procedure, the fluid delivery system and switcher must be set up according to established procedure.

Procedure

ACTION	RATIONALE
1. Wash hands thoroughly.	1. Careful hand washing is essential to prevent the spread of infection.
2. Place the patient in the Trendelenburg position.	2. This position minimizes the danger of air embolism when the catheter is opened.
3. Open a package of sterile gauze pads and saturate them with povidone-iodine solution.	
4. Clamp both sides of the subclavian catheter with bulldog clamps. *Do not use hemostats.*	4. Hemostats have teeth that cut the Silastic tubing. Bulldogs are smooth.
5. Remove the tape from the injection cap connections from both sides of the **Y**.	

ACTION	RATIONALE
6. Place a protective linen saver under the catheter and sterile gauze pads under the catheter connections.	
7. Don mask. The patient, if able, should also don a mask. If not, simply ask the patient to turn away from the catheter.	7. Masks help to control the spread of infection.
8. Don clean gloves.	
9. Wipe the injection caps over the **Y** connections thoroughly with the povidone-iodine–soaked sterile gauze pads.	
10. Wrap the remaining sterile gauze pad around the injection caps and let them soak for 2 minutes.	10. A 2-minute soak with the povidone-iodine solution is considered adequate in terms of disinfecting the area before the blood tubing is attached.
11. Unwrap the sterile gauze pad from the arterial side. Remove the cap from the arterial side and attach a 10-ml. syringe. Remove clamps, aspirate (and discard if clots present, then reaspirate), and flush the catheter.	11. Always aspirate first to ensure catheter patency.
12. Unwrap the soaked sterile gauze from the venous side. Remove injection cap and attach a 10-ml. syringe with the heparin prime. Unclamp, aspirate, inject and reclamp.	12. This provides systemic heparinization.
13. Remove the syringe from the arterial side of the catheter. Make sure that the arterial side of the catheter is securely clamped.	
14. Recheck the tubing for air bubbles and connect the arterial blood line to the arterial side of the catheter.	14. This prevents air embolus.
15. Place blood lines in the switcher and initiate single-access dialysis per established procedure.	15. This alternates blood flow through the venous and arterial sides of the access.
16. Turn on the blood pump to 100 ml./minute.	16. This starts blood moving through circuit.

ACTION	RATIONALE
17. Stop the blood pump and clamp the venous blood line when the blood has displaced the saline in the dialyzer.	
18. Remove the syringe from the venous side of the catheter.	
19. Inspect the venous blood line for air bubbles.	
20. Connect the venous blood line to the venous side of the subclavian catheter.	20. This completes the coupling.
21. Remove all clamps, turn on the blood pump, set all single-access settings as per established procedure.	
22. Tape *all* connections securely.	22. It is very important to minimize the danger of line separation.
23. Complete routine charting procedures, and record in the patient's chart.	

Precaution

Minimize recirculation or admixing of blood by following the procedures carefully. Recirculation or admixing of blood (10% to 24%) occurs because of the alternating of flows in common areas, e.g., access tubing, blood vessel, compliant blood lines. This results in decreased efficiency of dialysis, e.g., decreased clearances (BUN, creatinine).

Related Care

1. Understand transmembrane pressure (TMP). This is the total pressure (both positive and negative) exerted across a semipermeable membrane. Fluid loss is calculated by means of the following formula:

   UFF* x TMP = ml. to be removed/hr. x hrs. prescribed for dialysis
   = total ml. to be removed - anticipated oral and IV intake during dialysis
   = actual fluid loss

   This can be altered to some degree. Include any fluid prime or saline rinse.

2. Understand stroke volume (SV). SV is the volume of blood exchange per cycle. For adequate dialysis, the SV must be 6 ml. or greater. SV is calculated by counting the number of cycles in 1 minute and dividing that number into the blood pump speed.

_____

*Ultrafiltration factor of particular dialyzer used.

Complications

Emboli	Disequilibrium syndrome
Hepatitis	Medical complications
Catheter dislodgment/	Hypovolemia
displacement	Heparin allergy
Infection	

TERMINATING HEMODIALYSIS: SUBCLAVIAN CATHETER UNCOUPLING _____

Objective

To terminate hemodialysis therapy using a single-lumen subclavian catheter as temporary vascular access.

Special Equipment

Sterile gauze pads	Masks (2)
Povidone-iodine solution	Sterile disposable injection caps (2)
Alcohol prep pads	Normal saline solution for IV administration
Bulldog clamps	IV administration set
Clean gloves (1 pair)	

Procedure

ACTION	RATIONALE
1. Place the patient in the Trendelenburg position.	1. This position minimizes the danger of air embolism when the catheter is opened.
2. Open a package of sterile gauze pads and saturate them with povidone-iodine solution.	
3. Don clean gloves and mask. If able, the patient should also don a mask.	
4. Turn off the negative pressure if negative pressure is being applied.	

ACTION	RATIONALE
5. Turn off the blood pump and set all single-access settings as per established procedure.	
6. Remove blood lines from switcher.	
7. Tape the venous blood line up so that it is visible on the bed.	7. The venous line must be visible to observe air returning through it. Taping the line to the bed prevents the sudden return of blood due to gravity changes in pressure, as the blood line is fairly level.
8. Clamp the arterial blood line and the arterial side of the subclavian catheter.	
9. Remove the tape from the arterial connection.	
10. Separate the connection.	
11. Wipe the arterial catheter with a povidone-iodine–soaked sterile gauze pad, and wrap it so it can soak for 12 minutes.	11. This protects the arterial catheter from contamination as the extracorporeal circuit is being rinsed.
12. Connect IV of normal saline solution to arterial tubing. Open clamp on saline line and arterial blood line.	
13. Turn on blood pump at rate of 100 ml. until approximately 150 to 200 ml. of saline is infused.	
14. Turn off blood pump.	
15. Clamp arterial blood tubing, arterial catheter, and saline line.	
16. Disconnect saline line from arterial blood tubing.	
17. Open clamp on arterial blood tubing and turn blood pump on at 100 ml./minute. *Note*: Arterial side of subclavian catheter remains clamped.	
18. Return blood to patient until air reaches air detector alarm.	
19. Clamp venous blood line and venous side of the catheter when the rinse is complete.	

ACTION	RATIONALE
20. Wipe the venous side of the catheter with a povidone-iodine–soaked sterile gauze pad, then wrap it and let it soak for 2 minutes.	
21. Separate the connection carefully.	
22. Apply the new sterile injection caps to both sides of the catheter. Be careful not to contaminate the end of the caps that fit down into the catheter.	
23. Tape the connections securely with plastic tape.	
24. Flush catheter, including both branches, with solution, as ordered.	24. This maintains the patency of the catheter.
25. Perform subclavian dressing change per established procedure.	25. The dressing change should be done at least weekly.
26. Keep bulldog clamps on dressing at all times in case of inadvertent cap separation dislodgment.	
27. Complete postdialysis evaluation and record in patient's chart.	

Precautions

1. Place the patient in the Trendelenburg position every time the catheter is opened. Should a clamp fail there is a real danger of the patient's receiving an air embolism, which could be fatal.

2. Visually check the subclavian catheter each run for cracks or splits in the Silastic. Be especially aware of the areas where the clamps are applied.

3. Infuse heparin to keep the subclavian catheter patent between hemodialysis treatments if the catheter is not being flushed with continuous solution. A physician's order for dose and method of administration (i.e., constant, intermittent) must be obtained.
   Note: If the dressing loosens and the catheter appears to be working its way out during dialysis, *do not attempt* to push it back into the patient as this could result in a hemothorax, which could be life threatening. Positioning of the catheter with a guidewire should be done by the physician.

Related Care

Perform catheter care as per protocol for subclavian lines.

Complications

Catheter disonnection/dislodgment
Air embolism
Infection

REFERENCES

Anderson, R., and Steeno, M.: WBPTT and ACT clotting time methods for use in hemodialysis. AANNT J., 9:27–30, 1982.

Gutch, C.F., and Stoner, M.H.: Review of Hemodialysis for Nurses and Dialysis Personnel, 4th ed. St. Louis, C.V. Mosby, 1984.

Hanes, C., and Stephenson, T.: An alternate method of ultrafiltration. Nephrol. Nurse, 2:55–57, 1980.

Johnson, J., and McKinney, B.: An experience with biocompatible hemoperfusion in a pediatric overdose. Nephrol. Nurse, 5:8–10, 1983.

Larson, E., Lindbloom, L., and Davis, K.B. (eds.): Development of the Clinical Nephrology Practitioner: A Focus on Independent Learning. St. Louis, C.V. Mosby, 1982.

Linos, D. A., Mucha, P., Jr., and Van Heerden, J. A.: Subclavian vein, a golden route. Mayo Clinic Proc., 55:315–321, 1980.

Northwest Kidney Center: Hemodialysis Procedure Manuals. Seattle, 1983. (Unpublished.)

An Overview. In Flamenbaum, W., et al.: Nephrology: An Approach to the Patient with Renal Disease, Philadelphia, J.B. Lippincott, 1982.

Swedish Hospital Medical Center: Hemodialysis Manuals. Seattle, 1983. (Unpublished.)

PERITONEAL DIALYSIS

Sherri Dano-Adams, R.N.
Elaine Larson, R.N., Ph.D., FAAN and
Barbara Fellows, R.N., M.A., E.T.

Overview

Peritoneal dialysis, by the processes of osmosis and diffusion through the peritoneal membrane, removes end products of metabolism and excess fluid that accumulates in acute or chronic renal failure. To initiate peritoneal dialysis, a temporary or permanent catheter is inserted into the peritoneal cavity with the tip terminating in the true pelvis or vesicorectal fossa (Fig. 3–6). Dialysate is then instilled and removed repeatedly, insuring that a high mean diffusion gradient is maintained between body fluids and dialysate.

There are three phases to each dialysis exchange.

Inflow Phase. This is the time required to infuse the exchange volume, as determined by gravity or pump, catheter placement, size of tubing, and volume to be infused.

Diffusion Phase (Dwell Time). This is the time the dialysate solution remains in the peritoneal cavity before being drained. The diffusion time will vary with the clinical needs of the patient and the type of peritoneal dialysis employed.

Outflow Phase. This is the time required to recover the infused dialysate plus any excess fluid from the extracellular fluid space. Ideally, outflow volume should be equal to or greater than the inflow volume. Usually the patient has an excess of extracellular fluid volume as manifested by weight gain, hypertension, or peripheral edema, and needs to lose fluid dur-

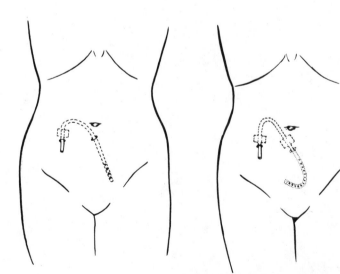

Figure 3-6. Schematic of peritoneal catheter tract. (From Tenckhoff, H.: Chronic Peritoneal Dialysis Manual. Seattle, University of Washington School of Medicine, 1974, p. 27. Reproduced by permission.)

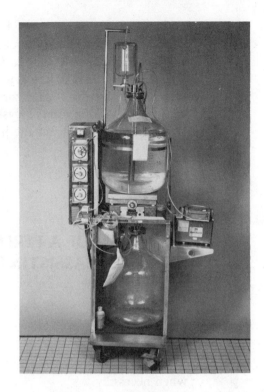

Figure 3-7. Peritoneal dialysis set-up; automated system.

ing the dialysis. A *positive balance* (greater total volume than initial volume) means that excess fluid has been removed from the patient. A *negative balance* (greater initial volume than total volume recovered) means that there is excess fluid retained by the patient.

Two methods of peritoneal dialysis are generally employed: intermittent peritoneal dialysis, whereby dialysate is exchanged by an automated cycle

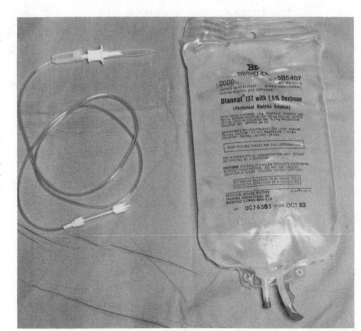

Figure 3-8. Solution bag and connecting tubing for continuous ambulatory peritoneal dialysis.

two to three times an hour (Fig. 3–7), and continuous ambulatory peritoneal dialysis, a continuous 24-hour a day treatment that requires changing the dialysate only four to five times during the 24-hour period (Fig. 3–8). The former system is the type of peritoneal dialysis mainly employed in the critical care setting, while continuous ambulatory peritoneal dialysis is generally used in long-term dialysis. For this reason, the procedures included in this section will focus on the intermittent peritoneal dialysis system.

INSERTION OF A PERITONEAL DIALYSIS CATHETER (ASSISTING WITH) _____

Objective

To monitor and support the patient during this procedure, assisting when necessary.

Special Equipment

Sterile surgical gown(s) and glove(s)
Caps
Masks
Sterile plastic draping sheet
Large draping towels (4)
Split eye drape
Povidone-iodine solution
Heparin 1:1000
Lidocaine 0.5% or 1% without epinephrine
Sterile gauze pads
Towel clips
Needles:
   One 25-gauge, two 20-gauge, 1½ inches long
   Two no. 20, 4 inches long
   One stainless steel short-bevel, 13- to 15-gauge,
      3 inches or longer
Syringes:
   One 5 ml.
   Two 20 ml.
Four hemostats
Curved Kelly clamp
Blade handle, no. 11 with 15 blades

Toothed thumb forceps
Needle holder
2-0 silk suture with cutting edge needle
2-0 or 3-0 gut or chromic suture with tapered needle
One large semicurved clamp, 9 inches
Peritoneal catheter supplies:
   Trocath
   Trocar
   Uterine sound
   Catheter
2 foot sterile latex rubber tubing with needle adapter and solution
   administration set attached
Sterile prewarmed dialysate

Procedure

ACTION	RATIONALE
1. Obtain and record patient's weight, temperature, blood pressure, pulse, respiratory rate, and abdominal girth.	1. This provides a baseline for comparison during dialysis.
2. Assess patient's abdomen for:	
A. Bowel distention; report to physician.	A. With bowel distention there is increased risk of bowel perforation.
B. Urinary bladder distention; empty bladder.	B. This decreases chances of bladder perforation.
C. Abdominal skin integrity for signs of local infection. If present:	C. This prevents introduction of organisms into the peritoneum from locally infected areas.
(1) Clean these sites with povidone-iodine or other antiseptic preparation.	
(2) Cover locally infected sites with a sterile dressing.	
(3) Report these to physician.	
3. Prepare peritoneal catheter insertion site.	3. This helps to control infection.
A. Shave abdomen from xiphoid to symphysis pubis.	
B. Perform a surgical abdominal scrub extending from xiphoid to symphysis pubis, over both flanks, and with particular attention to umbilicus.	B. The umbilicus harbors a greater number of organisms.

ACTION	RATIONALE
4. Place patient in supine position.	

5. Employ strict aseptic technique.
  A. Mask all persons in immediate area.
  B. Assist with sterile draping.	

6. Provide desired local anesthesia.	
7. Monitor patient's response during peritoneal dialysis catheter insertion.	
8. Inform patient of potential discomfort during advancement of catheter into peritoneal cavity.	8. This prevents sudden movement or jerking of the patient.
9. Monitor alteration in comfort level. A. Report sudden onset of pressure in bladder, epigastrium, or rectum.	A. Pressure in bladder indicates that the catheter should be pulled back slightly; pressure in the epigastrium suggests omental entanglement of the catheter; pressure in the rectal area indicates that the catheter tip is in the proper position.
B. Report continued discomfort in rectal area.	B. Continued rectal pain suggests that the catheter is in too far.

10. Prime patient's abdomen with fluid, as prescribed.
  A. Check priming solution for sterility; warm to body temperature.
  B. If bottle is warmed in a water bath, dry outside of bottle before it is inverted.
  C. Prime the inflow tubing with dialysate.
  D. Connect primed inflow tubing and monitor inflow volume of dialysate.
  E. Assess patient carefully for respiratory distress as well as abdominal discomfort.
  F. Measure amount of fluid instilled accurately.
	B. This prevents contamination of the sterile fluid.
	
	E. Large volumes of fluid in the abdominal cavity can cause respiratory insufficiency by limiting lung expansion.

11. Place the patient in a 45-degree position.	11. This enhances comfort and facilitates proper drainage.

ACTION	RATIONALE

12. Secure peritoneal dialysis catheter.

13. Apply dressing.

Precaution

Assess the patient frequently during the procedure for tolerance to supine position, hemodynamic alteration, respiratory status, and the like.

Related Care

1. Assess site for hemorrhage.
2. Assess patency of catheter.
3. Assess for fluid leakage at catheter exit; change dressings and clean site when moist.

Complications

Hemorrhage
Catheter occlusion
Bowel perforation
Bladder perforation

PERITONEAL DIALYSIS CATHETER SITE CARE _____

Objectives

1. To assess and clean exit site to prevent local and systemic infection or to detect early signs of it.
2. To maintain and assess skin integrity at the peritoneal catheter exit site.

Special Equipment

Protective bed pad
Tape
Plastic bag
Forceps

Face mask(s)
Povidone-iodine solution
Hydrogen peroxide solution
Sterile gauze pads

Procedure

ACTION	RATIONALE
1. Mask all persons in immediate area.	1. This aids in infection control.
2. Expose catheter site, using forceps to remove dressings around catheter.	
3. Inspect exit site for signs and symptoms of infection (purulence, redness, tenderness, induration).	
4. Remove dried blood with hydrogen peroxide.	4. Dried blood can serve as nutrient for bacteria.
5. Cleanse exit site gently with povidone-iodine solution. A. Begin around site. B. Work outward.	
6. Cleanse entire circumference of catheter with povidone-iodine solution; allow antiseptic to dry completely.	6. This prevents gauze dressings from sticking to the skin and allows maximum bacteriostatic effects to occur.
7. Secure peritoneal dialysis catheter on sterile gauze pad.	7. This avoids skin irritation and decreases risk of catheter contamination from skin.
8. Cover area with additional sterile gauze pads.	
9. Secure dressing, keeping areas of gauze exposed.	9. This allows skin to breathe and decreases risk of anaerobic bacterial growth; it also prevents bacterial contamination.

Precaution

Secure catheter position during site care.

Related Care

1. Perform peritoneal site care daily after first 48 hours, after each dialysis, whenever dressings are moist, or whenever exit site is exposed or contaminated.
2. Assess skin integrity daily.
3. Vary the position of the taped-down catheter with each dressing change.

Complications

Catheter displacement
Infection

MONITORING INTERMITTENT PERITONEAL DIALYSIS _____

Objectives

1. To ensure the proper composition and temperature of the dialysate and proper functioning of equipment.
2. To check proper functioning of equipment during peritoneal dialysis, taking corrective action as necessary.
3. To monitor peritoneal dialysis therapy and to assess the patient's physiologic and psychologic response to it.
4. To initiate appropriate adjustments in the dialysis according to the patient's physiologic response.

Special Equipment

Peritoneal dialysis log sheet
Skin scrub tray
Povidone-iodine solution
Mask(s)
Linen savers
Tape
Prewarmed dialysate
Peritoneal dialysis machine
Sterile gloves

Waste container
Patient assessment tools:
  Blood pressure cuff
  Stethoscope
  Sphygmomanometer
  Thermometer
  Scale
  Tape measure

Procedure

ACTION	RATIONALE
1. Check composition of dialysate on label with physician order, giving particular attention to the concentration of potassium and glucose.	1. Glucose in the dialysate increases osmotic pressure, drawing off extracellular fluid from the patient and increasing urea clearance. The potassium concentration of the dialysate is ordered in a concentration that will maintain the patient's serum potassium within a safe range.

ACTION	RATIONALE
2. Check dialysis machine and temperature of dialysate, which should approximate body temperature.	2. Urea clearance is maximized and body heat loss is minimized when dialysate is near body temperature.
3. Obtain patient's weight, blood pressure (supine and upright), pulse, respiratory rate, and temperature.	3. This provides a baseline for comparison during dialysis.
4. Palpate patient's abdomen. A. Note and record degree of any distention. B. Measure abdominal girth with tape measure.	4. This provides a baseline for comparison during dialysis. Fluid retention is often first noted in increasing abdominal girth.
5. Place dialysis log conveniently at bedside and complete predialysis information (patient's name, hospital number, date and time, vital signs, bath composition, additives, length of treatment).	
6. Determine and record on log the ordered volume to be infused with each cycle—usually 1500 to 2000 ml. for adults.	6. The volume infused will depend on patient size and tolerance. Exchange volumes of greater than 2 liters increase clearance only minimally. To improve dialysis efficiency, it is preferable to increase the number of cycles per hour rather than to increase the volume infused with each exchange.
7. Place bed in higher position.	7. This enhances gravity outflow and provides easy access to the patient.
8. Place protective pads under patient.	
9. Prepare machine and connect patient, using strict aseptic technique.	9. This minimzes the risk of infection.
10. Place patient in outflow cycle before initiating the inflow phase.	10. This assures that any residual fluid that may be in the patient's peritoneal cavity is drained prior to dialysate infusion, thus preventing overdistention of the abdomen.
11. Monitor inflow phase. A. Ensure that: (1) All clamps from inflow reservoir to patient are released. (2) Tubing is free of kinks, and automated system is functioning properly.	

ACTION	**RATIONALE**
B. Time inflow cycle and observe for flow obstruction.	B. The inflow phase is approximately 5 to 10 minutes, depending upon the volume to be infused and the height of the reservoir bottle. Slow inflow can result from external or subcutaneous tube kinking and internal catheter obstruction. This should be noted and corrected before dialysis is continued.
12. Monitor diffusion phase. A. Observe patient's response to fluid volume infused. Note any discomfort or respiratory distress.	A. Intolerance and discomfort during the diffusion phase may indicate too much fluid being infused, peritoneal infection, or adhesion formation.
B. Assess catheter site for fluid leakage or bleeding.	
13. Monitor outflow phase. A. Ensure that (1) All clamps from patient to outflow bottle are released. (2) Dialysis tubing is free of kinks. (3) Inflow clamping mechanism is activated.	
B. Observe the ease and speed of outflow drainage.	B. The dialysate fluid should normally drain by gravity in a steady stream. Initial outflow may be slow secondary to an air lock in the dialysis tubing, fibrin deposit at the internal end of the catheter, or an inadequate pool of fluid in the abdomen. If outflow is impeded, remove any air in the tubing, reposition the patient, give another small amount of inflow solution and again attempt to start outflow.
C. Repeat the outflow phase if less than 80% of the volume infused is not recovered.	C. This is to prevent abdominal distention and volume overload. Increasing the glucose concentration of the dialysate will increase the amount of fluid removed from the patient. This may be

ACTION	RATIONALE
	necessary if the patient has an increasing negative balance secondary to fluid absorption.
D. Note patient complaints of discomfort.	D. Pain on outflow may be due to increased suction during the outflow phase. If an outflow pump is being used, it may be necessary to change to gravity drainage, as this produces less suction.
E. Observe and record appearance of the outflow fluid.	E. Cloudy outflow fluid is a sign strongly suggestive of infection.
14. Calculate inflow and outflow volumes at end of each outflow cycle. A. Add amount of inflow fluid remaining and amount of fluid in outflow bottle to obtain total fluid volume.	
B. Subtract initial dialysate volume from sum of inflow and outflow volumes.	B. A positive balance indicates the *machine* has more volume than it started with. A negative balance indicates the *machine* has less volume than it started with. A positive balance means the patient is losing volume, whereas a negative balance means the patient is retaining volume.
15. Determine and record on log sheet the length of time for each phase. A. Inflow phase time will be variable, depending on the volume infused and the delivery system, either gravity or pump. B. Diffusion phase is ordered by the physician and is dependent on the clinical needs of the patient, usually 10 to 25 minutes. C. Outflow phase will vary with the volume infused and recovery by gravity or pump, usually 10 to 25 minutes.	
16. Monitor patient's vital signs, abdominal girth, and neurologic status frequently throughout the dialysis treatment.	16. With any dialysis patient, prompt recognition of change in status will prevent more serious complications.

Precautions

1. Monitor the patient's vital signs, abdominal girth, and mental status throughout the dialysis, since rapid fluid and electrolyte changes can occur during dialysis.
2. Observe patient for symptoms of insulin reaction. A high glucose content in the dialysate causes hyperglycemia, resulting in increased insulin production. When dialysis is discontinued rapidly, there is less time for the body to reach homeostasis.
3. Maintain sterility when handling the peritoneal catheter.
4. Monitor outflow carefully throughout the dialysis to ensure that fluid is not retained in the peritoneal cavity.
5. Assess patient for both hypervolemia and hypovolemia, as dialysis can produce rapid fluid shifts.
6. Assess for atelectasis, since dialysis encourages hypoventilation.

Related Care

1. Record exact time of initiation and termination of infusion, amount of solution infused and recovered, and total balance, color of outflow, and before and after dialysis weight.
2. Weigh wet dressings to estimate fluid lost: 1 gram = 1 ml.
3. Obtain a blood chemistry profile, which may include BUN, albumin level (because of protein loss), and electrolyte levels.
4. Utilize effective skin care and range of motion exercises.

Complications

Peritonitis	Dysrhythmias
Bowel, bladder, visceral perforation (mainly at the time of catheter insertion)	Hemorrhage
	Hyperglycemia
	Dehydration
Fluid and electrolyte imbalances	Mechanical defects

REFERENCES

Harrington, A.R., and Zimmerman, S.W. : Renal Pathophysiology. New York, John Wiley & Sons, 1982, pp. 211–224.

Peritoneal Dialysis Procedures. Seattle, University Hospital Nursing Services, 1982.

Popovich, R.P., et al.: Continuous ambulatory peritoneal dialysis. Ann. Intern. Med., 88:449–456, 1978.

Tenckhoff, H.: Chronic Peritoneal Dialysis. Seattle, University of Washington School of Medicine, 1974.

4

THE
NEUROLOGIC
SYSTEM

INTRACRANIAL PRESSURE
MONITORING

Marilyn M. Ricci, R.N., M.S.N., CNRN

Overview

INTRACRANIAL PRESSURE

The rigid intracranial compartment containing blood, brain, and cerebrospinal fluid (CSF) is normally in a state of pressure and volume equilibrium. An increase in the volume of one intracranial component must be accompanied by reciprocal changes in one or both of the other components so that total pressure remains constant (0 to 15 mm. Hg or 50 to 200 cm. H_2O). Fluctuations in pressure normally occur in response to the respiratory cycle, arterial pulsations, changes in intrathoracic pressure (cough, sneeze, Valsalva maneuver), and position changes.

The intracranial pressure (ICP) will remain within normal ranges as long as the compensatory mechanisms can accommodate for a volume increase (compliance). As intracranial volume increases and the compensatory mechanisms are exhausted or fail, ICP increases or intracranial hypertension occurs (sustained ICP of greater than 15 mm. Hg for more than 20 minutes). As ICP increases and cerebral autoregulation is lost, there is a concomitant decrease in cerebral perfusion pressure (MAP – ICP = CPP) with associated ischemia and hypoxia.

There is a direct relationship between elevations of ICP, brain stem dysfunction, and clinical neurologic changes. However, the clinical signs are not reliable in determining actual pressure elevations, detecting early intracranial hypertension, or determining the severity. Direct measurement is the only clinically reliable method of evaluating ICP.

TYPES OF INTRACRANIAL PRESSURE MONITORING

ICP monitoring is a continuous, direct measurement technique that utilizes an intracranial sensor, transducer, and recording device. The sensor transmits changes in ICP to a transducer; the mechanical impulses are converted to electrical impulses that are recorded on an oscilloscope or chart or both. Table 4–1 indicates the advantages and disadvantages of the various types of ICP monitoring.

Intraventricular. A small rubber or polyethylene catheter is introduced through a burr hole into the anterior horn of the lateral ventricle, usually on the side of the nondominant hemisphere. The catheter is connected via a stopcock and fluid-filled pressure tubing to a transducer, and to a monitor or recording device. The catheter may also be connected to an external ventricular drainage system to enable drainage of CSF and blood.

TABLE 4-1. Advantages and Disadvantages of Types of ICP Monitoring

INTRAVENTRICULAR	SUBARACHNOID	EPIDURAL
ADVANTAGES		
Ease of CSF sampling and drainage; reliability of measurement; access for determining volume-pressure response; and instillation of medications or contrast media.	Useful with small ventricles; no penetration of brain parenchyma; access for volume-pressure response and CSF sample.	Ease of insertion; low risk of infection since dura is not penetrated and there are no external connection sites; recalibration not necessary; sensor and ICP readings will not be altered by air or occlusion by blood.
DISADVANTAGES		
Difficulty in placement (small ventricles, midline shift); risk of damage to brain parenchyma; risk of infection; catheter occlusion with blood, brain tissue; need for realigning transducer with head and recalibration; ventricular collapse with rapid CSF drainage.	Unreliability at high ICP levels; and for compliance testing; requires intact skull; risk of infection; inability to withdraw CSF in a significant amount; need for realigning transducer and recalibration; risk of bleeding from insertion.	Questionable accuracy of measurement; inability to calibrate after insertion; inability to determine volume-pressure response or sample CSF; wave-form may become dampened by wedge effect from the dura.

Subarachnoid.   A hollow metal subarachnoid screw (bolt) is inserted through a ½-inch twist drill hole approximately 1 mm. beneath the dura into the subarachnoid space. The device is connected via a stopcock and fluid-filled pressure tubing to a transducer, and to a monitor and recorder. The device is placed behind the hairline on the side of the nondominant hemisphere.

Epidural.   A balloon radiotransmitter or a fiberoptic transducer is placed through a burr hole between the skull and dura. The adjacent dura must be free from the inner table to avoid a wedge effect and high, inaccurate pressures. The monitoring equipment will vary according to the type of device. (The transmitter or transducer may also be placed subdurally.)

Objectives

1. To detect early changes in ICP.
2. To assess ICP waves.
3. To detect impending cerebral damage secondary to increases in ICP.
4. To determine cerebral perfusion pressure (normal CPP $\geq$ 50 mm. Hg).
5. To determine intracranial volume-pressure responses (compliance).
6. To provide a guide for nursing interventions, e.g., positioning, suctioning.
7. To provide a guide for medical therapy, e.g., administration of diuretics, hyperventilation, barbiturate therapy, CSF drainage.

Special Equipment

PLACEMENT OF ICP MONITORING DEVICE

Disposable razor

Surgical caps, masks, and gowns

Sterile gloves

Sterile surgical towels

Disposable basin

Povidone-iodine scrub, solution, and ointment

Sterile 4-inch x 4-inch gauze sponges

Alcohol wipes

Local anesthetic (1% to 2% lidocaine (Xylocaine) with epinephrine)

Syringe with 25-gauge needle

Twist drill set

Suction setup

3-0 silk suture

Sterile 2-inch x 2-inch gauze sponges

Bone wax and Gelfoam

Tape (adhesive, silk) or Elastoplast for occlusive dressing

Light source

IV pole

MONITORING EQUIPMENT

Monitoring equipment (3-channel to enable simultaneous monitoring of ECG, ICP, arterial pressure)

Transducer, holder, and dome with stopcock

Pressure tubing

Three-way stopcocks/manifold with Luer-Lok syringes (1 ml., 10 ml.)

Monitoring device:

Subarachnoid screw, handle, and three-way stopcock with drainage bag (permits flushing of pressure tubing and irrigation of screw without opening to air)

Intraventricular catheter and stopcock with external ventricular drainage system

Sterile dead-end caps for stopcock ports

Vial of sterile normal saline without preservative and 20-ml. syringe

Level

Centimeter tape measure (unless the ventricular drainage system has a height scale)

Procedure

ACTION	RATIONALE
1. Prepare the monitoring system: A. Assemble the equipment according to type of device to be inserted.	

ACTION	RATIONALE
B. Fill the transducer dome, pressure line, and stopcocks with sterile saline without preservative (see "Hemodynamic Monitoring Single-Pressure Transducer System").	B. Preservative is irritating to the brain. Air in the line dampens the wave form and gives inaccurate pressure readings.
C. Apply caps or Luer-Lok syringes to stopcock ports as appropriate.	C. This maintains sterility.

      (1) For intraventricular monitoring a 10-ml. syringe should be used on the transducer.

      (2) For subarachnoid monitoring a 10-ml. and a 1-ml. syringe should be used on the transducer (Fig. 4–1).

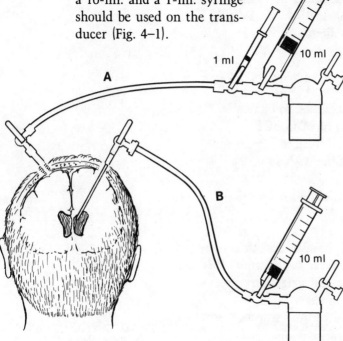

Figure 4-1. Intracranial pressure monitoring. *A*, Subarachnoid screw with 1 ml and 10 ml syringes for flush attached to transducer, or *B*, intraventricular catheter with 10 ml syringe for flush attached to transducer.

D. Place transducer in holder.

E. Calibrate the monitoring system.

2. Prepare the patient for the insertion of the monitoring device:	
A. Assist with the insertion of an arterial line.	A. This is necessary for recording cerebral perfusion pressures.
B. Place the patient in a supine position with the head of bed elevated 30 to 45 degrees or as ordered.	
C. Suction the patient prior to preparing the insertion site.	C. This facilitates maintaining the airway during the insertion procedure.

ACTION	RATIONALE
D. Wash hands for 3 minutes.	
E. Shave the insertion site.	E. This decreases the risk of infection and aids in securing an occlusive dressing.
F. Don mask and cap.	
G. Place a sterile towel under the patient's head and open another sterile towel.	G. Sterile technique and a sterile field decrease the risk of infection.
H. Don sterile gloves.	
I. Scrub the insertion site vigorously for 10 minutes with povidone-iodine scrub and rinse well with the solution.	
J. Place a sterile towel over the area until time for insertion.	
K. Record neurologic status and vital signs.	

3. Assist with the insertion of the monitoring device.

ACTION	RATIONALE
A. Don sterile gown and gloves.	A. All personnel in the area must wear mask, cap, gown, and gloves to decrease the risk of infection.
B. Stabilize the patient's head.	B. This facilitates placement.
C. Assist in placement of the device and establishing the monitoring and drainage systems.	
D. Reassure the conscious patient.	D. This eases anxiety and promotes cooperation.
E. Monitor neurologic status and vital signs.	
F. Record initial ICP readings.	F. This provides a baseline.
G. Apply povidone-iodine ointment and a small, sterile occlusive dressing at the site.	G. This prevents infection.

4. Set up the external drainage system when an intraventricular catheter is placed.

ACTION	RATIONALE
A. Secure the collection setup to an IV pole at the desired height (5 cm.—3 to 4 mm. Hg) from the foramen of Monro.	A. The ICP and CSF drainages are regulated by the height of the drip port in relation to the pressure source (approximately 1 inch above the ear). Positioning the drip site too high may increase ICP and positioning too low may cause excessive CSF drainage and ventricular collapse.

ACTION	RATIONALE

B. If the collection setup does not have a height scale, attach a centimeter measuring tape to the pole or device with the 0 at the drip port and the desired height measure 1 inch above the ear. Use a level to ensure accurate placement (Fig. 4–2).

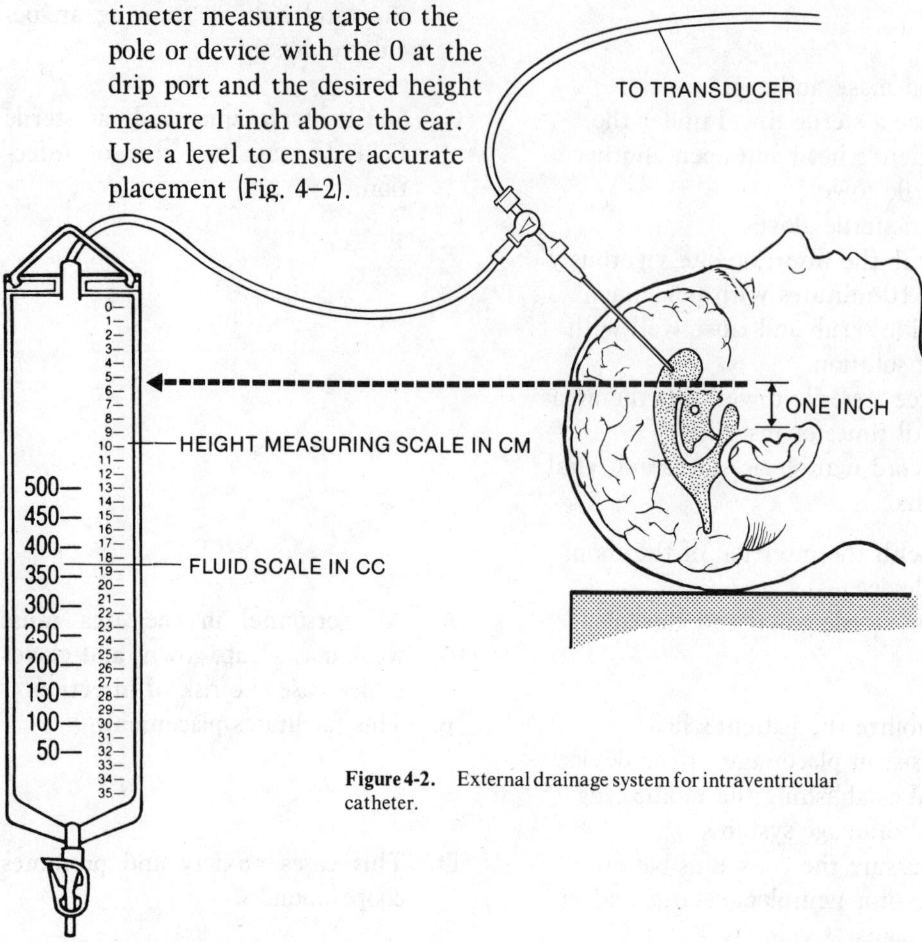

TO TRANSDUCER

ONE INCH

HEIGHT MEASURING SCALE IN CM

FLUID SCALE IN CC

Figure 4-2. External drainage system for intraventricular catheter.

C. Check to ensure all connections are secure. Apply tape as necessary to connections.

C. This prevents excessive CSF drainage and infection.

D. Avoid retrograde CSF flow by use of reflux valve or positioning of drainage system.

D. This prevents infection and increased ICP.

E. Mark the drainage system with time and date.

E. This enables rechecking catheter placement.

F. Record the length of the catheter from the insertion site (skull films may be ordered to check placement).

5. Maintain the monitoring system.
   A. Subarachnoid
      (1) Observe the ICP reading and pressure wave forms.

      (1) This allows for determination of the need to treat and the patency of system.

ACTION	RATIONALE
(2) Flush the system with 0.10 ml. sterile saline from the 1-ml. syringe every 6 to 8 hours or as ordered and when the wave form becomes dampened unless the ICP is elevated or the preirrigation pressure and wave form do not return within 2 minutes.	(2) Patency of system must be maintained. Irrigation is avoided when ICP is elevated or there is reduced compliance.
(3) Following instillation of saline, hold screw firmly, and open the stopcock to the drainage bag.	(3) The drainage bag permits drainage of excess fluid or blood without opening the system to air.
(4) Notify the physician if the fluid is blood tinged or if excessive drainage is present.	(4) Bleeding is a complication; usually there is no drainage. Excessive drainage is indicative of elevated ICP.
(5) Return stopcocks to monitoring position and observe for ICP reading and wave form.	(5) Preirrigation pressure and wave form will return unless there is poor compliance or the monitoring system is not patent.
(6) Check the system for leaks at all junctions of stopcocks and tubing every shift and as necessary.	(6) Maintaining a closed system decreases the risk of infection and air leaks.
(7) Flush air from the pressure tubing with saline by turning the stopcock at the screw off to the patient and on to the drainage bag.	(7) Air dampens the wave form and could cause an air embolus. The drainage bag enables flushing without opening the system.
(8) Use only Luer-Lok syringes and replace when empty. Fill with saline from a new vial or a reservoir using closed technique.	(8) This decreases the risk of infection.
(9) Disconnect the system *when absolutely necessary* by turning the stopcock at the screw off to the patient; use sterile gloves to disconnect the pressure tubing at the stopcock manifold; and close the pressure tubing/stopcocks with dead-end caps.	(9) Disconnection of the system increases the risk of infection.

ACTION	RATIONALE
(10) Reestablish the monitoring system, using new tubing and stopcocks to the stopcock at the screw.	
1. Intraventricular	
(1) Observe the CSF at the drainage port for fluctuation with the system open to drain (every hour).	(1) Fluctuation indicates proper placement, patency, and functioning of the intraventricular catheter. Occlusion of the system dampens the wave form, gives inaccurate ICP readings, and interferes with the ability to drain CSF to reduce elevated ICP.
(2) Mark the fluid level in the drainage bag with the time and date each shift. The CSF drainage may be calculated each shift with output totals.	
(3) Flush the pressure tubing to remove air, blood, and debris by turning the stopcock off to the patient. The flush solution will flow into the drainage bag so the amount used must be recorded and subtracted from the total drainage for the shift.	(3) NOTE: The ventricular catheter should be irrigated *only* by the physician.
(4) Check the monitoring system for air leaks and the drainage system for CSF leaks every shift and as necessary.	(4) Air dampens the wave form. CSF leak, may result in excessive drainage and collapse of the ventricles.
(5) Change or empty the drainage system when full, disrupted, disconnected, or not working as appropriate. Use strict aseptic technique at all times. Use sterile gloves, towel, a new drainage setup and antiseptic solution to cleanse the disconnect site when changing the system.	(5) This reduces the risk of infection.
(6) Disconnect the system *when absolutely necessary* by turning the stopcock at the catheter off to the patient or transducer as appropriate; use sterile gloves to disconnect the pressure tubing at the stopcock manifold; and close	(6) Disconnection of the system increases the risk of infection.

ACTION	RATIONALE
the pressure tubing/stopcocks with dead-end caps.	

6. Perform insertion site care.
   A. Cleanse the site with povidone-iodine solution, apply ointment and place split 2-inch x 2-inch gauze pads around the device, using strict aseptic technique. Use sterile gloves and scissors to split the gauze squares.
   B. Apply benzoin to the skin and tape to provide complete occlusion.
   C. Change the dressing and assess the insertion site for redness, swelling, and drainage every 24 to 72 hours or as ordered and as necessary. A patient who perspires profusely will need frequent dressing changes.
   D. Avoid disturbing the dressing or getting it wet.
   E. Inspect the dressing each shift to ensure that it is intact, occlusive, clean, and dry.

   A. This reduces the risk of infection.

   D. This reduces the risk of infection.
   E. A loose dressing may place traction on the ventricular catheter and displace it. A wet dressing may be indicative of a CSF leak or bleeding.

7. Obtain pressure measurements.
   A. Obtain and record ICP measurements every 15 minutes to 1 hour.

   B. Confirm the position of the transducer in relation to the pressure source prior to recording and treating for elevation of ICP. (The stopcock at the transducer must be level with the foramen of Monro.
   C. Obtain and record CPP every hour.
   D. Monitor pressure wave patterns (see Related Care).

   A. Trends are more significant than a single pressure in determining ICP elevations and poor compliance.
   B. Improper positioning results in inaccurate pressure readings.

   C. These measurements are an indication of cerebral blood flow.
   D. These wave patterns are an indication of loss of compliance, need to treat ICP, and patency of system (see the Trouble-shooting Guide under Related Care).

ACTION	RATIONALE
E. Record all events that result in a change in ICP, e.g., activities, therapeutic modalities, sleep.	E. This guides nursing activities and indicates responsiveness to treatment for increased ICP.
F. Record response to CSF drainage, duration opened to drain, and color of CSF.	F. This indicates effectiveness of CSF drainage and presence of bleeding.
G. Balance and recalibrate the system every 4 to 8 hours and when accuracy of ICP is questionable.	G. This ensures accurate ICP measurements.
H. If unable to obtain pressure measurement or the wave form is poor, trouble-shoot the system.	H. See Trouble-shooting Guide under Related Care.

8. Assist in discontinuing the monitoring system.

ACTION	RATIONALE
A. Provide 3-0 nylon suture with needle, sterile hemostat, and scissors. Provide a wrench to remove the screw.	
B. Apply povidone-iodine ointment and a small dressing to the insertion site for at least 24 hours.	B. This decreases the risk of infection.
C. Inspect the site for a CSF leak.	C. A CSF leak could be a source of infection.
D. Leave the wound open to air after 24 hours if there is no evidence of a CSF leak.	

Precautions

1. Use a 1-ml. syringe to introduce fluid into the intracranial compartment via the subarachnoid screw.
2. Note that if the ICP increases over 2 mm. Hg/second in response to a small amount of fluid, this is indicative of altered compensation or compliance.
3. Protect the monitoring device when positioning or moving the patient and when the patient is agitated.
4. Avoid rapid, prolonged drainage of CSF, which will result in collapse of the ventricles, damage to bridging cortical veins, and intracranial bleeding/hematoma.
5. Note that excessive loss of CSF in a patient with elevated ICP can alter the ICP dynamics and result in upward herniation of the brain stem and the cerebellum with subsequent dysrhythmias and respiratory arrest.
6. Maintain a closed system and avoid disconnections to reduce the risk of infection.
7. Avoid treatment of elevated ICP without accurate pressure measurements. Mean pressures may be used for assessment and guide to therapy

after determining that the monitoring system is working and the pressures are accurate.

Related Care

1. Monitor pressure wave forms (Fig. 4–3).
   A. *A Waves (also called Plateau or Lundberg Waves)*. These are large plateau-like formations that recur at intervals of varying lengths. They frequently reach greater than 50 mm. Hg (65 cm. H_2O) and last 5 to 20 minutes. They usually occur in patients with elevated baseline pressures (20 to 40 mm. Hg). In a series of A waves, both amplitude and duration increase. This is indicative of a decrease in compliance and probable vasomotor instability. Plateau waves may be accompanied by increased neurological deficits. These waves are an ominous sign and may have a catastrophic outcome; i.e., there is zero cerebral blood flow when MAP = ICP. Most of these waves seem to abort spontaneously, but they should always be treated, and measures should be taken to increase the compliance.
   B. *B Waves*. These waves are short-term oscillations that are lower in amplitude than A waves. They occur regularly at a rate of 0.5 to 2/minute and range from 20 to 50 mm. Hg. B waves tend to occur more frequently with decreased compliance. They correspond to changes in respirations (Cheyne-Stokes), and they may precede the appearance of an A wave.
   C. *C Waves*. C waves are rhythmic, rapid oscillations of pressure without any known clinical relevance. Pressures may be up to 20 mm. Hg at a rate of 6/minute.
2. Use all known nursing measures to prevent increased ICP.
   A. Preoxygenate before suctioning; suction briefly. Prevent excessive coughing.
   B. Position the patient with head elevated 30 to 45 degrees; avoid neck flexion.

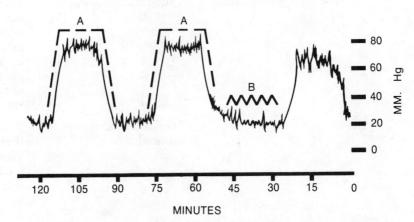

Figure 4-3. Ventricular fluid pressure variations: *A*, plateau waves; *B*, "B" waves.

  C. Avoid the use of the Valsalva maneuver (e.g., straining at stool).

  D. Decrease environmental noise.

 3. Administer specific therapeutic measures to control elevations of ICP.

  A. Fluid restrictions.

  B. Hyperosmolar agents: mannitol (Osmitrol), glycerol.

  C. Diuretics: Furosemide as alternative to hyperosmolar agent when serum osmolality is elevated.

  D. Glucocorticoids: dexamethasone (Decadron) most common.

  E. Hyperventilation (first 48 hours to decrease PCO_2).

  F. Hypothermia.

  G. CSF drainage.

  H. Barbiturate therapy: pentobarbital, thiopental.

  I. Thorazine or pancuronium (Pavulon) to decrease muscle activity.

TABLE 4–2. Trouble-shooting ICP Monitoring Systems

PROBLEM	CAUSE	SOLUTION
ICP wave-form dampened or absent.	Air between the transducer diaphragm and pressure source.	Eliminate air bubbles with sterile saline. Tighten connections.
	Occlusion of intracranial measurement device with blood, brain tissue, or compression by ventricular wall.	Flush intraventricular catheter or screw as directed by physician; 0.25 ml. sterile saline frequently used.
	Transducer connected incorrectly; loose connections.	Check connections and be sure appropriate connector for amplifier is in use.
	Incorrect gain setting for pressure or patient having plateau waves.	Adjust gain setting for higher pressure range.
	Trace turned off.	Turn power on to trace.
False high pressure reading.	Transducer too low.	Place the venting port of transducer at level of foramen of Monro. For every 1 inch the transducer is below the pressure source there is an error of approximately 2 mm Hg.
	Transducer incorrectly balanced.	With transducer correctly positioned, rebalance. Transducer should be balanced every 2 to 4 hours and prior to initiation of treatment based on a pressure change.
	Monitoring system incorrectly calibrated.	Repeat calibration procedures.

4. Test CSF for cells; culture.
5. Provide emotional support to patient and family members.
6. Prevent complications secondary to the monitoring system.
7. Trouble-shoot the system (Table 4–2).
8. Notify the physician of the following:
   A. When elevation of ICP does not respond to therapy.
   B. The monitoring system is not functional.
   C. Sudden elevations of temperature and leukocyte count.
   D. Deterioration of neurologic status.
   E. CSF leakage from insertion site.
9. Discontinue ICP monitoring when:
   A. There is no longer an indication for use.
   B. The line is no longer functional.

TABLE 4–2. Trouble-shooting ICP Monitoring Systems *(Continued)*

PROBLEM	CAUSE	SOLUTION
False high pressure reading *(Continued)*.	Air in system. Air may attenuate or amplify pressure signal.	Remove air from monitoring line.
False low pressure reading.	Complete occlusion.	Flush monitoring device.
	Air bubbles between transducer and CSF. Loose connections.	Eliminate air bubbles with sterile saline or Ringer's lactate. Tighten connections.
	Transducer level too high.	Place venting port of transducer at level of foramen of Monro. For every 1 inch the transducer is above level of pressure source there will be an error of approximately 2 mm Hg.
	Zero and/or calibration incorrect.	Re-zero and calibrate monitoring system.
Low ICP pressure	Collapse of ventricles due to overdrainage.	Check to make sure positive pressure of 15 to 20 mm Hg exists. If ventriculostomy is being used there may be inadequate positive pressure. Drain CSF slowly.
	Otorrhea and/or rhinorrhea.	Note that these conditions cause false low pressure reading secondary to decompression. Record correlation between drainage and pressure changes.

Complications

Infection
Hemorrhage/hematoma
Collapse of the ventricle
CSF leak from insertion site

REFERENCES

Mendelow, A.D. et al.: A clinical comparison of subdural screw pressure measurements with ventricular pressure. J. Neurosurg. 58:45–50, 1983.

Neurosurgical Intensive Care Unit Procedure Manual, Barrow Neurologic Institute of St. Joseph Hospital and Medical Center, Phoenix, AZ, 1983.

Ricci, M.: Intracranial hypertension: Barbiturate therapy and the role of the nurse. J. Neurosurg. Nurs., 11:247–252, 1979.

Ricci, M. (ed.): Core Curriculum for Neuroscience Nursing, 2nd ed. Am. Assoc. Neuroscience Nurses, Park Ridge, IL, 1984.

Riley, J.M.: Intracranial pressure monitoring made easy. RN, 44:53–57, 1981.

Smith, R.: Assessment skills for the nurse: Nervous system invasive neurological assessment techniques. In Hudak., C., et al. (eds.): Critical Care Nursing, 3rd ed. Philadelphia, J.B. Lippincott, 1982.

LUMBAR AND CISTERNAL
PUMBAR AND CISTERNAL
_____ PUNCTURES (ASSISTING WITH) _____

Marilyn M. Ricci, R.N., M.S., CNRN

Overview

A lumbar or cisternal puncture is the introduction of a hollow needle with a stylet into the subarachnoid space of the spinal canal. It is performed to gain information about the cerebrospinal fluid (CSF) to help diagnose, treat, or assess the progress of disease involving the central nervous system.

The lumbar puncture (Fig. 4–4) is performed at the level of L_{3-4} or L_{4-5} vertebral interspace to avoid damage to the spinal cord, which ends approximately at the L_{1-2} vertebral level. A cisternal puncture (Fig. 4–5) is the introduction of a short-beveled, hollow needle with a stylet through the midline above the spinous process of the second cervical vertebra and under the posterior rim of the foramen magnum into the cisterna magna (the space between the cerebellum and the medulla). As the needle is correctly placed in the subarachnoid space and the stylet is removed, drops of CSF will escape. The manometer is then attached to the needle, either directly or by using a three-way stopcock. Care must be taken to avoid sudden loss of the CSF. Normally the fluid moves up and down on respiration and moves freely upward on straining, coughing, and abdominal compression. After the CSF pressure measurements are completed, the fluid is allowed to drain off slowly until the desired amount has been obtained.

The contraindications to lumbar puncture are local inflammation or infection at the puncture site; clinical signs of increased intracranial pressure

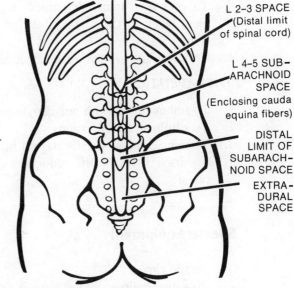

Figure 4-4. Lumbar puncture.

L 2–3 SPACE
(Distal limit
of spinal cord)

L 4–5 SUB–
ARACHNOID
SPACE
(Enclosing cauda
equina fibers)

DISTAL
LIMIT OF
SUBARACH-
NOID SPACE

EXTRA-
DURAL
SPACE

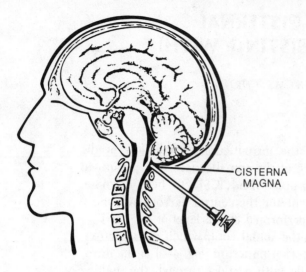

Figure 4-5.   Cisternal puncture.

CISTERNA MAGNA

until a mass lesion has been ruled out (fluid withdrawal from the spinal subarachnoid space produces a rapid pressure reduction that can precipitate herniation of the cerebellar tonsils and medullary compression); suspected intracranial mass lesions, e.g., brain tumor, posterior fossa tumors, subdural hematoma, brain abscess; and suspected spinal cord tumor (lumbar puncture may precipitate rapid progression of symptoms).

Objectives

DIAGNOSTIC

1. To measure CSF pressure.
2. To obtain CSF for visualization and laboratory analysis.
3. To perform "spinal dynamics" tests that could indicate partial or complete block in the CSF circulation as a result of a spinal cord or disc lesion.
4. To inject air, oxygen, or radiopaque substances for x-ray visualization.

THERAPEUTIC

1. To remove blood and purulent material from the subarachnoid space.
2. To administer medications.
3. To induce spinal anesthesia (via lumbar puncture only).
4. To drain CSF for the reduction of intracranial pressure in very select cases.

Special Equipment

Sterile gloves   Sterile gauze pads
20-gauge hollow needles with stylets   Povidone-iodine solution

Three-way stopcock
Manometer
Fenestrated drape
Three small test tubes with labels
Needles
Syringes

Alcohol sponges
Local antiseptic
Band-Aid
Razor (for cisternal puncture)
Light source

Procedure

ACTION	RATIONALE
1. Position patient in a lateral recumbent position with back at edge of bed. Complete positioning depends upon area of puncture (Figs. 4–6 and 4–7).	1. This keeps the plane of the patient's back perpendicular to the plane of the surface on which he is lying.
A. Lumbar: (1) Arch the back. (2) Flex knees tightly against abdomen. (3) Flex neck forward on chest. (4) Place small pillow under head.	A. This position widens the interspinous spaces and promotes easier entry into the subarachnoid space.
B. Cisternal: (1) Place head on small pillow with chin flexed onto chest.	B. This position makes the site accessible by bringing the brain stem and spinal cord forward in the spinal canal.

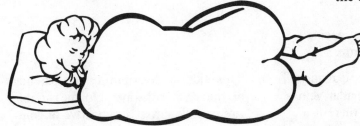

Figure 4-6. Alignment of vertebral column in a horizontal plane.

NECK FLEXED FORWARD   KNEES PULLED UP TO ABDOMEN

Figure 4-7. Position for lumbar puncture.

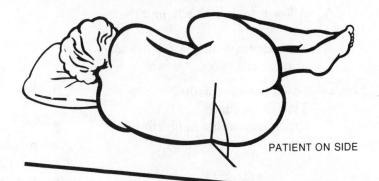

PATIENT ON SIDE

ACTION	RATIONALE
2. Help patient to maintain desired position during procedure by providing support behind head and knees, and keeping the "up" shoulder from falling forward. Stand on the side of the bed the patient is facing.	2. Support helps to prevent sudden movements and resultant trauma.
3. Prepare the skin site with povidone-iodine solution followed by alcohol.	3. This helps to prevent infection. Alcohol removes the povidone-iodine to avoid introducing it into the subarachnoid space.
4. Provide local anesthesia.	
5. Monitor patient's status during needle insertion and throughout the procedure.	5. The patient will feel pressure as the spinal needle is inserted and a stab of pain as the dura is penetrated. Pain radiating down the legs occurs if a spinal nerve root is irritated by the needle. Persistent pain or other sensations may require repositioning of the needle.
6. Help patient to straighten legs slowly after spinal needle is in appropriate position.	6. This prevents a false increase in intraspinal pressure due to muscle tension and abdominal compression.
7. Instruct patient to breathe normally and avoid straining.	
8. Attach manometer to spinal needle and read the opening pressure.	
9. Perform Queckenstedt test, if requested, by compressing both jugular veins for 10 seconds. Normally there is a rapid rise in pressure in response to compression and a rapid return to normal when compression in released.	9. This aids in determining the patency of the CSF pathway. No measurable rise or a slow rise is indicative of complete or partial subarachnoid block respectively. Breath-holding or straining causes failure of pressure to drop.
10. Collect specimens of fluid. A. Allow it to drop slowly into the test tubes. B. Place approximately 1 ml. in each of three test tubes.	
11. Label each test tube with: A. Type of specimen. B. Specimen number in order of sequence.	B. The sequence in which the specimens are obtained is essential for interpretation of laboratory results.
C. Patient's name.	

ACTION	RATIONALE

12. Apply a Band-Aid to the puncture site after needle is withdrawn.

Precautions

1. Maintain strict aseptic technique.
2. Instruct the patient to refrain from coughing, straining, or moving during the procedure, unless instructed to do so by the physician.
3. Be prepared to provide artificial ventilation and maintain a patent airway in the event of brain stem herniation as a result of removal of CSF.

Related Care

1. Instruct the patient to cooperate, breathe normally, and relax as much as possible.
2. Send the specimens of CSF directly to the laboratory, since changes that occur if the fluid is allowed to stand will alter the findings.
3. Observe opening and closing pressures, amount and character of the fluid, drugs if administered, tolerance, and patient's reactions.
4. Instruct the patient to lie flat for 4 or more hours following a lumbar puncture (usually ordered by the physician).
5. Encourage liberal intake of fluid, if the condition permits.
6. Assess changes in vital signs, neurologic status, headache, nausea/ vomiting, and redness, swelling, or drainage from the puncture site.

Complications

Tentorial and cerebellar tonsil herniation   CSF leak
Medullary compression   Infection
Respiratory arrest   Pain
Headache   Paraplegia
Nuchal rigidity

REFERENCES

American Association of Neuroscience Nurses: Core Curriculum for Neuroscience Nursing, 2nd ed. Chicago, American Association of Neuroscience Nurses, 1984.

Brunner, L., et al.: The Lippincott Manual of Nursing Practice, 3rd ed. Philadelphia, J.B. Lippincott, 1982.

Luckmann, J., and Sorrensen, K.: Medical-Surgical Nursing: A Psychophysiologic Approach, 2nd ed. Philadelphia, W.B. Saunders, 1980.

Mancall, E.L.: Alpers and Mancall Essentials of the Neurological Examination, 2nd ed. Philadelphia, F.A. Davis, 1981.

Mayo Clinic and Foundation: Clinical Examinations in Neurology. Philadelphia, W.B. Saunders, 1981.

HYPOTHERMIA
——————— AND HYPERTHERMIA ———————

Marilyn M. Ricci, R.N., M.S., CNRN

Overview

Hypothermia and hyperthermia are therapeutic modalities for maintaining total body temperature at a desired level. Hypothermia is utilized to reduce cellular metabolism, which results in a concomitant decrease in the oxygen requirement of the body tissues. Hyperthermia is utilized to increase and maintain body temperature at a normothermic level.

Hypothermia and hyperthermia equipment incorporates both cooling and heating systems. A pump circulates fluid (usually water) from the reservoir through the thermal blanket, which is either warmed or cooled by the circulating fluid. Most control units can regulate the temperature both manually and automatically. The automatic control system monitors the patient's temperature electronically and regulates cycling of the main unit within preset limits. A temperature sensing probe transmits information to the control system, which causes the machine to heat or cool fluid going to the thermal blankets.

Within critical care settings, these units may be portable or built in. Each unit has a control panel that contains control knobs, indicator lights, and thermometers to indicate the temperature of the circulating fluid and the patient's temperature. Safety features include an alarm system, back-up thermostats, and electrical safeguards. The tubing from the thermal blanket is connected to the unit at two hose couplings. Each unit usually is able to regulate several blankets.

The thermal blankets/pads are made of plastics and synthetic fabrics that are easily cleaned, lightweight to facilitate handling, pliable to fit body contours, firm to resist being pinched off, and smooth enough to avoid causing pressure areas. The blanket/pad may be either reusable or disposable.

Objective

To alter body temperature to a prescribed level by means of an elective clinical therapy.

Hypothermia
1. To lower excessively high temperatures secondary to cerebral trauma and febrile diseases.
2. To minimize tissue damage from diminished oxygen delivery when blood

flow to vital organs is reduced or interrupted (e.g., intracranial surgery or cardiac surgery).

3. To decrease metabolic activity, thereby reducing oxygen requirements (e.g., increased ICP, cerebral edema).

Hyperthermia

1. To warm a patient to as near normothermia as possible prior to obtaining an EEG for the determination of electrocerebral silence.

2. To rewarm the patient to normal body temperature following induced hypothermia.

3. To assist the patient to maintain normal body temperature, as in cases of spinal cord trauma, shock state, and surgery.

Special Equipment

Hypothermia and hyperthermia unit
Thermal blanket/pad
Rectal temperature probe or thermometer
ECG monitor
Indwelling urinary catheter (to facilitate monitoring
   of urinary output)

Procedure

ACTION	RATIONALE
1. Place a single sheet over mattress under thermal pad.	
2. Place one bath blanket on top of thermal pad, under patient. Additional thermal pads may be placed on top of the patient, if increased contact area is needed.	2. Always use a single layer of bath blanket between the patient and thermal pad to facilitate heat exchange and protect the patient's skin.
3. Tuck bath blanket that is on top of pad lightly under mattress.	3. Tight restrictions over the pad or creases in the pad impede the flow of fluid.
4. Place pillows, if needed under head or for positioning, under thermal pad rather than directly under patient.	4. Maximal contact between the patient's skin and the pad increases cooling and heating efficiency.
5. Attach hoses from thermal pad to machine. Be sure the hoses are not kinked or twisted.	

ACTION	RATIONALE
6. Check that reservoir in machine is filled with appropriate solution (distilled water or an antifreeze solution, as recommended by the manufacturer) to level indicated.	
7. Prepare equipment according to manual or automatic mode. Plug into wall outlet.	
8. Prior to starting the machine, take vital signs and assess conscious level, pupils, motor function, and skin condition.	
A. Manual control:	
(1) Place temperature dial at "start" and push manual button to activate machine.	
(2) Dial desired thermal pad setting.	
(a) Hypothermia:	(a) Running the machine at the 40° F. setting for long periods will increase the possibility of ischemia of the pressure areas and freeze burns of the skin. The reset temperature allows for the tendency of the patient's temperature to drift downward.
(i) Place the temperature dial at 40° F. for approximately 5 minutes.	
(ii) Then reset temperature control to 1° F. above the desired temperature.	
(b) Hyperthermia:	
(i) Place temperature control at 100° F. for approximately 5 minutes.	
(ii) Then reset temperature to a setting of 1° F. below the desired temperature.	
(3) Adjust temperature setting of thermal pad to attain desired temperature of patient.	
(4) Monitor patient's temperature every 15 minutes until desired temperature has been reached.	(4) Usually it takes 3 to 4 hours to bring a patient's temperature to the desired range when using one thermal pad.
(5) Adjust temperature setting of thermal pad to maintain a stable body temperature.	(5) Usually a 20^0- to 25^0 F. differential between the pad and body temperatures will maintain a stable hypothermic state.

ACTION	RATIONALE

B. Automatic control. The cooling or heating process is controlled by the patient's body temperature, via a rectal probe.

(1) Place temperature dial at "start," and push manual button to activate machine.

(2) Dial desired thermal pad setting.

    (a) Hypothermia: Place temperature control at 40° F. for 5 minutes.

    (b) Hyperthermia: Place temperature control at 100° F. for 5 minutes.

(3) Reset temperature to 1° F. above (hypothermia) or below (hyperthermia) the desired patient temperature.

(4) Depress automatic control button.

(5) Insert lubricated tip of temperature probe about 4 inches into patient's rectum and tape it securely in place. (An axillary probe may be used if rectal insertion is contraindicated.)

(6) Insert metal jack at other end of probe into patient probe adapter on machine.

(7) Obtain rectal temperature of patient by depressing appropriate button on control panel.

(8) Check that electronic control meter is giving accurate readings of patient's temperature.

    (a) Take patient's rectal temperature manually.

    (b) Move temperature control dial to settings 3° F. above and below actual patient temperature. The "cool" and "heat" indicators should go on appropriately.

(6) The thermostatic control will heat or cool the fluid circulating through the thermal pad according to the patient's temperature as monitored by the rectal probe.

Precautions

1. Use hypothermia cautiously in patients with impaired circulation because of the possibility of severe tissue damage.
2. Prevent shivering, which occurs during initial cooling and rewarming phase, since it can increase metabolic rate, body temperature, oxygen usage, and circulation; cause hyperventilation; and may produce hypoglycemia. Shivering appears first in the masseter muscles, then in the neck and pectoral muscles, and finally in the long muscles of upper and lower extremities. Administer medications to prevent shivering, as prescribed.
3. Reduce or stop the procedure within 1° to 3° F. of the desired level, since temperature may "overshoot" or "drift" 1° to 2° F. after the desired temperature has been reached.
4. Evaluate the patient's clinical status during hypothermia in view of an anticipated depression of sensorium, respirations, cardiac output, renal output, and other vital functions.
   A. Avoid temperature decrease exceeding 1° F. per 15 minutes to avoid premature ventricular contractions.
   B. Monitor parameters of cardiac dynamics.
   C. Maximal reduction of heart rate usually occurs with the initial temperature drop.
5. Be alert for cardiac insufficiency due to rapid surface rewarming.
6. Be prepared for an alteration in the metabolism of drugs during hypothermic and hyperthermic states. A cumulative effect may occur during rewarming.
7. Avoid any sudden sharp rise in temperature.
8. Avoid puncturing the thermal blanket with pins.
9. Check the equipment for leaks, kinks, twists, and mechanical and electrical failure.

Related Care

1. Monitor vital signs, neurologic status, color of lips, and capillary refill at least every 30 minutes, and urinary output every hour.
2. Protect skin integrity by repositioning, applying lotion, and massaging bony prominences at least every 30 to 60 minutes. Wrap distal extremities with towels to decrease incidence of frank shivering and preserve skin integrity.
3. Maintain a patent airway by positioning, suctioning, and avoiding oral intake when the gag and swallow reflexes are depressed.
4. Protect the patient's eyes in the absence of the corneal reflex and when eye secretions are decreased.
5. Reduce circulatory stasis by doing range of motion exercises and avoiding restrictive bands.

Complications

Frostbite/fat necrosis
Focal tissue necrosis
Hypersensitivity to cold
Ventricular fibrillation and cardiac dysrhythmias
Acidosis (metabolic or respiratory, or both)
Oliguria/anuria
Embolization
Hyperpyrexia
Ileus
Cold diuresis

REFERENCES

American Association of Neuroscience Nurses: Core Curriculum for Neuroscience Nursing, 2nd ed. Park Ridge, American Association of Neuroscience Nurses, 1984.
Beaumont, E.: Hypo/hyperthermia equipment. Nursing '74 4:34, 1974.
Hudak, C., et al.: Critical Care Nursing, 3rd ed. Philadelphia, J.B. Lippincott, 1982.
St Joseph's Hospital and Medical Center: Nursing Procedure Manual. Phoenix, St. Joseph's Hospital and Medical Center, 1983.

SKELETAL TRACTION
───────── OF THE CERVICAL SPINE ─────────

Marilyn M. Ricci, R.N., M.S., CNRN

Overview

Skeletal traction is a means of external fixation that is used to immobilize the cervical vertebral column for the prevention of damage to the underlying spinal cord and spinal nerves. The placement of cervical tongs or a halo ring into the skull with the application of traction at the desired weight will enable reduction of the fracture/dislocation and maintenance of the anatomical alignment of the vertebral column.

Cervical tongs consist of a stainless steel body with a sharp pin attached on each end (Fig. 4–8). The method and location of placement of each type of tong vary slightly, but the care is essentially the same.

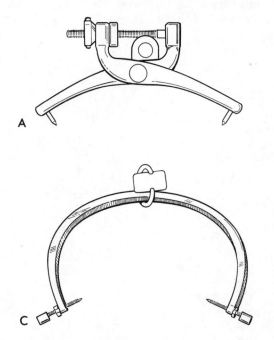

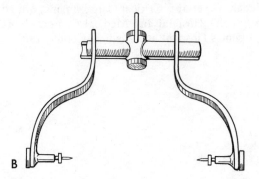

Figure 4-8. All three types of cervical tongs consist of a stainless steel body with a pin about 1/8 inch (0.3 cm) in diameter with a sharp tip attached to each end. *(A),* Crutchfield tongs are placed about 5 inches (12.7 cm) apart in line with the long axis of the cervical spine. *(B),* The pins on the Vinke tongs are placed at the parietal bones, near the widest transverse diameter of the skull, about 1 inch (2.54 cm) above the helix. *(C),* The pins on the Gardner-Wells tongs are farther apart, with the pins inserted slightly above the patient's ears.

For insertion of *Crutchfield tongs* an incision is made exposing the skull. Two holes are drilled into the outer table with a twist drill. The tongs are placed and the screws are tightened until there is a firm fit. *Vinke tongs* are inserted in a similar manner. The points of *Gardner-Wells tongs* are pressed against the scalp and advanced until the spring-loaded mechanism indicates that the correct pressure is being exerted. Tilting the tongs back and forth seats the pins in the outer table of the skull. The points are angled in the direction of pull of the weights to decrease the possibility of tong displacement.

After the tongs are inserted the traction is applied by extending a rope from the center of the tongs over a pulley and attaching the desired amount of weight. X-rays are taken immediately and at frequent intervals to evaluate the effectiveness of the reduction and alignment. Excessive traction may produce distraction of the vertebra with stretching and damage to the underlying neural elements.

The *halo device* consists of a metal ring that fits around the patient's head and is attached to the skull by four pins. Two posterolateral and two anterolateral pins are threaded through holes in the ring, screwed into the outer table at 90-degree angles, and locked in place. There are no scalp incisions or drill holes. Direct traction may be applied to the cervical spine in a similar manner as the tongs, or stabilization may be achieved by attaching the device to a body jacket/vest.

Procedures for insertion of an external fixation device, maintenance of the desired traction, and tong or pin care are presented. Because the objectives, precautions, related care, and complications are similar, they are presented only once and identified as general.

Objectives: General

1. To align the cervical vertebrae following injury.
2. To reduce a fracture, dislocation, and/or locked facets of the cervical spine.
3. To minimize movement of a potentially unstable vertebral column.
4. To prevent additional damage to the bony elements, ligaments, spinal cord, and spinal nerves by providing stability of the cervical spine.
5. To stabilize the vertebrae and decrease pain and discomfort.
6. To immobilize the vertebral elements until healing has occurred.
7. To permit safe turning, repositioning, and skin and pulmonary care.
8. To prevent infection at the pin sites or halo fixation points by performing site care each shift.

INSERTION OF AN EXTERNAL FIXATION DEVICE (ASSISTING WITH) _____

Special Equipment

Tongs or halo device (with software, hardware, and tools)
Razor or clippers or both
Local anesthetic, e.g., 1% lidocaine
Povidone-iodine scrub, solution, and ointment
Syringe and needles for anesthetic
Surgical gloves
Traction assembly with desired weights
Crutchfield and Vinke tongs:
    Sterile twist drill set
    Scalpal with blades
    Suture

Procedure

ACTION	RATIONALE
1. Trim and shave the selected pin sites.	1. Visibility of the skin sites facilitates care and prevention of infection.
2. Cleanse the pin sites with povidone-iodine solution.	
3. Assist in the preparation of the anesthetic and the equipment.	
4. Set up the traction assembly.	4. Traction is to be applied immediately after the insertion of the tongs/halo crown.
5. Hold the patient's head and neck stable during the insertion procedure. A cervical collar or sandbags may be used.	5. Securing the head facilitates placement of the device and decreases risk of further damage to the underlying neural elements.
6. Assist with the application of the traction at the desired weight, or the halo vest.	6. Immediate and continuous immobilization aids in prevention of further neurological damage.
7. Record the procedure, including the amount of weight applied and the patient's response to the procedure.	7. This serves as baseline data since additional weights are added or removed to achieve the desired vertebral alignment and fracture reduction.

MAINTENANCE OF THE DESIRED TRACTION _____

1. Check the tongs every 4 hours initially and then at least every shift to determine placement and tightness. Notify the physician if they are loose or slip out. Do not move the patient until tongs are secure.	1. The tongs may not be finally seated until 24 hours following insertion. Loose tongs may slip out of place and may require readjustment to maintain the desired effect.

ACTION	RATIONALE
2. Immobilize the head and neck in neutral position with sandbags if the pins pull out, and remove the weights gently. Manual traction may be applied if necessary.	
3. Check the traction assembly every 4 hours, and after turning or transporting the patient or after other movement. Be sure the weights are hanging freely, the rope is in place on the pulley, the knot on the rope is not against the pulley, and the direction of the pull and the patient's head and body are in correct alignment.	3. When the weights are resting on an object, and the traction is released, malalignment and additional spinal cord damage could occur. The weight of the traction may pull the patient up in bed until the knot at the tongs rests against the pulley, releasing the traction. The patient may require being pulled down in bed frequently.
4. Gently add or subtract weights as ordered. Apply weights slowly and carefully to avoid sudden jerking movements. Sedatives may be required to achieve muscle relaxation.	4. The amount of traction is determined by the purpose of the procedure and the muscular status of the patient. Immobilization is achieved by 5 to 15 pounds, depending on whether there is bony displacement. Reduction of a fracture dislocation may require application of up to 60 to 80 pounds in 10-pound increments.
5. Assess the patient frequently for neurologic changes as the weights are changed or the patient is moved. X-rays will be repeated frequently as the weights are increased.	5. Excessive traction will distract the spine and produce neurologic impairment. Insufficient traction may result in bony compression of neural elements.
6. Use five people to lift a patient. One person should be at the head to stabilize the neck, maintain the traction manually, and coordinate the move. The other four people handle the patient as *one* unit, avoiding twisting. A mobilizer may also be used.	6. A patient may be safely lifted and moved up in bed or from one bed to another using a four-person synchronous lift with a fifth person at the head. The amount of traction and the patient's position must be maintained throughout the procedure.
7. Inform the patient of all activities and ask the patient to report any discomfort or changes in sensation.	7. An informed patient will be able to cooperate and avoid sudden movements.
8. Record the status of the tongs, traction, and patient's response to change in weights and position, and to moving.	

TONG OR PIN CARE

Special Equipment

Hydrogen peroxide
Sterile normal saline
Povidone-iodine ointment (unless otherwise specified)
Cotton-tipped applicators
Sterile 2-inch x 2-inch gauze squares
Sterile gloves
Optional:
>   Povidone-iodine–soaked gauze squares
>   Iodoform gauze

Procedure

ACTION	RATIONALE
1. Remove the dressing from each pin site.	1. The use of a dressing depends on the type of tongs and physician preference. A dressing will be applied when a pin site is infected.
2. Inspect the pin sites each shift and as necessary for bleeding, CSF leak, swelling, redness, and purulent drainage. Note any complaints of pain at the pin sites.	2. The pins may perforate the inner table and dura, which causes a CSF leak. Contamination of the pin sites causes infection and subsequent swelling and pain.
3. Clip or shave the hair around the pin sites as necessary.	3. Inspection and pin care are difficult when the hair is present. Hairs may become twisted around the pins and promote infection.
4. Cleanse the area around each pin with hydrogen peroxide during each shift. Use a separate applicator for each site.	4. The removal of crusts and old ointment aids in preventing infection. Cross contamination can occur, and all pin sites may become infected.
5. Rinse each area thoroughly with normal saline and dry well.	5. Hydrogen peroxide is irritating to the skin.
6. Use applicators to apply the ointment or sterile gloves to wrap gauze around the pins. Check with physician regarding preferences.	

| ACTION | RATIONALE |

7. Record the condition of the sites, the presence of drainage or swelling, and the method of care site.

Precautions: General

1. Never remove or reduce the amount of traction without a physician's order when the patient is being treated for a fracture or dislocation or both.
2. Avoid sudden movements of the traction device, the patient, or the bed.
3. Check the tongs, traction, bolts, and other devices whenever the patient has been moved or repositioned.
4. Support the head and neck and maintain the traction whenever the patient is moved. *Do not release the traction.*
5. Note that pain and motor or sensory losses may be caused by overreduction of the fracture and incorrect alignment.
6. Maintain the patient in a neutral or slightly hyperextended position to provide the maximum benefit from the traction.
7. When moving a patient up in bed or from one bed to another, use a four-person synchronous lift with a fifth person at the head to stabilize the head and neck, maintain the traction manually, and coordinate the move. Do not begin the move until each person's role and position have been determined and everyone is ready.
8. When using a turning frame, use at least two persons to ensure patient safety and reassure the anxious patient.
9. Assess cranial nerves VI, IX, and XII, which may become damaged from the pin placement.
10. Note that hypoventilation and cardiovascular instability may occur as a result of paralysis of the respiratory musculature and loss of sympathetic innervation respectively.
11. Avoid hyperextension of the neck in a cardiopulmonary resuscitation situation. Use the jaw thrust method and maintain the head and neck in a neutral position.
12. Keep a wrench taped to the front of the halo vest at all times to remove the front of the vest in the event of cardiac arrest.

Related Care: General

1. Assess the patient for changes in motor, sensory, and pulmonary function at frequent intervals (every 1 to 2 hours) immediately after the traction has been applied, when the weights are changed, and when the patient is moved.

2. Administer mild analgesics to control headache, spasm of the neck muscles, and discomfort at the pin sites or halo-fixation points. Avoid medications that cause respiratory depression.

3. Avoid contamination of the pin sites from the patient's hands or accidental spilling of fluids.

4. When a small rolled towel is placed under the back of the neck to achieve the desired vertebral alignment, keep the roll in place at all times, and replace immediately when it becomes soiled or wet. A diagram may help to ensure correct placement.

5. Turn and reposition the patient at least every 2 hours to help prevent pulmonary and skin problems. Use log-rolling technique, a turning bed, or frame to maintain alignment and prevent flexion, hyperextension, and rotation of the cervical spine.

6. Maintain an adequate airway, blood oxygenation, and perfusion pressures because the injured spinal cord is susceptible to additional insult from hypoxia and hypotension.
   A. Monitor respiratory and cardiovascular parameters every 2 hours and as necessary.
   B. Report signs of respiratory insufficiency, e.g., dyspnea, tachypnea, abnormal blood gases, and the subjective feeling of the patient's "not getting enough air."
   C. Assist the patient to clear the airway by suctioning and manual coughing.
   D. Encourage deep breathing or the use of the incentive spirometer every 2 hours to prevent atelectasis and increase vital capacity.
   E. Maintain patency and humidification of endotracheal or tracheostomy tube as necessary.
   F. Note that mechanical ventilation may be needed in the event of respiratory failure from paralysis or fatigue of the respiratory musculature. This may not occur until 24 to 72 hours post injury.
   G. To prevent aspiration use a nasogastric tube until bowel sounds have returned.
   H. Note that placing the patient in prone position on a turning frame may further compromise pulmonary function.
   I. Use chest physiotherapy to facilitate effective pulmonary function.
   J. Use support hose and leg exercises to decrease hypotensive effects of peripheral vasodilatation and venous pooling.
   K. Administer low doses of dopamine to maintain a blood pressure of at least 80/50.
   L. Avoid fluid overload which will cause spinal cord edema.
   M. Administer atropine if the heart rate is less than 48 per minute. (Bradycardia may be precipitated by suctioning and position change.)
   N. Monitor for dysrhythmias and give medication if necessary.

7. Inspect the skin of the entire body, and give skin care every 2 hours to maintain skin integrity. Padding, pressure mattresses, and sheepskin may be used to prevent skin breakdown. Check the edges of the halo vest by inserting a finger to determine if it is too tight.

8. Monitor bowel sounds during each shift. Use a nasogastric tube to prevent stomach dilation and aspiration, which impair pulmonary function. It may be necessary to measure abdominal girth.

9. Assess extremities for changes in size, color, and temperature. Measure the calf and thigh circumferences to detect swelling from deep-vein thrombosis; heparin may be administered for prevention and control. Apply antiembolus stockings, and perform range of motion exercises to the lower extremities every 4 hours.

10. Anticipate perceptual disturbances and restlessness due to immobilization, sensory deprivation, and the environment. Reinforce orientation to reality and provide diversional activities, e.g., radio, TV, prism glasses, mirrors.

Complications: General

Infection at the pin site(s)
Neurologic damage due to excessive traction
Malalignment
Erosion of the bone at the pin sites

REFERENCES

Hickey, J.: The Clinical Practice of Neurological and Neurosurgical Nursing. Philadelphia, J.B. Lippincott, 1981.

Howard, M., and Corbo-Pelaia, S.: Halo traction: A review of acute care. Am. J. Nurs. 82:1839–1843, 1982.

St. Joseph's Hospital: Nursing Procedure Manual. Phoenix, St. Joseph's Hospital and Medical Center, 1983.

Snyder, M. (ed.): A Guide to Neurological and Neurosurgical Nursing. New York, Wiley, 1983.

5

THE
GASTROINTESTINAL
SYSTEM

MANAGEMENT OF
UPPER GASTROINTESTINAL
HEMORRHAGE

Barbara Buss Fugleberg, R.N., B.S.N., CCRN,
Elaine Brogdon, R.N., M.N.,
Kathy Mossing, R.N., M.A., M.B.A., and
Barbara Tabor, R.N., B.S.N., CEN

Overview

Gastrointestinal bleeding can be an insidious process with few manifestations, or it can present with massive hemorrhage. In some cases it may be necessary to pass a nasogastric tube to observe and test aspirate to determine if bleeding is or has been present. Active bleeding may be nonsurgically controlled by irrigating the gastrointestinal tract with iced saline solution to constrict the arteries by hypothermia, by applying pressure locally with balloon tamponade, or by constricting the bleeding vessels through local or systemic infusion of vasopressin (Pitressin).

NASOGASTRIC TUBE INSERTION

Overview

Nasogastric tubes are used to assess gastrointestinal function, detect complications, treat problems, administer medications, provide feedings, and decompress the stomach and duodenum. For these purposes the stomach is intubated with either a single-lumen Levin tube or a double-lumen sump tube. The sizes most frequently used for adults are 16 and 18 Fr.

The Levin tubes are either rubber or plastic and are approximately 48 inches in length. Marker rings are located at 18-, 22-, 26-, and 30-inch points; lumen size ranges from 10 through 18 Fr.

Sump tubes are of clear plastic, constructed much the same as Levin tubes. The unique feature of the sump tube is its second lumen, which serves as a decompression vent to prevent blockage of the suction lumen by large particles or gastric mucosa.

Objectives

1. To determine the site, freshness, and amount of gastrointestinal bleeding.
2. To test aspirate for frank blood (or guaiac) or acidity.
3. To administer antacids.
4. To lavage stomach, when necessary.

Special Equipment

Nasogastric tube
Water-soluble lubricant
50-ml. irrigating syringe
Emesis basin
Tape
Glass of water/straw

Ice
Suction source
Stethoscope
Rubber band
Safety pin

Procedure

ACTION	RATIONALE
1. Position patient, using one of the following:	
A. Left lateral position.	A. This facilitates passage of the tube into the cardia of the stomach.
B. Trendelenburg position.	B. This is indicated for hypotensive, comatose patients.
C. Sitting position.	C. This decreases gag reflex and makes swallowing easier.
2. Place nasogastric tube on ice or refrigerate.	2. This stiffens the tube for easier insertion, especially if the patient is intubated.
3. Lubricate tube.	3. This lessens irritation of the mucosa.
4. Place 50-ml. irrigating syringe on end of tube.	
5. Measure length of tube to be passed.	
A. Measure from bridge of nose to ear lobe to xiphoid process.	A. This measurement is the approximate length of the tube needed to reach the stomach.
B. Indicate this length by placing tape at that point on tube.	

ACTION	RATIONALE
6. Determine which nostril is more patent.	6. Choose the nostril with the best air flow.
A. Ask the patient if he has ever had nasal surgery, trauma or a deviated septum.	
B. Occlude one nostril at a time while the patient breathes through the nose.	
7. Insert tube.	
A. Pass tube gently into the nasopharynx.	
B. If resistance is met rotate the tube slowly, aiming downward and toward the closer ear.	B. Avoid pressure on the turbinates, which may cause bleeding or pressure.
C. Advance tube firmly and steadily while patient is swallowing.	C. Swallowing facilitates passage of the tube.
D. Offer sips of water from a glass when tube reaches posterior nasopharynx.	D. In the alert patient, this minimizes gagging and facilitates passage of the tube.
E. Flex the patient's head on his chest. Pass tube until tape mark is reached and secure to nose with tape.	E. This opens the esophagus and facilitates passage in the intubated patient.
8. Withdraw tube immediately if any change in respiratory status is noted.	8. This may indicate placement in the bronchus.
9. Test for tube placement, using one or more of the following techniques.	
A. Obtain gastric content by aspirating with 50-ml. syringe.	
B. Auscultate with stethoscope over gastric area while 50 ml. of air is inserted into tube.	B. If tube is properly placed, a rush of air should be heard.
C. Place end of tube in glass of water to check for bubbling.	C. Bubbling indicates tube is in the bronchus, and immediate withdrawal is necessary.
D. Obtain order for x-ray to confirm placement.	D. The absence of bubbling does not confirm placement.
10. Connect tube to suction, or continue with gastric lavage (see "Gastric Lavage").	

ACTION	RATIONALE

11. Secure tube to patient's gown.
   A. Tie a slipknot around the tube with a rubber band.
   B. Pin the rubber band to the patient's gown.
	11. This prevents tugging on the tube when the patient moves.

Precautions

1. Assess for coiling in oral pharynx or esophagus and then for tube patency if patient gags or vomits around the tube.
2. Assess for possible tube placement into the lungs if patient becomes cyanotic or dyspneic.
3. Maintain airway with frequent suctioning if oral secretions persist.

Related Care

1. Maintain patency of the tube by irrigation and repositioning.
2. Observe drainage for changes.
3. Keep a record of the amounts of intake and output.
4. Restrain or sedate patient, if indicated, to prevent removal of the tube and possible aspiration of the gastric contents.
5. Record size and type of nasogastric tube inserted and type of suction used.
6. Connect Salem sump tubes to continuous suction. Connect Levin tubes to intermittent suction.

Complications

Aspiration	Nasal mucosa erosion
Electrolyte imbalance	Trauma to gastric mucosa
Hyperventilation	Reflux esophagitis
Bradycardia	

REFERENCES

Brunner, L.S., and Suddarth, D.S. (eds.): Lippincott Manual of Nursing Practice, 3rd ed. Philadelphia, J. B. Lippincott, 1982, pp. 392–395.

Erickson, R.: Tube talk. Nursing 82, 12:55–62, (July) 1982.

Luckmann, J., and Sorensen, K.: Medical-Surgical Nursing: A Psychophysiologic Approach, 2nd ed. Philadelphia, W.B. Saunders, 1980.

McConnell, E.: Ten problems with nasogastric tubes and how to solve them. Nursing 79, 9:78–81, 1979.

Strange, J.M.: An expert's guide to tubes and drains. RN, 46(4):35–42, 1983.

GASTRIC LAVAGE

Objectives

1. To control upper gastrointestinal bleeding by vasoconstriction of gastric vessels, using hypothermia.
2. To remove any toxins, large blood clots, or old blood from the stomach.

Special Equipment

Large-bore (32 Fr.) Ewald tube or 18 Fr. Salem sump tube
Large 2- to 3-liter inflow bottle
Large-bore inflow and outflow tubing, connected to the
    inflow bottle with **V**-connector
Iced normal saline solution
Outflow bottle
50-ml. aspirating syringe
Lubricant
Large pair of hemostats for clamping tubing

Procedure

ACTION	RATIONALE
1. Set up lavage equipment (Fig. 5–1).	
2. Insert Salem sump or Ewald tube (see "Nasogastric Tube Insertion" for details of tube advancement).	
3. Obtain gastric specimen.	3. This is used for diagnostic purposes.
4. Siphon initial gastric contents into outflow bottle.	4. Initial emptying of the stomach decreases chance of vomiting and possible aspiration.
5. Fill inflow bottle with iced normal saline solution, with inflow tubing clamped.	5. Normal saline solution is isotonic; this prevents decreased osmolarity. Ice is used to cause vasoconstriction in the stomach.
6. Open inflow tubing, starting with 250-ml. inflow rate.	6. An initial 250-ml. amount checks the patient's tolerance for adding extra fluid to the stomach and facilitates emptying the stomach contents.

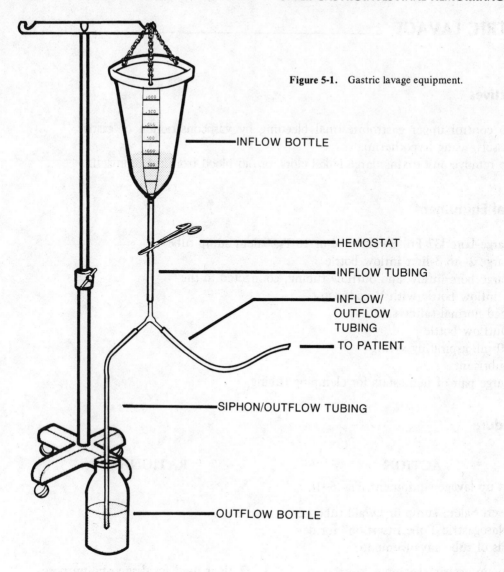

Figure 5-1. Gastric lavage equipment.

INFLOW BOTTLE

HEMOSTAT

INFLOW TUBING

INFLOW/ OUTFLOW TUBING

TO PATIENT

SIPHON/OUTFLOW TUBING

OUTFLOW BOTTLE

ACTION	RATIONALE
7. Increase inflow amount to 500 ml. as soon as possible.	7. 500 ml. of fluid are needed to flatten the rugae of the stomach.
8. Infuse and siphon out solution repeatedly, using large syringe or siphoning set up.	
9. Measure inflow and outflow amounts.	9. These amounts should be equal; inflow should not exceed outflow or distention will occur.
10. Lavage until clear.	10. This assures adequate "washout" of the stomach.

Precautions

1. Suction oral cavity frequently during procedure to prevent possible aspiration and enhance patient comfort.
2. Assess for tube patency, including coiling in oral pharynx or esophagus, if patient vomits around the tube.
3. Assess tube placement into the lungs if the patient becomes cyanotic or dyspneic.
4. Maintain airway with frequent suctioning if oral secretions persist.

Related Care

1. Maintain patency of tube through irrigation and repositioning.
2. Observe drainage for changes.
3. Keep a record of the amounts of intake and output.
4. Restrain patient, if indicated, to prevent removal of the tube and possible aspiration of the gastric contents.
5. Record size and type of nasogastric tube inserted.

Complications

Aspiration	Nasal mucosa erosion
Electrolyte imbalance	Trauma to gastric mucosa
Hyperventilation	Reflux esophagitis
Bradycardia	Hypothermia, if using
Chills	iced saline
Shock	

REFERENCES

Brunner, L.S., and Suddarth, D.S. (eds.): Lippincott Manual of Nursing Practice, 3rd ed. Philadelphia, J. B. Lippincott, 1982, pp. 890–891.
Hamilton, H.K., and Rose, M.B. (eds.): Procedures. Springhouse, PA, Intermed Communications, 1983, pp. 551–553.
Luckmann, J., and Sorensen, K.: Medical-Surgical Nursing: A Psychophysiologic Approach, 2nd ed. Philadelphia, W.B. Saunders, 1980.

SENGSTAKEN/BLAKEMORE TUBE

Overview

Bleeding from gastric and esophageal varices can be controlled by applying local pressure to the bleeding sites. This is accomplished by the insertion

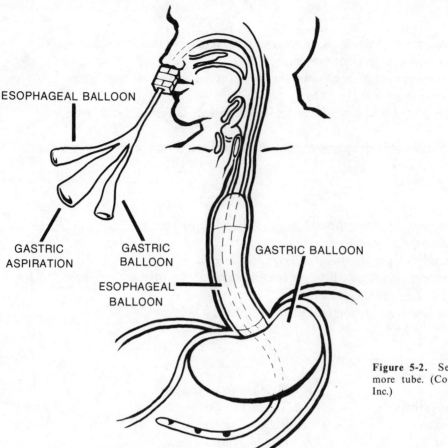

ESOPHAGEAL BALLOON

GASTRIC
ASPIRATION

GASTRIC
BALLOON

ESOPHAGEAL
BALLOON

GASTRIC BALLOON

Figure 5-2. Sengstaken-Blakemore tube. (Courtesy of Davol, Inc.)

of the triple-lumen, double-balloon, 20 Fr. red rubber Sengstaken/Blakemore tube. One lumen is used for gastric aspiration, one for inflating the esophageal balloon, and one for inflating the gastric balloon (Fig. 5–2). An additional modification is recommended—that is, the use of an accessory nasogastric tube to remove oral secretions draining into the esophagus and prevent aspiration. After insertion and inflation of the balloons, traction is applied to prevent advancement into the stomach.

Objective

To control massive bleeding from esophageal varices via nonoperative management, using esophagogastric balloon tamponade.

Special Equipment

Sengstaken/Blakemore tube
Accessory 18 Fr. nasogastric tube

Suction source
Sphygmomanometer
50-ml. aspirating syringe
Lidocaine or cocaine
Topical spray
Oral mouthpiece
Sponge rubber cube
Four rubber-tipped hemostats
Two suction setups
2½-ft. rubber tubing (blood pressure tubing size)
Water-soluble lubricating jelly
Catcher's mask, football helmet with mouth guard, or 1- to 2-lb.
   weights.
Scissors
Y connector
Adhesive tape

Procedure

ACTION	RATIONALE
1. Place patient in left lateral position.	1. This facilitates gastric balloon introduction into the cardia of the stomach.
2. Prepare tubes.	
A. Hold air-filled balloons under water to test for air leaks.	A. This assures proper function.
B. Lubricate both balloons and lower parts of Sengstaken/Blakemore tube with water-soluble jelly.	B. This decreases trauma to mucous membranes.
C. Tape the 18 Fr. nasogastric tube alongside Sengstaken/Blakemore tube, level with top of esophageal balloon.	
D. Connect accessory esophageal tube to low continuous suction.	D. This prevents secretions from accumulating in the esophagus
3. Attempt to empty stomach and esophagus with Ewald tube lavage, prior to insertion (see "Gastric Lavage").	3. This minimizes the possibility of aspiration.
4. Measure length of tube to be passed.	
A. Place the balloon at the xiphoid.	
B. Measure the distance between the nose and the xiphoid.	
C. Note the mark on the side of the tube.	

ACTION	RATIONALE
5. Anesthetize posterior pharynx and nostrils topically.	5. This decreases the discomfort caused by tube passage.
6. Insert tube (see "Nasogastric Tube Insertion").	
A. Pass Sengstaken/Blakemore tube, with balloons deflated, through nasopharynx into stomach to at least 50-cm mark or 10-cm. beyond the mark measured on the tubing. (A guidewire into the gastric lumen may facilitate tube insertion.)	A. This decreases the possibility of inflating the gastric balloon in the esophagus.
B. Aspirate gastric tube lumen.	B. This verifies gastric positioning and helps to avoid regurgitation during tube manipulation.
C. Insert plastic bite block or airway, if oral route is used.	C. This prevents biting of the tube.
7. Confirm tube placement.	
A. Aspirate stomach contents from the gastric port.	
B. Auscultate over the stomach with a stethoscope while injecting air into the gastric port.	
C. Obtain abdominal x-ray after injecting balloon with 20-ml. of air.	C. The visible outline of the partially inflated balloon can be seen.
8. Inflate gastric balloon, using 50 to 250 ml. of air, and double-clamp inlet immediately distal to opening.	8. This prevents air leaks.
9. Withdraw tube until resistance is encountered.	9. This engages gastric balloon at the cardioesophageal junction.
10. Maintain gentle tension on tube by:	
A. Taping to a cube of sponge rubber as it emerges from the nasal orifice; or	A. This fixes position of the tube at the cardioesophageal junction. The sponge also minimizes pressure on the nostril caused by the traction.
B. Applying gentle traction with 1 to 2 lbs. of pull and small sponge taped on tube; or	
C. Fixing the tube to a baseball catcher's mask or a football helmet with mouth guard worn by patient.	

ACTION	RATIONALE
11. Lavage stomach (see "Gastric Lavage").	11. This prevents clotted blood from plugging tube. Immediate evacuation of stomach contents allows for subsequent evaluation of gastric tamponade effectiveness.
A. Irrigate until clear through gastric inlet.	
B. Then connect gastric end to continuous or intermittent suction.	
12. Inflate esophageal balloon if bleeding is not controlled by gastric tamponade.	
A. Connect 2½-ft. rubber tubing from esophageal inlet via **Y** connector to sphygomanometer (Fig. 5–3). Observe baseline pressure and *not* transient peak pressure.	A. This permits periodic checking of esophageal balloon pressure. With proper position, pressure will vary with respirations and esophageal contractions.

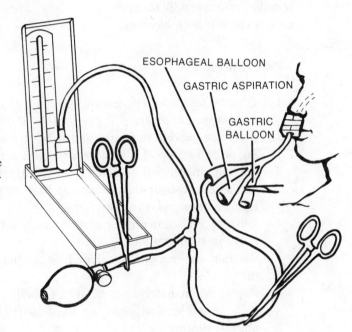

ESOPHAGEAL BALLOON

GASTRIC ASPIRATION

GASTRIC BALLOON

Figure 5-3. Sengstaken-Blakemore tube connected to a sphygmomanometer. (Courtesy of Davol, Inc.)

B. Inflate to 30 to 45 mm. Hg pressure.	B. The lowest pressure necessary to stop bleeding is used.
C. Double-clamp with rubber-tipped hemostat.	C. This prevents air leaks.
D. Check to see if patient complains of substernal pressure.	D. Complaint of substernal pressure as higher pressures are reached is not uncommon.
13. Switch accessory nasogastric tube suction from constant to low intermittent suction.	

ACTION	RATIONALE
14. If bleeding continues after esophageal balloon pressure is maintained at 45 mm. Hg., inflate gastric balloon with air gradually up to 400 ml.	14. Prolonged maintenance of high pressure causes mucosal ulceration within a few hours.

15. Maintain tamponade for 72 hours.
   A. Release esophageal balloon pressure and relax traction on gastric balloon 12 to 24 hours prior to withdrawal.
   B. Observe for rebleeding, and should bleeding recur, reestablish esophageal pressure.
   C. Transect tube with scissors and remove Sengstaken/Blakemore tube if there is no rebleeding.

C. This ensures balloon deflation prior to removal.

Precautions

1. Observe for persistent gastric bleeding; this indicates possible gastric erosions or peptic ulcer.
2. Maintain balloon pressures and tube position to prevent persistent bleeding or pulling up of the balloon to the trachea.
3. Suction pharyngeal secretions frequently to prevent aspiration. If alert and able to cooperate, the patient may be provided with a dental suction tip to suction his own secretions.
4. Observe for ineffective gastric lavage and stomach emptying that may result in regurgitation.
5. Restrain the patient if agitated or confused, to prevent removal of the tube.
6. Report immediately symptoms of sudden back pain, upper abdominal pain, unstable vital signs, or fluid in the chest that may indicate esophageal rupture.

Related Care

1. Maintain ongoing evaluation of coagulation factors.
2. Use and care for nasogastric tube, as indicated in "Nasogastric Tube Insertion."
3. Lavage stomach every 30 to 60 minutes.
4. Monitor balloon pressures every 30 to 60 minutes.
5. Reposition the Sengstaken/Blakemore tube, when necessary, to maintain optimum effect and prevent complications.
6. Elevate head of bed or place head of bed on 6- to 8-inch blocks.
7. Provide frequent oral care.

8. Maintain a prophylactic pulmonary regimen.
9. Maintain an accurate intake and output record.
10. Keep patient under constant surveillance.
11. Tape scissors within clear view and easy reach.

Complications

Rupture or laceration of esophagus
Necrosis or erosion of esophagus or stomach
Aspiration
Asphyxiation
Prolonged bleeding

Supplier

Davol, Inc.

REFERENCES

AACN Clinical Reference for Critical-Care Nursing. (M.R. Kinney, ed.). New York, McGraw-Hill, 1981, pp. 701–703.

Blakemore, A.H. (ed.): Instructions for Passing the Esophageal Balloon for Control of Bleeding from Esophageal Varices. New York, Davol, Inc.

Brunner, L.S., and Suddarth, D.S. (eds.): Lippincott Manual of Nursing Practice, 3rd ed. Philadelphia, J. B. Lippincott, 1982, pp. 457–459.

Hamilton, H.K., and Rose, M.B. (eds.): Procedures. Springhouse, PA, Intermed Communications, 1983, pp. 534–540.

MESENTERIC ARTERY LINE AND VASOPRESSIN (PITRESSIN) INFUSION

Overview

Portal vascular system bleeding may be identified and located by angiography. Vasopressin (Pitressin) infusion may be selected as the treatment of choice; it may be administered systemically via a peripheral intravenous line or, preferably, by a local infusion. The latter is accomplished by catheterizing the superior mesenteric artery or one of its branches through the femoral artery under fluoroscopy.

Objective

To induce splanchnic arteriolar vasoconstriction and decreased portal blood flow by use of vasopressin in patients with esophageal varices.

Special Equipment

Infusion pump and administration tubing
500 ml. normal saline solution, or 500 ml. 5% dextrose in water
Vasopressin (Pitressin) 20 units/vial

Procedure

ACTION	RATIONALE
1. Monitor patient response while line is inserted via femoral artery, under fluoroscopy.	1. Visualization is necessary for accurate placement in superior mesenteric, celiac, left gastric, or gastroduodenal artery.
2. Prepare solution. A. Add 100 units vasopressin to 500 ml. 5% dextrose in water or to 500 ml. normal saline solution (provides 0.2 units/ml.). B. Label admixture.	
3. Prime IV administration tubing and infusion pump tubing, removing all air.	3. This prevents infusion of air and possible air embolism.
4. Prepare infusion pump. Guidelines for infusion rates are: A. Intra-arterial: 0.1 to 0.4 units/min. (60 drops/ml. = 30 to 120 drops/min. with 6 to 24 units/hour). B. Peripheral IV: 20 units/100 ml. 5% dextrose in water infused over 10 to 20 minutes every 3 to 4 hours (approximates 5 units/hour).	4. An infusion pump is necessary to maintain a constant accurate flow rate and, in the case of arterial infusion, to overcome arterial pressure.
5. Assess effectiveness of infusion by decreased or stoppage of bleeding.	
6. Wean patient from vasopressin infusion. A. Taper off over 24 hours and then infuse plain 5% dextrose in water for 24 hours at a keep-open rate.	6. Immediate withdrawal of the drug may precipitate hemodynamic instability or renewed bleeding or both.

ACTION	RATIONALE

B. Administer vasopressin at a rate of:
   (1) 0.2 unit/ml./min. for 24 hours.
   (2) 0.1 unit/ml./min. for 48 hours.
   (3) 0.05 unit/ml./min. for 12 hours.
   (4) Plain 5% dextrose in water or normal saline solution, 1 ml./min. for 24 hours.
C. Remove catheter the fifth day.

Precautions

1. Use extreme care to prevent dislodging the arterial catheter, as arterial bleeding and hemorrhage may result. In addition, clotting or compromised circulation of the leg used for catheter insertion may occur.
2. Stabilize the IV catheter securely. If the solution infiltrates, immediately remove the IV line to avoid tissue sloughing.
3. Keep the leg straight that is used for arterial line insertion; restrain if necessary.

Related Care

1. Assess for infection or clot formation at the cutdown site.
2. Assess frequently for IV patency (systemic) and possible infiltration.
3. Assess the leg used for insertion of the arterial catheter for changes in pulses, temperature of extremity, and mottling.
4. Evaluate frequent blood pressures for trends indicating development of hypertension.
5. Attach the patient to a cardiac monitor and observe for development of dysrhythmias and myocardial ischemic changes.
6. Secure line with tongue blade and keep in direct vision.

Complications

ADH effect; water and sodium retention
Decreased splanchnic blood flow, including hepatic artery and renal artery vasoconstriction and subsequent damage
Coronary artery vasoconstriction in systemic administration

REFERENCE

Berk, J.L., and Sampliner, J.E. (eds.): Handbook of Critical Care Medicine, 2nd ed. Boston, Little, Brown, 1982, pp. 45–46.

——— GASTRIC LAVAGE IN OVERDOSE ———

Barbara Buss Fugleberg, R.N., B.S.N., CCRN,
Elaine Brogdon, R.N., M.N.,
Kathy Mossing, R.N., M.A., M.B.A., and
Barbara Tabor, R.N., B.S.N., CEN

Overview

Gastric lavage in the overdosed patient is indicated when the patient has central nervous system depression or inadequate gag reflex or when vomiting is contraindicated.

Objectives

1. To remove poisons, life-threatening overdoses of medication, and irritating substances from the stomach quickly and efficiently.
2. To obtain a specimen for analysis.

Special Equipment

Large 2- to 3-liter inflow bottle
Large-bore inflow and outflow
    tubing connected to inflow
    bottle with **V** connector
Large-bore 32 Fr. Ewald tube
Outflow bottle
50-ml. aspirating syringe
Lubricant

Hemostats
ECG recorder
Cardiac monitor
IV line with 5% dextrose in water
Saline irrigating solution
Charcoal tablets (10 to 15)
Magnesium citrate (340 ml.)
Restraints

Procedure

ACTION	RATIONALE
1. Obtain vital signs.	1. This is done to detect hypotension or cardiac dysrhythmias.
2. Attach patient to cardiac monitor.	2. This monitors for dysrhythmias and bradycardias.
3. Start IV line with 5% dextrose in water at a keep-open rate.	3. This provides access for emergency drug administration.
4. Draw samples for blood work (usually electrolyte levels and toxicology screen; in addition, determinations of alcohol and arterial blood gas levels may be indicated).	4. These are used for baseline studies, to detect levels of toxins in the blood stream, and to document respiratory status.

ACTION	RATIONALE
5. Obtain ECG.	5. This will detect any cardiac abnormalities.
6. Assess gag reflex.	6. If absent, the patient may need to be intubated to prevent aspiration.
7. Place patient in left lateral, Trendelenburg, or sitting position.	7. See ratioanles under "Nasogastric Tube Insertion."
8. Assess heart rate prior to insertion of Ewald tube.	8. If heart rate is below 100, atropine 0.4 mg. is given IV to block vagal response and prevent bradycardia during passage of the tube.
9. Place padded tongue blade in mouth.	9. This prevents the patient from biting on the tube.
10. Place lubricated Ewald tube in mouth and pass tube to black ring (approximately 20 inches) into stomach. See "Nasogastric Tube Insertion" for specifics of tube advancement.	
11. Lavage stomach (see "Gastric Lavage").	
12. Administer the following, if prescribed, after lavage is completed:	
A. Charcoal (10 to 15 tablets), liquefied and instilled into tube.	A. Charcoal helps to absorb any remaining toxins.
B. Magnesium citrate (340 ml.).	B. This encourages peristalsis and elimination.

Precautions

1. Maintain suicide precautions (e.g., remove any remaining pills from patient area; keep in restraints after lavage) if patient is suicidal.
2. Maintain airway by suctioning excess oral secretions if the patient is comatose.
3. Insert a nasogastric tube after the Ewald tube is removed as a precaution against vomiting if the patient is comatose and not intubated.
4. Place the patient in four-point restraints and a waist restraint, if necessary. Restraint is necessary for most patients to prevent them from pulling out the Ewald tube.

Related Care

1. Maintain a clear oral airway throughout procedure.
2. Assess neurologic, respiratory, and cardiovascular status.

3. Observe for any sign of trauma to the patient.
4. Obtain medical history regarding pharmacologic profile.
5. Obtain samples for repeat electrolyte determinations to monitor for electrolyte imbalance, especially potassium depletion, if more than 20 liters of normal saline solution are used.
6. Catheterize the patient during the procedure, if comatose, to monitor output more closely.
7. Request a psychiatric consultation as part of follow-up care.

Complications

Aspiration	Hypertension
Respiratory arrest	Hypotension
Cardiac dysrhythmias	Acidosis
Renal failure	Coma
Hepatic failure	Delirium
Seizures	Pulmonary edema
Urinary retention	Bleeding disorders
Hyperthermia	

REFERENCES

Brunner, L.S., and Suddarth, D.S. (eds.): Lippincott Manual of Nursing Practice, 3rd ed. Philadelphia, J. B. Lippincott, 1982, pp. 890–891.

Oderda, G.M., and Schwartz, W.K.: General management of the poisoned patient. Crit. Care Q. 4(4):2–15, 1982.

Rumack, B.H., and Peterson, R.G.: Poisoning: Prevention of absorption. Top. Emerg. Med. 1(3):13–18, 1979.

____ PARACENTESIS (ASSISTING WITH) ____

Barbara Buss Fugleberg, R.N., B.S.N.,
Elaine Brogdon, R.N., M.N.,
Kathy Mossing, R.N., M.A., M.B.A., and
Barbara Tabor, R.N., B.S.N., CEN

Overview

Withdrawal of fluid from the abdominal cavity may be required for diagnostic or therapeutic purposes. After a history of trauma, this may help to determine intra-abdominal bleeding. In other cases, samples of ascitic or abdominal fluid may be obtained for composition analysis. Paracentesis may also be necessary to relieve dyspnea or urinary frequency caused by large amounts of accumulated fluid, which places pressure on the diaphragm and bladder, respectively.

Objective

To introduce a needle or catheter into the peritoneum to remove accumulated fluid for laboratory studies or to decompress the abdomen.

Special Equipment

Sterile gauze pads
Povidone-iodine solution
Tape
Cotton swabs
Local anesthetic
2-ml. syringe and 25-gauge
    needle
Scalpel blade and handle
Normal saline solution for injection
Paracentesis needle or catheter or both

50-ml. syringe
Sterile collection container
Sterile drapes
Ringer's lactate solution
Sterile specimen container(s)
Sterile gloves
Foley catheterization tray (if
    needed)
Suture material
Suction source

Procedure

ACTION	RATIONALE
1. Have the patient void (or catheterize patient, if necessary) before procedure is begun.	1. This prevents bladder distention and possible nicking of bladder with needle.

ACTION	RATIONALE

2. Position the patient:
   A. Upright, on side of bed, supported; *or*
   B. Flat in bed.	

3. Prep area with povidone-iodine solution.	3. The procedure should be performed under sterile technique.
4. Provide local anesthetic for introduction at puncture site.	4. This eliminates some of the pain of large-bore needle introduction.

5. Assist with insertion of trocar.
   A. A needle with obturator is introduced, with sterile precautions, through a stab incision in midline below the umbilicus.
   B. Obturator is removed.
	
	B. This allows introduction of drainage tube and removal of fluid.

6. Introduce solution and drain fluid.
   A. Inject small amount of saline.
   B. Apply small amount of suction.
   C. Drain blood or ascitic fluid through tube into sterile container by gravity.
   D. Obtain only as much fluid as necessary to decrease abdominal pressure or to obtain samples for laboratory studies.
   E. Lavage peritoneum with 1 liter of Ringer's lactate solution, in trauma.
	A. This maintains patency.
	
	D. Removal of 1 to 1.5 liters can cause hypotension and shock.
	
	E. This enables the color of the return to be determined for assessing intra-abdominal injury.

7. Reposition patient side to side (optional).	7. This helps to obtain extra fluid that may be accumulated in pockets on either side.
8. Monitor patient response during trocar removal.	
9. Apply sterile dressing to incision site.	

10. Send fluid for:
   A. Laboratory studies (WBC's, bile, intestinal or pancreatic juices, proteins, and cultures).
   B. RBC determination. (Test for RBC's and blood is negative if newsprint can be read through the solution.)	

Precautions

1. Remove fluid slowly to prevent hypovolemia and hypotension.
2. Catheterize the patient or have him void prior to procedure. If bladder is distended it may be punctured.

Related Care

1. Monitor blood pressure, pulse, and respiratory status preparacentesis and frequently postparacentesis for indications of developing hypotension.
2. Observe the size of the trocar wound; if it is large, it may require suturing.
3. Assess incision site for bleeding several times during the first 30 minutes after paracentesis.
4. Measure abdominal girth to identify possible internal bleeding and/or further accumulation of ascitic fluid; do this at least once daily.
5. Assess for scrotal edema or peritoneal fluid leakage.
6. Record patient data and response to procedure.

Complications

Hypotension	Protein depletion
Hemorrhage	Encephalopathy
Infection	

REFERENCES

Brunner, L.S., and Suddarth, D.S. (eds.): Lippincott Manual of Nursing Practice, 3rd ed. Philadelphia, J. B. Lippincott, 1982, pp. 455–458.
Hamilton, H.K., and Rose, M.B. (eds.): Procedures. Springhouse, PA, Intermed Communications, 1983, pp. 527–529.

PERITONEAL LAVAGE
(ASSISTING WITH) _____

Barbara Buss Fugleberg, R.N., B.S.N., CCRN

Overview

Blunt abdominal injuries may produce severe retroperitoneal injuries without significant physical signs. A negative paracentesis tap, however, does not rule out the presence of intra-abdominal injury. Peritoneal lavage can detect free blood in the peritoneal cavity.

Objectives

1. To determine the presence of free blood in the peritoneal cavity by instilling a balanced saline solution into the cavity.
2. To obtain fluid for examination.

Special Equipment

Foley catheter set (if needed)
Nasogastric tube
Suction machine
Shave prep kit
Povidone-iodine solution
IV pole
Macrodrip IV tubing
1 liter of balanced saline solution (i.e., Ringer's lactate or normal saline)
Peritoneal dialysis tray
Sterile gloves
3-ml. syringe with 25-gauge 1-inch needle
Local anesthetic
20-cc syringe
14-gauge 8-inch intracatheter
Extension tubing
Masks
Suture material
Drainage bag with tubing (i.e., urine collection bag)
Sterile 3-way stopcock
Sterile latex tubing, 2-inch
Sterile gauze pads
Antibiotic ointment
Tape

Procedure

ACTION	RATIONALE
1. Have patient void or catheterize patient before procedure.	1. This decreases the chances of bladder perforation.
2. Record vital signs and abdominal girth.	2. This provides a baseline for postprocedure comparison.
3. Obtain baseline abdominal films.	3. Air may enter the abdomen during the procedure and cause confusion in later abdominal films.
4. Insert nasogastric tube and connect to suction (see "Nasogastric Tube Insertion").	4. This decreases the chances of bowel perforation.
5. Prepare insertion site. A. Shave prep the abdomen from the umbilicus to the pubic area. B. Perform povidone-iodine prep.	5. The procedure should be performed under sterile technique.
6. Place patient in supine position.	
7. Set up three-way irrigation system. A. Attach macrodrip IV tubing to the liter of sterile balanced saline solution and flush out all air. B. Connect three-way stopcock to the male end of the IV tubing. C. Connect extension tubing to the opposite end of the stopcock. D. Attach latex tubing to the end of the extension tubing. E. Insert drainage tubing into the latex tubing. F. Maintain sterility of the third port of the stopcock.	A. This prevents instilling air into the abdomen.
8. Assist the physician with the insertion of the intracatheter into the abdomen (see "Paracentesis [Assisting with]").	
9. Remove sterile cap from the third port of the stopcock and hold for the physician to attach the intracatheter.	9. This completes the three-way irrigation system.
10. Instill 1000 ml. of solution into the peritoneal cavity at a rate of 10 to 20 ml./kg. over a 15-minute period. A. Turn stopcock off to the drainage bag.	

ACTION	RATIONALE

B. Open roller clamp on the IV tubing.

C. Close roller clamp on the IV tubing when infusion is complete.

11. Roll patient side to side, unless contraindicated.

11. This facilitates obtaining fluid or blood that may accumulate in pockets on either side.

12. Open drainage system.
    A. Turn stopcock off to the IV solution.
    B. Unclamp the roller clamp on the extension tubing, if present.
    C. Allow fluid to drain from the abdomen into the drainage bag.

13. Record amount and character of drainage.

14. Send fluid to laboratory for analysis.
    A. RBC determination. (Test for RBC's and blood is negative if newsprint can be read through the solution.)
    B. Laboratory studies (amylase, bile, culture, and Gram stain).

15. Apply sterile dressing after the physician removes the catheter and sutures the incision.

Precaution

Warm the solution to minimize discomfort and chills.

Related Care

1. Monitor blood pressure, pulse, and respiratory status throughout and after the procedure.
2. Assess incision site for bleeding.

Complications

Bleeding from incision site
Bleeding secondary to laceration of blood vessels

Visceral perforation
Respiratory distress, arrest
Chills

REFERENCES

AACN: Clinical Reference for Critical–Care Nursing. (M.R. Kinney, ed.). New York, McGraw-Hill, 1981.
Hamilton, H.K. (ed.): Procedures—The Nurse's Reference Library. Springhouse, PA, Intermed Communications, 1983, pp. 529–531.

STOMA/FISTULA MANAGEMENT

Carolyn A. Tamer, R.N., E.T.

Overview

Ostomy or fistula management has three aims: skin care, containment, and odor control. Because many variables are present in the acute care setting, a basic method of practice is described in handling each ostomy/fistula and will usually be different from that taught to the patient for self-care.

The three major types of procedures—colostomy, ileostomy, and urostomy—require specific stoma care. The stoma is created by the part of the ileum or colon that is brought out to and made flush with or raised above the abdominal wall. The nature of the discharge depends upon the portion of the intestinal tract that is used to create the stoma.

Colostomies may involve a surgical opening of the colon through the abdominal wall. Placement may be made in the ascending, transverse, descending, or sigmoid colon. The stoma may be a temporary measure, involving loop or double-barreled procedures, or may be permanent. Care of the descending or sigmoid colostomy is contingent upon the expected discharge from the stoma. Under normal conditions only flatus is passed, and drainage will be absent for approximately 1 week postoperatively. A transverse colostomy is generally a loop ostomy or, less commonly, a double-barreled ostomy. The loop ostomy stoma is maintained postoperatively outside the abdomen for approximately 2 weeks by a stomal support consisting of either a rod or an **X**-shaped bridge (Figs. 5–4 and 5–5). Opening of the loop ostomy may be delayed for several days and, in that case, will require only a dressing. The double-barreled ostomy allows complete separation of the healthy bowel from

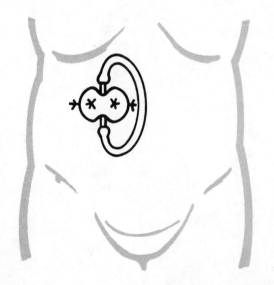

Figure 5-4.   Transverse colostomy with rod and tubing.

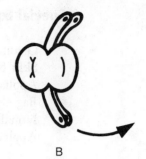

Figure 5-5. Loop colostomy with Hollister bridge. *A,* Sutures hold bridge in place; *B,* sutures removed and bridge folded in half, ready to be slipped out.

A

B

diseased or injured portions. Occurrence of fecal discharge is unpredictable, and it may be liquid to soft in nature, depending upon oral intake.

An ileostomy is usually a permanent procedure that discontinues use of the colon and rectum (which may be removed). The terminal ileum is everted and sutured, usually on the right side of the abdomen, to make a spout-type stoma. The discharge is liquid to paste-like and has a high enzyme content that is caustic to the peristomal skin.

Urostomies may involve ileal or colon loop procedures (ileal conduit, ileal bladder, and Bricker pouch) or cutaneous ureterostomies. These urinary diversions are generally permanent. They function immediately and require containment beginning in the operating room.

Fistula or drain sites do not always have caustic drainage but do often require frequent dressing changes. Drainage containment can be effectively and efficiently accomplished by application of a skin barrier and bag. In addition, the skin is protected, patient comfort is improved, and output can be measured.

Ostomy/fistula care is a clean procedure, not usually sterile. After the skin is cleansed, a skin barrier should be applied for protection before placing of the bag. Examples include Skin Prep Spray, Stomahesive, Colly-Seel, Crixilline, or karaya. The ostomy bag to be applied over the skin barrier should be drainable, adhesive backed, transparent, and odor proof. Adhesive-backed bags are more reliable, will not shift, and may not require the use of an appliance belt.

OSTOMY/FISTULA CONTAINMENT _____

Objectives

1. To contain the discharge efficiently.
2. To permit observation of the stoma/fistula.

Special Equipment

Ostomy bag	Soap and water
Skin barrier	Face cloth and towel
Appliance deodorant	Protective bed pad
Bag closure, elastic or clamp	Clean gauze pads
Nonallergic tape—2-inch	Straight drainage collection set
Appliance belt (if needed)	

COLOSTOMY/ILEOSTOMY/UROSTOMY

Procedure

ACTION	RATIONALE

1. Place protective bed pad under patient.

2. Prepare skin.
    A. Wash peristomal skin gently with mild soap and warm water.
    B. Rinse thoroughly and pat dry.
    C. At this point, if bagging a urostomy, apply gauze pads as wick.

3. Measure stomal diameter.

4. Select and prepare most appropriate skin barrier.
    A. Cut hole in wafer, washer, or gasket to fit stoma.
    B. Cut separate holes in a large piece of skin barrier (and ostomy bag) if there is 2 to 8 cm. of skin between double-barreled colostomy stomas.
    C. Then, using a spray, apply twice, allowing to dry between applications (Fig. 5–6).

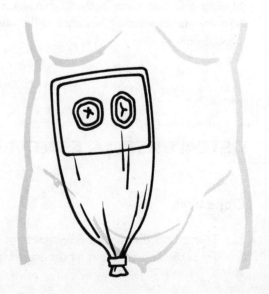

Figure 5-6. Double-barreled colostomy stomas, both stomas covered by pouch.

ACTION	**RATIONALE**
5. Stretch karaya ring (if used) enough to hug base of stoma securely; moisten one side, allow to become tacky, and then apply around stoma.	5. These substances adhere best in moist areas and protect the skin while permitting healing.

  A. Apply ring under double-barreled colostomy stomas with rod stomal support. Both stomas and rod support are covered by pouch (Fig. 5–7).

  B. Apply over an ×-shaped stomal bridge.

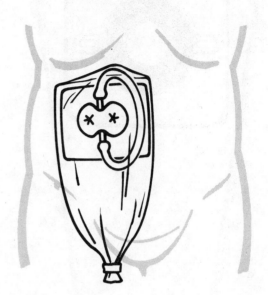

Figure 5-7. Ease the pouch over rod and tubing, being careful to have opening cut to fit closely over stoma.

| 6. Draw stoma size onto adhesive backing of ostomy bag, and cut out an opening approximately 1/8 inch to 1/4 inch larger than karaya ring (Fig. 5–8). Choose bag with precut hole, if available (Fig. 5–9). | 6. This provides leeway for skin barrier to melt away without exposing adhesive backing of the bag. |

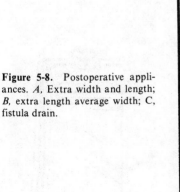
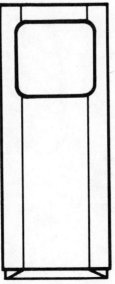
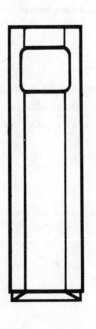
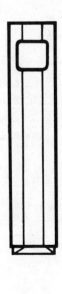

Figure 5-8. Postoperative appliances. *A,* Extra width and length; *B,* extra length average width; *C,* fistula drain.

A   B   C

ACTION

RATIONALE

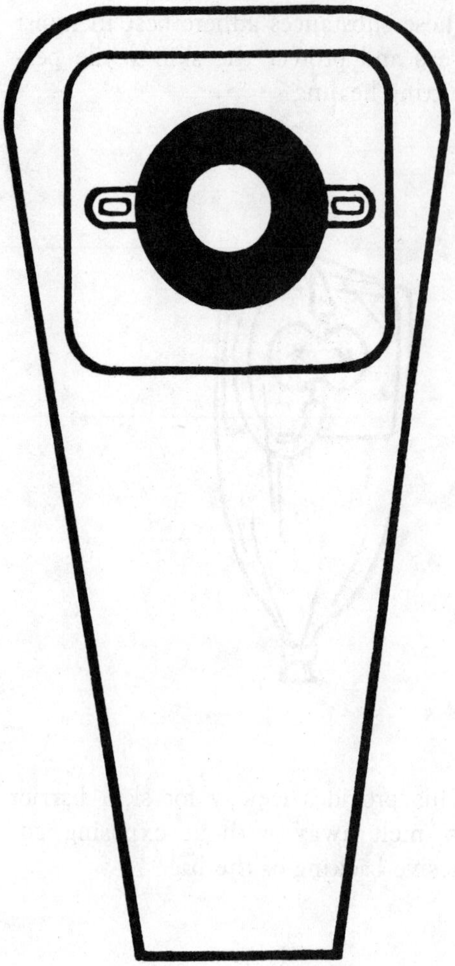

Figure 5-9. Example of presized, open-ended drainable pouch. Must be ordered according to size of stoma.

7. Remove protective backing of adhesive portion of ostomy bag, cut into half- or quarter-sections, and replace (Fig. 5–10).

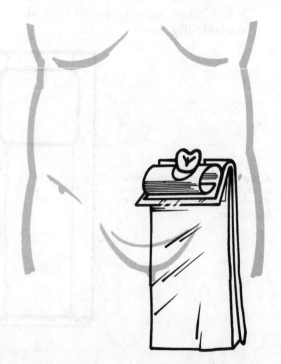

Figure 5-10. Applying large piece of adhesive. Lower half is already adhering; upper half is ready for removal of paper backing.

ACTION	**RATIONALE**
8. Apply bag.	
A. Place hand inside ostomy bag and apply sideways over skin barrier.	A. Sideways application permits increased ease of drainage and emptying.
B. Remove protective backing in half- or quarter-sections, starting with bottom side, and secure each section to skin barrier (Fig. 5–11).	B. This permits seal-tight adherence and prevents leakage.

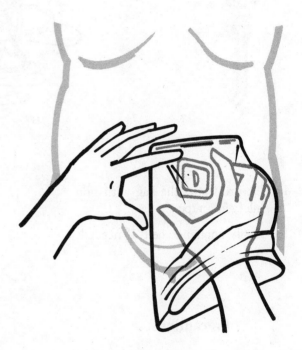

Figure 5-11. Sealing adhesive around stoma.

ACTION	**RATIONALE**
C. Hold clean gauze pads in hand over stoma, if discharge is liquid.	
9. Apply karaya powder around edge of stoma and karaya ring and to seam in ring.	9. This helps to protect exposed skin and may strengthen weak areas in karaya seal.
10. Instill deodorant and close bag with elastic or clamp.	
11. Attach bag to straight drainage set, if discharge is liquid in large amount (Fig. 5–12).	11. This allows accurate output measurement, eliminates the need for frequent emptying, and lessens the chance of bag leaking from overfill.

ACTION   RATIONALE

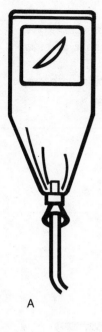

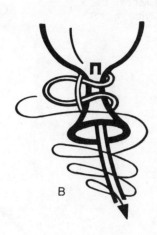

Figure 5-12.   Attaching drainage bag to constant drainage when dealing with large quantity of liquid. *A,* Pouch attached to constant drainage tube; *B,* method for attaching tube using a rubber band around junction of pouch and tube — pull rubber band tightly, securing it with a small piece of tape.

A   B

12. Picture-frame the bag with non-allergenic tape.

13. Apply appliance belt, if needed.

12. This provides additional support.

13. This may add an increased sense of patient security and aid in maintaining the seal.

Precautions

1. Observe for deviations of stoma color from characteristic dark pink to red.
    A. Blanching or lightening may indicate interference with circulation.
    B. Dark red to purple may indicate damage to the stoma's blood supply.
2. Observe for stomal edema as well as for bleeding from the peristomal area or the stoma.
3. Use a bag that can be emptied, cleaned, resealed, and left in place for several days. Repeated removal of appliances increases the risk of skin irritation or damage.
4. Exercise care when removing an appliance from a suture line. Avoid pulling the sutures, and do not contaminate the incision with the bag contents.
5. Do not tape a leak from beneath the adhesive backing. Leaking discharge will be trapped, resulting in excoriation of the skin.
6. Assess for tension on the stoma due to edema, mesenteric pull, position of skin folds, or position of the patient. Extra tension on the stomal sup-

port could damage the bowel nerve or blood supply. The patient may have to sit in a reclining position to avoid placing tension on the stoma.

7. Never twist or turn a stomal support; this puts torsion on the bowel.

8. Insure that the appliance belt is applied correctly. It must remain even with the bag tabs. If it rides up or down the bag may cut the stoma or pull up from the skin, causing leakage. Tight belts may cause cutaneous or stomal pressure ulcers. If applied improperly, a belt can predispose a patient to a prolapsed stoma or parastomal hernia.

9. Press the bag adhesive gently but firmly to form a seal, and be especially careful that it has no wrinkles.

10. Do not allow mucus or drainage to get under the skin barrier, since this will prevent a good seal.

Related Care

1. Use warm water or a mild solvent to permit easier removal of the appliance. Wash any solvent used from the skin to avoid irritation. Expose the skin to the air for several minutes before applying additional adhesive.

2. Measure intake and output accurately in case of potential electrolyte imbalances.

3. Use two or three appliances if there is a wide area of skin between stomas or fistulas. If the margins of skin between sites are narrow, apply one large bag over the openings (Fig. 5–13).

4. Attach the bag to a straight drainage collection set at night to avoid having to wake the patient.

5. Use a template as a pattern for cutting the adhesive-backed opening in the bag.

6. Change the bag every 1 to 2 days if no skin protection is used, or every 4 to 5 days if a skin barrier is used or whenever leakage is noted.

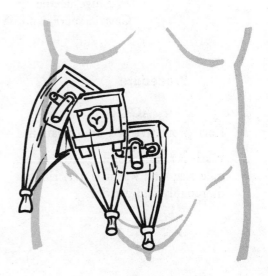

Figure 5-13. Ileostomy appliance flanked by two fistulas that have drains and pouches. This prevents excoriation by containing the fistula drainage.

7. Apply the appliance belt loosely enough so that two fingers can be easily inserted under it.

8. Apply an additional karaya ring around the stoma if the stoma recedes into the skin folds when the patient stands or sits.

Complications

Edema

Lacerations

Pressure ulcers

Prolapsed stoma

Parastomal hernia

Excoriated skin

Infection

FISTULA/DRAIN SITE CARE _____

Objectives

1. To cleanse the skin surface surrounding the fistula/drain.
2. To prevent skin irritation, excoriation, and infection from drainage material.
3. To measure drainage output accurately.

Special Equipment

See equipment. for "Ostomy/Fistula Containment."

Sterile gauze pads

Sump tube

Optional:

    Thoracic catheter

    15-gauge needle

    Gastric suction pump

Procedure

ACTION	RATIONALE
1. Place protective pad under patient.	
2. Wash peristomal skin gently with mild soap and warm water; rinse thoroughly and pat dry.	

ACTION	RATIONALE
3. Apply Skin Prep Spray or Skin Prep Wipe and a sterile dressing to a site when drainage is less than 200 ml./day.	3. Skin Prep is an excellent skin barrier that can be applied under dressings to prevent irritation, when bagging is not necessary.
4. Apply adhesive-backed bag and a skin barrier if drainage is greater than 200 ml./day (see "Ostomy/Fistula Containment").	4. This provides accurate output, protects the skin, and eliminates dressing changes.
5. Attach bag to constant drainage if fistula or drain site drains more than 800 ml./day.	5. The bag is less likely to fall off or leak from weight and permits measuring the output.
6. Attach bag. A. Attach bag to sump suction (e.g., Shirley or Salem) if fit is precarious and if bagging around an existing tube; or	A. Suction improves fluid flow away from the fistula/drain and reduces reflux while the air vent in the sump tube reduces the force being exerted on the site, allows an elastic closure to be put around the existing tube or bottom of the bag while the suction tube picks up the drainage, and eliminates the need to empty the bag frequently.
B. Attach drainage bag to suction system using a 28 Fr. thoracic catheter with a 15-gauge needle, inserted as an air vent, if drainage is too thick for sump tube.	B. The thoracic tube has a single large chamber that is less likely to become obstructed or require flushing.

Precautions

Same as precautions for "Ostomy/Fistula Containment."

Related Care

Same as related care for "Ostomy/Fistula Containment."

Complications

Same as complications for "Ostomy/Fistula Containment."

COLOSTOMY IRRIGATION _____

Overview

A sigmoid colostomy is generally the only ostomy to be irrigated regularly. It is generally ordered in the acute setting, to relieve constipation or to prepare the patient for radiologic studies or surgery. If the patient in the acute care setting has not been regulated previously with this technique, the nurse may have to assume the responsibility for providing this care.

Objectives

1. To empty the colon.
2. To cleanse the lower gastrointestinal tract.
3. To prevent intestinal obstruction.

Special Equipment

Colostomy irrigation set
Irrigation reservoir
1000 ml. tepid tap water
   or other ordered solution
Cone tip or catheter
Irrigation sleeve
Belt
Bag closure or elastic
Lubricant
Bed pan or commode
Toilet paper
Protective bed pad
Equipment for colostomy care (see special equipment for
   "Ostomy/Fistula Containment").

Procedure

ACTION	RATIONALE
1. Fill irrigating reservoir with 1000 ml. tepid water or other solution prescribed.	1. Using too little solution does not stimulate a good evacuation.
2. Hang irrigating reservoir with solution 45 to 50 cm. (18 to 20 inches) above stoma.	
3. Remove existing bag from patient if irrigation sleeve is provided.	

ACTION	RATIONALE
4. Attach irrigation sleeve snugly to patient with belt from set.	4. This helps to control odor and splashing.
5. Lubricate irrigating tip; allow some solution to flow through catheter.	
6. Instill irrigation fluid using cone-tip method or catheter.	
A. Insert cone tip 1 to 2 cm. (½ to ¾ inch) into stoma and hold with firm, gentle pressure; or	A. The cone-tip shape acts as a natural dam, holding the water in the colon until its removal.
B. Insert catheter gently about 10 to 15 cm. (4 to 6 inches); move it in and out slowly while allowing solution to flow.	B. This cleanses and clears the terminal end of the colon up to 15 cm. (6 inches). The slowly flowing solution helps to relax the bowel and facilitates passage of the tube.
7. Allow long drainage sleeve to hang in bed pan or commode during evacuation, which may take up to 1 hour.	7. This prevents soiling of the patient or bed linen.
8. Remove sleeve, rinse, and dry for reuse (if reusable).	
9. Wash and dry skin; apply clean bag (see "Ostomy/Fistula Containment").	

Precautions

1. If cramping occurs, stop the flow of solution, and allow the patient to rest before progressing. Painful cramps may be caused by too rapid flow or too much solution.
2. Do not finger-dilate any stoma. Dilation may cause tearing of mucosa and skin, leading to infection, fibrosis, and stricture formation.
3. Be sure the belt fits snugly to prevent leakage.

Related Care

1. Insert the catheter 10 to 15 cm. (4 to 6 inches) through a baby bottle nipple to develop a cone tip. Insert the tube into the stoma up to the nipple hub, and hold firmly against the stoma while running the fluid in.
2. If all fluid is not evacuated, insert catheter and siphon off the remainder.
3. Place the patient on a bed pan or commode if the distal limb of a loop or double-barreled ostomy is to be irrigated, since the fluid will exit through the rectum.

Complications

Colon perforation
Lacerations
Retention of irrigation fluid

OSTOMY/FISTULA SKIN CARE _____

Objectives

1. To prevent peristomal tissue damage caused by stomal/fistula discharges.
2. To treat damaged peristomal tissue effectively and promote healing.

Special Equipment

Mild soap	Antacid
Warm water	Telfa gauze
Face cloth and towel	Karaya powder
Skin barrier	

Procedure

ACTION	RATIONALE
Prevention of Leakage	
1. Cleanse skin, using mild soap and warm water; rinse and pat dry thoroughly.	
2. Apply skin barrier (e.g., Stomahesive or Skin Prep Spray) as preventive measure.	2. This provides protection between the skin and adhesive.
A. Only when it leaks; or	
B. If using Stomahesive, by the seventh day; or	B. Change by the seventh day as a hygienic measure.
C. If using a karaya substance (e.g., Colly-Seel), every 2 to 4 days.	C. Karaya substances are water soluble and do not always last as long as Stomahesive.
3. Shave area before applying ostomy appliance, if body hair is present.	

ACTION	RATIONALE

Treatment of Mild Irritation (skin not broken, only reddened)

1. Cleanse skin, using mild soap and warm water; rinse and pat dry thoroughly.

2. Use skin barrier that ensures a good seal.
   A. Use Sween skin care cream daily prior to application of bag, instead of spray or water; or
   B. Use Skin Prep Spray or Wipes.

3. Keep an adequate supply of nonsterile sponges at hand to soak up drainage.

2. This prevents the skin from being disturbed for several days.

Treatment of Moderate Irritation (skin red with some broken areas)

1. Wash skin with mild soap and warm water; rinse thoroughly and expose to air for a few minutes.

2. Paint area with thin coat of decanted antacid. (Note: Do not shake the bottle.)
   A. Allow hydroxide suspension (e.g., Amphojel or Maalox) to settle in bottle.
   B. Pour off thin liquid on top.
   C. Use pasty liquid on bottom.
   D. Fan painted area dry.

2. This soothes the irritated skin and helps prevent the karaya powder from stinging.

3. Sprinkle karaya powder lightly over antacid, applying additional coats if it darkens as it soaks up moisture from weeping skin.

3. This dries the skin.

4. Spray lightly with Skin Prep Spray, let dry, spray again.

4. This provides a new surface on which to apply a clean bag.

5. Apply clean bag over Skin Prep Spray.

6. Change daily, and repeat skin treatment until healed.

ACTION	RATIONALE

Treatment of Severe Irritation (skin weeping, may have small ulcerated spots)

1. Follow steps 1 to 4 under "Treatment of Moderate Irritation." Step 4 may need to be repeated several times as skin continues to weep.

1. This allows the skin to become as dry as possible.

2. Use Skin Prep Spray when karaya no longer darkens.

3. Cover ulcerated spots with small amount of karaya powder and tiny piece of Telfa gauze.

3. This helps to absorb the moisture.

4. If skin is severely injured, perform treatment every 12 hours until condition improves, then every 24 hours.

5. Omit steps 3 through 5 when condition sufficiently improves; use only Stomahesive.

Precautions

1. Avoid the use of normal saline solution, alcohol, or hydrogen peroxide, as these agents can irritate and cause drying of the skin.
2. If the skin barrier or adhesive cannot be removed easily do not scrub the skin, as this can irritate the skin severely and provide a site for infection.
3. *Never* use benzoin compounds on irritated skin to improve the adhesiveness of the bag. Benzoin compounds contain aloes that are harmful to the skin and, since benzoin does not dry, it can cause continued damage.
4. Do not miss a treatment, since the skin can quickly become more irritated than previously if it is neglected.
5. Avoid using creams or ointments because they prevent the bag from adhering.

Related Care

1. See related care for "Ostomy/Fistula Containment."
2. Treat for *Candida* by spreading a very light coat of mystatin (Mycostatin) powder to the affected area with a fingertip daily until the skin clears. Then spray the area with Skin Prep, and apply the bag.

OSTOMY/FISTULA ODOR CONTROL _____

Objective

To control odors caused by containment of stomal/fistula discharges.

Special Equipment

Air freshener	Mouthwash
Appliance deodorant	Distilled vinegar
Warm water	

Procedure

ACTION	RATIONALE
1. Rinse open-ended bags with: A. Lukewarm water and mouthwash solution; *or* B. Distilled vinegar solution—60 ml. vinegar to 1 liter water.	1. This cleans and deodorizes the bags.
2. Use new bag, if necessary.	
3. Use room air freshener spray.	3. This reduces embarrassment.
4. Use an appliance deodorant after emptying and cleaning bag.	4. This continuously deodorizes the bag contents during use.
5. Carefully wash and dry the skin between changes of the appliance (see "Ostomy/Fistula Containment").	
6. Do not make holes in the bag.	6. This defeats the use and purpose of the bag.
7. Use a disposable bag.	7. This reduces all aspects of maintenance.

Precautions

1. Excessive rinsing and cleaning of the bag can weaken the skin seal, resulting in leakage.
2. Follow manufacturer's directions for use of appliance deodorants.

OBTAINING A URINE SPECIMEN FOR CULTURE AND SENSITIVITY FROM AN ILEAL LOOP STOMA _____

Objective

To obtain a sterile urine specimen for culture and sensitivity.

Special Equipment

Catheterization set
Protective bed pad
Culture container
Urostomy bag
Containment equipment (see special equipment for "Ostomy/Fistula Containment")

Procedure

ACTION	RATIONALE
1. Place protective bed pad under patient.	
2. Remove urostomy bag.	
3. Don sterile gloves and cleanse stoma site with same solution and technique used for catheterizing a urinary meatus; drape accordingly.	
4. Put drainage end of catheter in culture container.	
5. Insert catheter tip gently into stoma 10 to 15 cm. (4 to 6 inches).	
6. Hold culture container lower than stoma.	6. This facilitates urine flow by gravity.
7. Have patient cough if no urine flows.	
8. Pinch catheter with fingers and remove from stoma.	
9. Release pinch, thus siphoning a few drops.	

ACTION	RATIONALE
10. Record on the patient's chart if there was a residual greater than 5 to 10 ml.	10. Higher residuals indicate poor function.
11. Indicate that specimen was obtained by catheter.	
12. Apply clean bag.	

Precaution

Use caution when catheterizing the urostomy stoma so as not to injure the stoma site. Do not force the catheter.

Related Care

See related care for "Ostomy/Fistula Containment."

Complications

Perforation
Injury to anastomosis leading to internal urine leak

Suppliers

Hollister, Inc. (Disposable pouches; skin gel; deodorizer and germicide)
Mason Laboratories (Colly-Seel)
Perma-Type Company, Inc. (Fresh Tabs deodorant)
Pettibone Labs, Inc. (Ostobon deodorant)
E.R. Squibb and Sons, Inc. (Stomahesive; Mycostatin powder)
Sween Corporation (Sween cream; Hex-On spray)
United Surgical Corporation (Skin Prep Spray and Wipes;
    Bongort bags; Banish deodorant)

REFERENCES

AACN   Clinical Reference for Critical-Care Nursing (M.R. Kinney, ed.). New York, McGraw-Hill, 1981.
Brunner, L.S., and Suddarth, D.S. (eds.): Lippincott Manual of Nursing Practice, 3rd ed. Philadelphia, J. B. Lippincott, 1982, pp. 426–433; 517–518.
Heindel, M: How to protect your ostomy patients from post-op skin problems. R.N., 41(1):43–45, 1978.
Lenneberg, E. S., and Weiner, M.: The Ostomy Handbook. United Ostomy Association.
Taylor, V.: Meeting the challenge of fistulas and draining wounds. Nursing 80, 10:45–51 (June), 1980.

6

THE
HEMATOLOGIC
SYSTEM

BLOOD AND BLOOD COMPONENT
——————— ADMINISTRATION ———————

Ruth M. DeLoor, R.N., M.S.N., C.S., and
Mary Jo Schreiber, R.N., M.S.N., CCRN

Overview

Improved diagnostic techniques and increased knowledge of transfusion therapy have enabled specific blood components needed by the patient, such as platelets, clotting factors, plasma, and granulocytes, to be identified. With sophisticated equipment available for separating blood into its cellular and fluid parts, it is now possible to obtain these components in large quantities. An understanding of blood and blood component therapy, together with nursing responsibilities when transfusion therapy is prescribed, is important to the critical care nurse. The classification of blood and blood components for clinical use, a brief description, and some important uses follow.

WHOLE BLOOD

Whole blood may be either stored or fresh. In either case, it is drawn from a donor and collected in plastic bags (usually polyvinylchloride) containing citrate compounds to prevent coagulation (ACD—acid citrate dextrose [rarely used] or CPD—citrate phospate dextrose). If CPD-adenine (CPDA-1) is used, whole blood may be stored for 35 days after collection. Fresh whole blood is infused within 24 hours. Whole blood may be kept at 1° to 6° C. for up to 21 days after collection; when stored properly it contains all the normal constituents of fresh whole blood. Both fresh and stored blood must be typed and cross-matched before transfusing.

Stored Whole Blood (SWB). SWB is used to increase the oxygen-carrying capacity and circulating volume of the blood. The most common clinical indication for its use is replacement of acute blood loss to avoid hypovolemic shock. Because of the increased complexity of blood component therapy and a limited supply of SWB, both indications should be present when SWB is ordered.

Fresh Whole Blood (FWB). The use of FWB is indicated for the infusion of platelets and clotting factors in addition to the indications for SWB if blood components are not available. Because of severe limitations in the availability of FWB, other blood component therapy is used more frequently. Blood less than 5 days old also insures adequate red blood cell content of 2,3-diphosphoglycerate (2,3-DPG).

RED BLOOD CELLS (RBC's)

RBC's constitute the blood component remaining after most of the plasma is removed from whole blood. RBC's provide the same oxygen-carrying capacity as whole blood but in smaller volume. Therefore, RBC's reduce the risk for circulatory overload. There are three general types of RBC's, and all require typing and cross-matching.

Packed Red Blood Cells. Packed RBC's are prepared by removal of supernatant plasma sedimentation from or centrifugation of whole blood; this results in a unit containing 250 to 300 ml., with a hematocrit of 70%. When RBC's are prepared from a single plastic bag they should be used within 24 hours. RBC's prepared in double plastic bags, using a closed system, are viable for as long a period as an original container of whole blood.

The use of packed RBC's is indicated to increase oxygen-carrying capacity or for correction of anemia by transfusion. Increased use can allow effective production of other blood components through fractionization of plasma.

Fresh-Frozen Red Blood Cells. The technique of fresh-freezing RBC's prolongs the shelf life of RBC's and is used for storage of rare blood types, autotransfusion, patients who are a high risk for transfusion reactions, and immunodeficient patients.

The cells are frozen within 6 days of phlebotomy and stored for long periods. Fresh-frozen RBC's must be deglycerolized (washed) before administration; they are essentially free of WBC's, plasma proteins, and irregular antibodies.

Leukocyte-Poor Red Blood Cells. Leukocyte-poor RBC's are prepared from whole blood by the removal of supernatant plasma and the "buffy coat" of leukocytes, which results in 80% to 90% removal of total leukocytes. Leukocyte-poor RBC's are also called "buffy"-poor RBC's. Washed RBC's are also considered leukocyte poor. Patients who have repeated transfusions, febrile reactions to transfusions, and demonstrable leukocyte antibodies are considered for leukocyte-poor RBC transfusion. Proper screening is required, because of the difficulty in preparation, as are typing and cross-matching.

PLATELET CONCENTRATE

Platelets should be type-compatible with the individual patient. Three methods of preparation produce (1) single-donor platelets, (2) random pool platelets, and (3) a single-donor platelet pool. Single-donor platelets are prepared by centrifugation of fresh whole blood within 4 hours after collection and contain approximately 30 ml. of platelet concentrate, with an average number of 5×10^{10} platelets. Random pool platelets are prepared with platelet concentrates obtained from multiple donors (usually 4 or 8 units per bag) and pooled into a single unit. A single-donor platelet pool is obtained from a single donor by manual pheresis (2 to 4 units) or cell separation (4 to 8 units). Four to eight units are usually prescribed.

Platelets are used in cases of thrombocytopenia caused by lack of platelet production or misuse of platelets. The frequency of use depends upon the half-life of the transfused platelets, which can be 2 days or less. In transfusion reactions due to HLA antigen formation, platelet survival may be only a few hours. When one is infusing multiple units of platelets, either single donor or in a random pool, the risk of side effects such as chills, fever, and allergic reactions is increased. Hepatitis risk is the same as for whole blood. HLA matched platelets can be obtained if multiple transfusions and reactions are anticipated.

FRESH-FROZEN PLASMA (FFP)

Fresh-frozen plasma is obtained from whole blood. It contains albumin, globulins, coagulation factors, water, and electrolytes. The plasma is collected by plasmapheresis or separated from a unit of whole blood and frozen within 4 hours after initial donation. The exact amount of plasma is recorded on each unit bag; each unit contains approximately 200 ml. plasma. Fresh-frozen plasma is used primarily for plasma coagulation deficiencies and antibodies and must be used for infusion of viable factors V and VIII. Viability of the factors in fresh frozen plasma is 1 year. Plasma must be typed specifically for each patient; however, cross-matching and Rh compatibility testing are not necessary. Because fresh-frozen plasma requires 30 minutes to thaw, the blood bank must be notified early to facilitate preparation.

FACTOR VIII

Factor VIII (antihemophilic globulins) is a component of fresh plasma that has been processed and frozen to prevent denaturation. Preparations include:

Cryoprecipitated Antihemophilic Factor (Cryo). Cryo is prepared from FFP; traces of all plasma constituents are present, and it contains factors VIII and I (fibrinogen). The exact amount of factor VIII varies in each unit. Multiple units are usually administered, with an average of 100 units per bag. Cryo may be stored frozen for 1 year. It is used in classical hemophilia or in von Willebrand's disease as prophylaxis against spontaneous hemorrhage and treatment of hemorrhage. Cryo must be typed specifically for the patient, and the risk of hepatitis is present.

ANTIHEMOPHILIC FACTOR (AHF)

AHF is prepared in dried form and contains an assayed amount of AHF. Indications for use are the same as for cryo, but, because the amount of AHF is known precisely and it is easier to prepare, its use may be preferred. There is a risk of hepatitis.

GRANULOCYTE TRANSFUSION (WBC)

WBC's are obtained by plasmapheresis from an HLA-compatible donor. Preparation of granulocytes by cytopheresis requires expensive technology, close professional supervision, and 2 to 4 hours of the donor's time, creating a very high ratio of cost-to-effectiveness. With proper refrigeration WBC's may be stored for 24 hours without loss of effectiveness. WBC's are indicated for patients with decreased WBC count, usually secondary to radiation therapy or chemotherapy for malignant disease.

NORMAL SERUM ALBUMIN 25%

Normal serum albumin 25% is prepared from pooled human plasma and heat treated at 60° C. for 10 hours to decrease the risk of hepatitis. It contains 25% protein, with approximately 96% albumin, 135 mEq. sodium, and small amounts of chloride and potassium. Indications for use include shock, burn therapy, and hypoproteinemia. Normal serum increases intravascular volume by increasing colloid osmotic pressure and is therefore not indicated for the treatment of overall dehydration. It is available in 20-, 50-, and 100-ml. vials and does not require typing and cross-matching.

PLASMA PROTEIN FRACTION

Plasma protein fraction is prepared from pools of human plasma and is heated at 60° C. for 10 hours to decrease the risk of hepatitis. Situations such as shock or burns, in which the patient needs replacement of the intravascular volume, are examples of cases indicating the use of plasma protein fraction. Since hypotensive episodes may accompany rapid infusion of plasma protein fraction because of the presence of vasoactive kinins, it is not recommended for rapid treatment of hypovolemic shock. Each vial contains 250 to 500 ml., composed of approximately 5% protein, 83% albumin, 17% alpha and beta globulins, 110 mEq. sodium, 50 mEq. chloride, and a small amount of potassium.

Advances are constantly being made in procuring, processing, storing, and infusing blood and blood components. This overview is intended as a basis for encouraging continued learning and respect for the properties of human blood and its safe handling and administration. One procedure is offered as a useful approach for blood and blood component administration, and technical details specific to each blood component are presented in Table 6–1.

TABLE VI-I   Blood and Blood Component Administration Guide

BLOOD COMPONENT	ACTION(S)	ADMINISTRATION/ FILTER SET	INFUSION RATE	SELECT INSTRUCTIONS
Whole blood (WB)				
Stored WB	Increases blood volume and oxygen-carrying capacity of the blood.	Blood filter (170 microns)	2-4 hr.	Gently but thoroughly mix WB by inverting bag several times to give a uniform suspension before administration. Infuse very slowly for first 15 min.; observe patient for adverse reactions. Adjust infusion rate to infuse in 2 hr., unless patient's condition warrants slower infusion. Infusion should not take longer than 4 hr.
Fresh WB	Same as for stored WB; also provides platelets and clotting factors.	Component filter	2-4 hr.	Same as for stored WB. If FWB is being used for viable platelets, use a component/ platelet infusion administration set so that the platelets will be adequately maintained and transfused.
Red Blood Cells (RBC's)				
Packed RBC's	Increases oxygen-carrying capacity of the blood.	Blood filter	2-4 hr.	Same as WB, except do not mix. When RBC's are prepared from a single plastic bag, they must be transfused within 24 hr. RBC's prepared in double plastic bags using a closed system have the same dating period as an original container of whole blood.
Fresh-frozen RBC's	Same as for packed RBC's.	Blood filter	2-4 hr.	Same as for packed RBC's.
Leukocyte-poor RBC's	Same as for packed RBC's.	Blood filter	2-4 hr.	Same as for packed RBC's.
Platelet Concentrate	Increases platelet count; aids clot formation.	Component filter	Rapidly	Store at room temperature, and administer within 24 to 72 hr. of preparation. Infuse concentrate rapidly, within 15 to 30 min. Check label on container, which specifies the number of units.
Fresh Frozen Plasma (FFP)	Raises clotting factor level.	Blood or component filter	Rapidly	Requires 30 min. to thaw, notify blood bank early to facilitate preparation. Thus must be given within 6 hr. of thawing.

TABLE VI-I Blood and Blood Component Administration Guide

BLOOD COMPONENT	ACTION(S)	ADMINISTRATION/ FILTER SET	INFUSION RATE	SELECT INSTRUCTIONS
Factor VIII				
Cryoprecipitated antihemophilic factor (cryo)	Raises factor VIII and XIII levels, prevents and controls bleeding in hemophilia A, hypofibrinogenemia.	Component filter	Rapidly	May not be refrozen. Administer rapidly, approximately 4 units (60 ml.) in 15 min.
Antihemophilic factor (AHF)	Same as for cryo.	Component filter	Rapidly	Refrigerate with diluent until used. Use within 60 min. of preparation; administration should be completed 3 hr. after mixing.
Granulocyte Transfusion (WBC)	Raises leukocyte level.	Platelet filter	2 to 6 hr. (varies with each bag)	May be refrigerated for up to 24 hr. without loss of effectiveness. Clear only with sodium chloride. Infuse over a 2- to 6-hr. period; this depends upon the number of units in bag. Assess for infusion reaction; decrease infusion rate and call physician for orders. (Elevated temperature, rash and chills are expected reactions.)
25% Normal Serum Albumin	Increases intravascular volume.	Special administration set with vial	Adjusted according to clinical response	Considered compatible with common IV solutions. Infuse carefully; adjust rate according to clinical response. This should be used cautiously in patients who are susceptible to volume overload. Because of the high osmotic power of this preparation, it can increase intravascular volume rapidly and result in congestive heart failure or pulmonary edema. Also, in patients with trauma or postoperative wounds bleeding may increase with the rise in intravascular pressure.
Plasma Protein Fraction	Increases intravascular volume and protein level.	Component filter	Adjusted according to clinical response	Compatible with most parenteral IV solutions. Infuse carefully, according to clinical response.

Microaggregate filters (20-40 microns) may be utilized in blood/blood component administration.

Potential Advantages:
1. Reduces febrile transfusion reactions.
2. Can be used for transfusion of multiple units (up to 10).
3. Can be used for transfusing all blood components.

Potential Disadvantages:
1. Increased cost for single unit transfusion.
2. Decreased flow rate with some types of microaggregate filters.

Objectives

1. To ensure preservation of blood and select blood components during transfusion therapy.
2. To provide safe transfusion therapy through selected patient assessment and nursing interventions.

Special Equipment

Venipuncture equipment:
   Tourniquet
   18-gauge or 19-gauge needle or catheter
   Sterile gauze dressing
   Povidone-iodine swab applicators
   Povidone-iodine ointment
   Tape
250 ml. normal saline solution, isotonic,
   for IV administration
IV administration set, appropriate for blood
   or blood component being infused
Transfusion requisition
Blood or blood product
IV standard
Blood pressure cuff
Stethoscope
Thermometer

Procedure

ACTION	RATIONALE
1. Collect the specimen for cross-matching.	
A. Draw blood in tubes according to blood bank instructions.	

B. Label tubes carefully with:
   (1) Patient's full name.
   (2) Date.
   (3) Hospital identification number.
	B. An error in the proper labeling of the specimen or in the completion of the requisition form could result in the patient receiving the wrong blood or blood component unit.

2. Order prescribed blood or blood component.	
A. Validate for physician's order.	
B. Complete appropriate requisition form with such information as: (1) Patient's first and last name.	

ACTION	RATIONALE

(2) Patient's identification number.

(3) Name of requesting physician.

(4) Blood or blood component to be administered.

(5) Amount of blood or blood component to be administered.

(6) Date and time of administration.

(7) Previous transfusion reaction history.

C. Facilitate specimen transport to blood bank with completed blood requisition.

3. Prepare patient.

A. Obtain vital signs.

    A. This provides baseline data.

B. Position patient confortably.

C. Secure patent venous route for administration of blood or blood component.

(1) Use 18- or 19-gauge needle or intracatheter.

    (1) This allows easy flow of blood and causes less destruction of RBC's.

(2) Use only isotonic saline solution IV before, during, and following administration of blood or blood components.

    (2) Certain IV solutions, including 5% dextrose in water, contain no electrolytes and can cause hemolysis of the erythrocytes.

(3) Use sterile, pyrogen-free transfusion filter set with pore size of approximately 170 to 180 micrometers. (Special filters, with approximately a 20-micrometer pore size for microaggregates, may be required for certain patients; this is specified on the transfusion label of the blood or blood component unit.)

    (3) Blood, RBC's, platelets, granulocytes, fresh-frozen plasma, and cryoprecipitate administration require a filter to prevent fibrin clots and particulate debris from infusing. Pore size of the filter and surface area, arrangement of the filter, and drip chamber affect the infusion rate. Microaggregates can develop in stored blood; they have been implicated as a possible cause of shock lung. Patients who are massively

ACTION	RATIONALE
	transfused or who are undergoing cardiopulmonary bypass may warrant the use of special filters.
(4) Prime transfusion administration system; check system for absence of air.	(4) The entire filter should be completely covered and the ball should be free floating to preserve blood components during the filtration process.
(5) Maintain slow infusion of isotonic saline solution IV.	(5) This secures a patent venous route.

4. Obtain blood or blood component.
   A. Match patient identification form to unit of blood or blood component supplied by blood bank personnel. Note that only one unit is issued at a time, unless handling more than one unit concurrently on the same patient.
   B. Sign proper form for release of blood or blood component.

    A. Improper refrigeration increases the risk of complications. It is essential that only monitored blood bank unit refrigerators are used to store blood at a constant temperature.

    B. This certifies that information is accurate, and blood is released for transfusion to the appropriate patient.

5. Check blood or blood component, verifying identification data.
   A. Check chart for physician's order.
   B. Inspect the blood or blood component unit for abnormal color or appearance.
   C. Check unit of blood or blood component, requisition form, and patient's identification band to match:
      (1) Patient's name.
      (2) Patient's identification number.
      (3) Unit number.
      (4) ABO and Rh type.
      (5) Expiration date.
   D. Ask patient to identify himself.
   E. Check all data at patient's bedside. Two staff members should check data together; one of these should be an R.N. or physician.

5. The majority of hemolytic transfusion reactions are due to errors in giving the wrong blood or blood component to a patient.

ACTION	RATIONALE
F. Sign blood requisition form.	
G. Return blood or blood component to blood bank immediately if any discrepancy is noted.	
6. Administer blood or blood component, as prescribed by physician:	
A. Read blood or blood component unit label for general and specific cautions and instructions.	A. This ensures safe administration; individualized cautions and instructions may be required.
B. Assess clinical condition of patient.	B. This serves as baseline date, which should include vital signs (BP, T, P, R).
C. Attach blood or blood component unit to primed solution administration system, maintaining sterility of system.	
D. Infuse slowly for first 15 minutes, observing patient for adverse reactions.	D. Most hemolytic reactions occur in the first 15 minutes.
E. Adjust infusion rate based on clinical condition of patient and blood product being transfused (see Table 6–1).	
F. Assess the patient closely. Vital signs should be monitored throughout the transfusion according to the patient's condition and therapy given.	
7. Discontinue blood or blood component after completion of transfusion.	
A. Flush line with sodium chloride solution IV.	
B. Resume parenteral infusion, as ordered, or discontinue IV.	
8. Complete transfusion form.	8. The transfusion record is a legal document, and copies must be retained in the chart and blood bank.
· A. Indicate presence or absence of suspected reaction.	
B. Return laboratory copy of transfusion record with blood bag to blood bank.	
C. File one copy of transfusion record in patient's medical record.	
9. Record all nursing intervention, including patient response to the transfusion, on the patient's medical record.	

Precautions

1. Use fresh blood; monitor for hyperkalemia with blood nearing the end of the expiration period.
2. Monitor serum calcium levels. Multiple blood transfusions offer potential risk for hypocalcemia, since citrate binds calcium. Calcium gluconate is often prescribed after every second or third unit of blood.
3. Warm blood to body temperature or use a blood warmer during massive transfusion therapy, or as instructed specifically on the blood unit label (see "Blood Warming").
4. Do not add medication directly to the blood or blood component prior to or during a transfusion; if needed, it may be given separately. Medications in high concentrations or with a wide range in pH may in themselves cause hemolysis when injected into the blood tubing.
5. Do not allow the blood or blood components to stand longer than 30 minutes at room temperature prior to administration. The risk of complication increases with the length of time blood is out of the refrigerator.
6. Infuse blood and blood components in less than 4 hours because the longer the blood is left at room temperature the greater is the danger of bacterial proliferation and RBC hemolysis. If the blood must be infused for longer than 4 hours, many blood banks split the unit into two smaller units to be infused consecutively. If the unit is split the blood must be infused within 24 hours.
7. Never store blood in a refrigerator that has not been approved by the blood bank.

Related Care

1. Monitor changes of vital signs taken periodically during blood and blood component administration, and for the effect of changes on the patient.
2. Monitor the infusion rate and the patient's response to therapy. As the filter becomes saturated with debris and microaggregates, the infusion rate is slowed.
3. Assess for symptoms and signs of early transfusion reactions. Monitor the patient closely during the first 15 minutes or the first 50 ml. of the transfusion. Hemolytic reactions can occur early in the transfusion; the reaction may be proportional to the amount of blood infused (see "Transfusion Reaction").
4. Assess for oliguria, hemoglobinuria, shock, and jaundice as late transfusion reactions (see "Transfusion Reaction").
5. Perform site care, as prescribed by physician (see "Invasive Site Care").
6. Change the blood administration set after every unit of blood is infused, or every 24 to 48 hours if the administration set is not used for blood or blood component administration.

Complications

Air emboli	Hemolytic transfusion reactions
Allergic reactions	Hyperkalemia
Alloimmunization	Hypocalcemia
Bacterial contamination	Hypothermia
Bleeding diathesis	Microemboli
Circulatory overload	Shock
Febrile nonhemolytic	Viral hepatitis
transfusion reactions	Death

REFERENCES

American Association of Blood Banks: The Technical Manual of the American Association of Blood Banks, 8th ed., Philadelphia, J.B. Lippincott, 1981.

Microaggregate filtration (editorial), Transfusion, 23:89, 1983.

Miescher, P.A., and Jaffe, E.R.: Transfusion problems in hematology. Semin. Hematol., 18:2 (April), 1981.

Mollison, P.L.: Blood Transfusion in Clinical Medicine. Boston, Blackwell, 1983.

Pall Biomedical Products Corporation Brochure for the Ultipor SQ405 Blood Transfusion Filters. Glen Cove, NY, 1981.

Procedures. The Nurse's Reference Library. Nursing 83 Books. Springhouse, PA., Intermed Communications, 1983.

Rutman, R., and Miller, W.: Transfusion Therapy Principles and Procedures. Rockville MD, Aspen Systems Corporation, 1982.

Schned, A.R., and Silver, H.: The use of microaggregate filtration in the prevention of febrile transfusion reactions: Transfusion, 21:675–681, 1981.

Silver, H. (ed.): Blood, Blood Components and Derivates in Transfusion Therapy. A Technical Workshop. Washington, American Association of Blood Banks, 1970.

Wenz, B.: Microaggregate blood filtration and the febrile transfusion reaction. Transfusion, 23:95–98, 1983.

TRANSFUSION REACTION

Ruth M. DeLoor, R.N., M.S.N., C.S., and
Mary Jo Schreiber, R.N., M.S.N., CCRN

Objectives

1. To recognize and facilitate prompt nursing interventions should a transfusion reaction be suspected.
2. To enhance prompt determination of a potential transfusion reaction by providing specimens for analysis and maintaining collaboration with support services during which critical changes might occur.

Special Equipment

Transfusion reaction form
Thermometer
Blood pressure cuff
Stethoscope
IV administration set
Urine specimen container
Blood specimen containers (one each for clotted and
anticoagulated blood samples)

Procedure

ACTION	RATIONALE
1. Monitor patient closely while first 50 ml. are being transfused. Assess patient for apprehension, headache, back pain, chills, fever, dyspnea, cyanosis, urticaria, hypotension, nausea/vomiting, and rash.	1. Hemolytic reactions can occur early in the transfusion.
2. Monitor for changes or vital signs taken periodically during transfusion administration and effect of changes on patient.	
3. Assess for oliguria and jaundice after transfusion therapy.	3. These are late signs.
4. Facilitate prompt nursing interventions.	
A. Stop blood administration immediately.	A. The transfusion reaction may be proportional to the amount of blood infused.

ACTION	RATIONALE
B. Maintain patent IV route using a slow infusion of normal saline solution IV.	B. This provides a route for further IV medications or fluids.
C. Notify physician immediately of potential transfusion reaction.	C. The physician will decide whether the symptoms warrant a follow-through with the subsequent steps of this procedure. The physician should specify whether the IV is to be left in place and what fluids are to be infused.
D. Notify blood bank immediately of potential transfusion reaction.	D. The blood bank will outline the laboratory tests necessary for evaluating and defining the reaction.
E. Take the following to blood bank. (1) Partially used blood container and IV administration set. (2) Post-transfusion clotted and anticoagulated blood specimen. (3) Post-transfusion urine sample. (4) Completed copies of transfusion and transfusion reaction records.	E. Grouping, typing, and crossmatching procedures using both pre-transfusion and post-transfusion specimens of the recipient's blood will be repeated. A direct Coombs' test on the recipient's blood will be performed immediately and may be repeated in 24 hours. Bilirubin studies are also usually done. A Gram stain and culture are done on the blood container and tubing.
F. Perform clinical check of labels for potential errors.	F. This ensures that the correct blood unit has been given to the correct patient.
G. Start 24-hour urine collection.	G. Urine is collected for determination of heme pigments, granular casts, and the presence or absence of RBC's.
H. Monitor patient's vital signs immediately and every 15 minutes, or as often as indicated by severity of reaction.	H. The patient presents a potential risk for hypotension and shock.
I. Assess for oliguria or anuria, using continuous intake and output.	I. Hemoglobin may precipitate in kidney tubules and offer high risk for renal failure.
J. Administer medication as prescribed.	J. Antihistamines and antipyretics are frequently ordered in febrile or allergic transfusion reactions.

Precautions

1. Clarify acceptable parameters with the physician regarding reaction symptoms. If a transfusion reaction is anticipated, as in a leukemia patient, prophylactic antihistamines or antipyretics may be given prior to administration, or as needed with the occurrence of symptoms, as prescribed by the physician.
2. Administer oxygen, epinephrine, and sedatives, as prescribed by the physician for hemolytic transfusion reaction.
3. Monitor for circulatory overload, especially in patients with a medical history of cardiac dysfunction or anemia.
4. Monitor for febrile and allergic reactions.

Related Care

1. Maintain accurate documentation regarding blood or blood component administration, amount infused, and sequence of symptoms for ongoing clinical investigation.
2. Monitor for delayed hemolytic transfusion reactions.
3. Note that transfusion reactions must be reported to the Bureau of Biologics of the Food and Drug Administration.

Complications

Hypotension	Alloimmunization
Delayed hemolytic reaction	Allergic reaction
Shock	Sepsis
Viral hepatitis	Respiratory arrest
Renal dysfunction	Cardiac arrest

REFERENCES

Miescher, P.A., and Jaffe, E.R.: Transfusion problems in hematology. Semin. Hematol. *18:2* (April), 1981.

Mollison, P.L.: Blood Transfusion in Clinical Medicine. Boston, Blackwell, 1983.

Procedures. The Nurse's Reference Library. Nursing83 Books. Springhouse, PA, Intermed Communications, 1983.

Rutman R., and Miller, W.: Transfusion Therapy Principles and Procedures. Rockville, MD, Aspen Systems Corporation, 1982.

Silver, H. (ed.): Blood, Blood Components and Derivates in Transfusion Therapy. A Technical Workshop. Washington, D.C., American Association of Blood Banks, 1970.

AUTOTRANSFUSION

Ruth M. DeLoor, R.N., M.S.N., C.S., and
Mary Jo Schreiber, R.N., M.S.N., CCRN

Overview

Autotransfusion is used to reduce the risk of transfusion reactions, delayed hemolysis, and isoimmunization. It is often indicated for cases involving high frequency antigen states, rare cell types, or difficult cross-matching due to multiple antibiodies.

Objective

To remove, preserve, and transfuse blood or blood components from/to the original donor as a prescribed therapy for selected patients.

Special Equipment

Sterile blood recovery system, with
   suction device
Filters, with pore size of 170 micrometers
Sterile collecting container with anticlotting agent
Blood administration set

Procedure

ACTION	RATIONALE

1. Determine appropriate procedure for autotransfusion.
  A. Follow selected protocols by blood bank and as prescribed by physician. These include:
    (1) Phlebotomy with anticoagulating agent in vacuum container.
    (2) Modified blood recovery system during surgery or postoperatively with mediastinal drainage after open heart procedures.
  B. Ensure that blood is collected with sterile system in less than a 4-hour period.
	B. This reduces the potential for bacterial growth.

ACTION	RATIONALE
2. Facilitate transport of blood or blood components for storage/freezing, as prescribed by physician.	2. Storage of blood in the liquid state is used on a short-term basis. If a large volume of blood is needed, red cells are preserved by freezing for long-term storage.
3. Administer patient's reclaimed blood or blood components as prescribed (see "Blood and Blood Component Administration").	
4. Assess patient's hemodynamic status closely before, during, and after autotransfusion.	

Precautions

1. See precautions for "Therapeutic Phlebotomy," "Blood and Blood Component Administration," and "Transfusion Reaction."
2. Monitor closely for prevention of air emboli and microemboli; use filters as prescribed.
3. Do not transfuse blood that has been collected over a period longer than 4 hours.

Related Care

1. Check that the informed consent of the patient has been obtained, and check for the physician's order when autotransfusion involves blood collection.
2. See related care for "Therapeutic Phlebotomy," "Blood and Blood Component Administration," and "Transfusion Reaction."

Complications

Potassium intoxication	Emboli
Sepsis	Circulatory overload
Vascular trauma	

REFERENCES

American Association of Blood Banks: The Technical Manual of the American Association of Blood Banks, 8th ed., Philadelphia, J.B. Lippincott, 1981.

Emminzer, S., et al.: Autotransfusion: current status. Heart Lung, 10:83–87, 1981.

Mathewson, M.A.: Autotransfusion. Crit. Care Update, (Feb.), 1982.

Mollison, P.L.: Blood Transfusion in Clinical Medicine. Boston, Blackwell, 1983.

Procedures. The Nurse's Reference Library. Nursing 83 Books. Springhouse, PA, Intermed Communications, 1983.

Thurber, R.L., and Haver, T.M.: Autotransfusion and blood conservation: Curr. Prob. Surg., 19:97–156, 1982.

——————— BLOOD WARMING ———————

Ruth M. DeLoor, R.N., M.S.N., C.S., and
Mary Jo Schreiber, R.N., M.S.N., CCRN

Overview

Blood warming is used in such unusual circumstances as massive transfusions, rates above 50 ml./min., more than 2 units of blood given consecutively, exchange transfusions of the newborn, patients with potent cold agglutinins, or patients whose body temperature is 35 to 38° C. (95 to 100° F.).

Objective

To administer blood safely by a blood-warming technique.

Special Equipment

Blood-warming coil	Blood
Water bath	Blood administration set
Water bath thermometer	Normal saline solution, IV

Procedure

ACTION	RATIONALE
1. Prime blood-warming coil after blood unit and administration set have been attached; close distal clamp.	
2. Submerge blood coil into a 37° C. (99° F.) water bath (Fig 6–1).	2. This procedure applies to a blood-warming coil using heated water; devices are also available for controlled water baths or dry-heat warmers. Note that dry-heat warmers, microwaves, and radiowaves may cause gross hemolysis; their use requires close temperature monitoring and quality control measures.

ACTION   RATIONALE

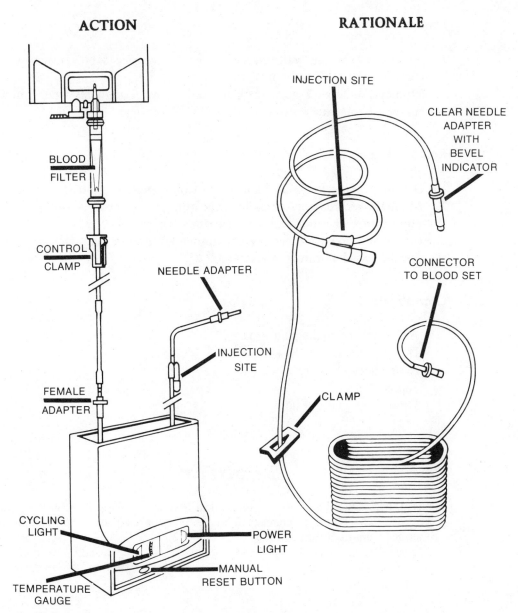

Figure 6-1. Water bath and blood-warming coil. (Courtesy of McGaw Laboratories, Irvine, CA.)

3. Perform blood transfusion as usual.
    A. Obtain patient's temperature prior to blood transfusion.
    B. Assess patient's status continuously.

4. Monitor water bath temperature range; maintain between 35 and 38° C. (95 and 100° F.).

4. Hemolysis may occur if blood is subjected to temperatures greater than 40° C. (104° F.).

5. Flush blood coil thoroughly with normal saline after transfusion. The coil holds approximately 50 ml. of blood.

Precautions

1. Ascertain that the warming device has undergone a preventive maintenance check within the institution.
2. Do not submerge **Y** adapter or any other connection sites when immersing blood coil into water bath.

Related Care

1. See related care for "Blood and Blood Component Administration."
2. Maintain records appropriately, indicating use of blood-warming therapy, temperature of water bath, and patient's temperature.
3. Follow additional protocols as recommended by the manufacturer for the specific blood-warming device used.

Complications

Activation of cold agglutinins
Hemolysis
Microshock
Sepsis
Equipment malfunction

REFERENCES

Mollison, P.L.: Blood Transfusion in Clinical Medicine. Boston, Blackwell, 1983.
Procedures. The Nurse's Reference Library. Nursing 83 Books. Springhouse, PA, Intermed Communications, 1983.

USE OF A BLOOD PUMP

Ruth M. DeLoor, R.N., M.S.N., C.S., and
Mary Jo Schreiber, R.N., M.S.N., CCRN

Objective

To infuse whole blood or packed RBC's rapidly when blood volume and oxygen-carrying capacity need to be increased immediately.

Special Equipment

Blood pump
Blood and blood administration set

Procedure

ACTION	RATIONALE
1. Prepare blood for administration (see "Blood and Blood Component Administration").	
2. Invert and insert a plastic, nonvented blood or solution container, with recipient set attached, through lower opening of mesh panel on blood pump apparatus.	
3. Check security of connections and complete insertion of total solution container into blood pump apparatus; suspend infuser by fabric strap.	
4. Inflate to desired pressure on gauge for pressure infusion; do not exceed 300 mm. Hg.	4. Overinflation may damage infuser and potentially increase hemolysis.
5. Adjust infusion rate by recipient set clamp.	
6. Maintain pressure infusion by squeezing bulb pump as blood is infused.	
7. Remove empty blood container by opening air valve to deflate infuser rapidly.	

ACTION   RATIONALE

8. Maintain continuous patient assessment as outlined in procedure for "Blood and Blood Component Administration."

Precautions

1. Check for blood bag rupture due to instrumentation.
2. Check for blood contamination due to leak in system.
3. Determine if air is trapped in the system. This could result from pumping blood when there is air in the bag. To prevent this, the pump should be deflated before the bag is completely empty.
4. Note that infusing blood under pressure coupled with the use of small tubing or needle could cause hemolysis.

Related Care

1. Monitor patient's status and effect of rapid transfusion continuously.
2. Check accuracy of the blood pump. Failure of the needle gauge to return to zero may indicate that the accuracy of the gauge has been impaired. Accuracy of the gauge may diminish with extensive use or age.
3. See related care for "Blood and Blood Component Administration."

Complications

Air embolism
Volume overload
Infiltration

REFERENCES

Procedures. The Nurse's Reference Library. Nursing 83 Books. Springhouse, PA, Intermed Communications, 1983.

Rutman, R., and Miller, W.: Transfusion Therapy Principles and Procedures. Rockville, MD, Aspen Systems Corporation, 1982.

7

THE
INTEGUMENTARY
SYSTEM

WOUND MANAGEMENT:
CLEAN WOUNDS

Sandra J. Pfaff, R.N., B.S.N.

Overview

Wound healing is a three-phase process of reestablishing the continuity of cellular and anatomic structures; it may be characterized as follows:

I Inflammatory phase: Leaking of circulating blood substances into wound; migration of polymorphonuclear neutrophil leukocytes, lymphocytes, macrophages, and antibodies into wound; bacterial proliferation in wound.

II Proliferative phase: Development of granulation tissue; migration and proliferation of epithelial and endothelial cells.

III Remodeling phase: Cell production and death; collagen production and absorption; capillary formation and obliteration; filling in by fat cells.

Factors that affect wound healing may be classified as intrinsic (host) and extrinsic (iatrogenic). Intrinsic factors may include nutritional status, diabetes, shock, acidosis, hepatic or renal failure, certain cancers (lymphosarcoma, multiple myeloma, chronic lymphocytic leukemia), remote infection, and bacterial flora. Extrinsic factors may include surgical technique, devitalized tissue, hematoma, seroma, dehiscence, steroid therapy, chemotherapy, and irradiation of the wound area.

Nursing responsibilities extend beyond the wound and dressing, encompassing all the intrinsic and extrinsic factors affecting wound healing. Cognizance of these factors, early recognition of alterations in the patient's condition, and prompt intervention are vital for wound healing. Preoperative nursing assessment should identify existing adverse host factors. Intervention should be directed toward controlling host factors preoperatively to reduce their impact during surgery. Preoperative and postoperative patient placement and personnel assignments may play a role in cross-colonization and cross-infection, particularly for patients who are at high risk for acquisition of infection.

Objectives

1. To promote wound healing through preoperative and postoperative nursing management of factors that affect wound healing.
2. To reduce the risk of delayed wound infection through aseptic wound cleansing and dressing changes.
3. To assess the condition of the wound and intervene appropriately when alterations or problems occur.

Special Equipment

Mineral or baby oil	Plastic bag
Hydrogen peroxide solution	Sterile gauze pads
Sterile normal saline solution	Tape
Tincture of benzoin	Cotton swabs
Gloves	

Procedure

ACTION	RATIONALE
1. Wash hands thoroughly with an antimicrobial agent.	
2. Loosen tape edges with mineral or baby oil if extremely adherent to skin.	2. This decreases trauma to skin and pain.
3. Remove tape by pulling it straight away from skin and toward wound.	3. This decreases pain and injury to new tissue and substrata.
4. Don clean glove over dominant hand.	
5. Remove dressing slowly, pulling gently from side to side toward the wound. If the dressing adheres to the wound, loosen the dressing by pouring a small amount of saline onto it at the point of adherence.	5. This prevents injury to new tissue and substrata.
6. Discard dressing and glove in plastic bag.	
7. Remove tape residue with mild soap and water.	7. This helps to prevent skin breakdown.
8. Assess and record: A. Wound condition (note erythema, bruising, pain, swelling). B. Drainage (note color, odor, consistency, amount). C. Skin condition (note erythema, induration, pain, blistering, skin temperature, and turgor).	
9. Cleanse the wound. A. Dry wounds:	

ACTION	RATIONALE
(1) Cleanse wound and surrounding skin with mild soap and warm water, using gentle circular motion that starts at the incision and moves outward away from the wound.	(1) This cleanses and stimulates circulation.
(2) Rinse and dry in the same manner.	
(3) Assess wound and skin condition.	
B. Draining wounds:	
(1) Don sterile glove on dominant hand.	
(2) Cleanse wound.	(2) This loosens and removes organic debris.
(a) Use sterile gauze pad saturated with normal saline or hydrogen peroxide solution.	
(b) Start at incision and work outward, using gentle circular stroke.	
(c) Use new sterile gauze pad for each stroke.	
(3) Cleanse deep narrow areas and suture sites with cotton swabs saturated with normal saline or hydrogen peroxide solution.	
(4) Rinse with saline-soaked sterile gauze pad; dry with sterile gauze pad.	
(a) Start at incision and work outward, using gentle circular stroke.	
(b) Use new sterile gauze pad for each stroke.	
(5) Assess and record wound and skin condition and drainage; differentiate between hard and fluctuant swelling.	

10. Dress the wound.
    A. Don sterile glove on dominant hand, or hold sterile forceps in dominant hand.

ACTION	RATIONALE
B. Apply dressings, touching them only with glove or forceps. Avoid dragging dressing across skin to wound.	
C. Apply tincture of benzoin to skin around dressing, as needed.	C. This toughens and protects damaged or fragile skin and promotes tape adherence.

Precautions

1. Use solutions in unit-dose or small-capacity containers supplied to each individual patient.
2. Never use cotton balls, since loose fibers can act as foreign bodies.
3. Use unpowdered gloves, since powder particles can act as foreign bodies.

Related Care

1. Integrate the following concepts into clean wound care.
    A. Dressings are used to support, immobilize, protect from trauma and contamination, absorb drainage, promote granulation and debridement, and provide an esthetic appearance. After the first 24 to 48 hours, dressings should be used only for esthetic reasons or protection from trauma.
    B. Wet dressings enhance wicking of organisms; therefore, dry dressings are preferred.
    C. The choice of dressing supplies and the size of the dressing are based on wound size, drainage, and protection needs. They must be secure enough to immobilize but loose enough to promote air circulation. Tape should be selected according to skin condition, allergies, frequency of dressing changes, and anticipated length of time dressings will be needed.
    D. Wound cleansing and dressing changes should occur when particulate matter in the air is at a low level, before or well after cleaning (i.e., housekeeping) activities, and with a limited number of persons present.
    E. Removal of rings and watches and careful hand washing prior to any procedure are essential.
2. Monitor nutrition, hydration, and other intrinsic factors.
3. Perform dressing changes of other wounds (surgical, decubitus, intravascular or intra-arterial puncture sites, tracheostomy) as separate procedures, using separate supplies. The cleanest wound should be dressed first.

Complications

Wound infection
Wound dehiscence

REFERENCES

Bruno, P.: The nature of wound healing. Nurs. Clin. North Am., *14*:667, 1979.
Centers for Disease Control: Guidelines for Prevention of Surgical Wound Infection. USPHS, CDC, 1982.

WOUND MANAGEMENT: CONTAMINATED WOUNDS

Sandra J. Pfaff, R.N., B.S.N.

Overview

All wounds, both clean and contaminated, are colonized by the patient's endogenous resident dermal and transient epidermal flora. The terms "clean-contaminated" or "contaminated" apply when organisms other than endogenous skin flora are likely to be present—e.g., in cases involving surgery of the gastrointestinal, pulmonary, or reproductive tracts, presence of drains, open or traumatic wounds, or colonization by exogenous organisms. The risk and incidence of infection and dehiscence in contaminated wounds exceeds that of clean wounds.

The terms "pathogenic" and "nonpathogenic" are misleading: any organism present in numbers greater than 10^5 is a potential cause of infection. Prevention depends upon controlling both the numbers of organisms that reach the wound and factors that enhance microbial growth. Infected wounds are much more likely to dehisce than are noninfected wounds.

Direct transmission by the hands of personnel is the primary source of cross-contamination. Hand washing is the single most important aspect of prevention. Adjuncts to control of cross-contamination are proper patient placement and proper handling and disposal of contaminated fomites.

Procedures for the management of wounds with drains, open wounds, wound irrigation, and wound cultures are presented. Because the objectives, precautions, related care, and complications are similar for all four procedures, they will be presented only once, identified as "general."

Objectives: General

1. To promote wound healing and reduce the risk of infection through nursing management of the contaminated wound.
2. To contain and manage infected and noninfected wound drainage, thereby reducing the risk of cross-contamination.
3. To intervene promptly and appropriately when infection is suspected.

Special Equipment: General

Tape
Sterile gauze pads

DRESSING WOUNDS WITH DRAINS _____

Special Equipment

Drainage bags
Karaya blanket
Montgomery straps
Hydrogen peroxide solution

Sterile normal saline solution or
    iodophor solution or both
Mask (if wound is infected)
Sterile safety pin
ABD pads

Procedure

ACTION	RATIONALE
1. Remove soiled dressing (see "Wound Management: Clean Wounds"), and replace Montgomery straps, as needed. Avoid dislodging drains, drainage bags, or drainage suction tubing.	
2. Replace crusted or rusty safety pin in Penrose drains.	
3. Cleanse wound and drain site. A. Use separate, hydrogen-peroxide soaked, sterile gauze pads, and cotton swabs. B. Follow with normal saline or iodophor cleansing or both.	3. This reduces the risk of cross-contamination, provides removal of organic debris, and stimulates circulation.
4. Change sterile gloves.	
5. Apply slit gauze around drain, or apply or replace drainage bag (based upon amount of drainage and skin condition). Ensure that hole in karaya blanket or adhesive backing of drainage bag is large enough to prevent occlusion of drain but small enough to expose a minimum of skin to drainage.	5. This draws drainage away from skin.
6. Apply sterile gauze pads separately to incision and drain site.	6. This draws drainage up into ABD pads.
7. Apply ABD pad over both sites, or overlap two or more ABDs to cover both sites. Apply so that air can circulate (Fig. 7–1).	

ACTION   RATIONALE

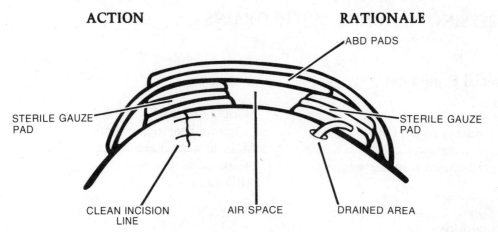

Figure 7-1.   Clearcut ways to speed healing. (Reprinted with permission from the August issue of *Nursing 75*. ©
Copyright 1983, Springhouse Corporation. All rights reserved.)

8. Secure dressing with tape or
   Montgomery straps.

9. Assess and record:
   A. Wound, drain site, and skin con-
      dition.
   B. Amount and characteristics of
      drainage.

DRESSING OPEN WOUNDS

Special Equipment

> Wide mesh gauze (plain or impregnated with
>   petroleum jelly or an antimicrobial agent)
> Iodophor or plain fine mesh gauze packing
> Sterile forceps or gloves
> Hydrogen peroxide solution
> Sterile normal saline solution
> Antimicrobial cream
> Irrigation equipment

Procedure

ACTION	RATIONALE
1. Remove soiled dressing slowly, pulling gently from side to side.	1. This provides gentle debridement.

ACTION	RATIONALE
2. Remove soiled packing slowly with sterile forceps.	2. This provides gentle debridement.
3. Irrigate wound gently with hydrogen peroxide solution, followed by sterile normal saline. Solution should flow from cleanest area to least clean area and thence into collecting basin from irrigation set.	3. This removes organic debris.
4. Cleanse skin. A. Use hydrogen peroxide solution. B. Then use normal saline solution to rinse. C. Dry thoroughly.	
5. Pack deep wounds with iodophor or plain fine mesh gauze, using sterile forceps, as prescribed by physician.	
6. Apply wide mesh gauze moistened with normal saline or gauze impregnated with petroleum jelly or an antimicrobial agent, using sterile forceps or sterile glove, as prescribed by physician.	6. This prevents drying and scabbing of the wound and reduces pain when gauze is removed.
7. Apply dry, nonocclusive dressing: secure in place.	
8. Change dressing every 4 to 6 hours, if using saline method.	
9. Assess and record: A. Condition of wound edges, subcutaneous and granulation tissue, and skin. B. Amount and characteristics of drainage.	

WOUND IRRIGATION

Special Equipment

Small plastic barrier drape with adhesive backing
8 Fr. red rubber catheter
Gown and mask (if wound is infected)

Protective bed pads
Bulb syringe
Safety pin
Irrigation solution
Sterile gauze pads

Procedure

ACTION	RATIONALE
1. Protect bed linens.	
2. Apply plastic barrier drape. A. Remove a 1-inch strip of paper backing from one edge of adhesive plastic barrier drape. B. Secure barrier drape to patient's skin between wound and Montgomery straps so that drape covers straps.	B. This protects the Montgomery straps.
3. Position patient so solution will flow in desired direction.	
4. Place free end of barrier drape into solution receptacle.	
5. Don sterile glove on nondominant hand.	5. and 6. The dominant hand controls the pressure of solution instillation; the gloved hand manipulates sterile items.
6. Attach red rubber catheter to tip of bulb syringe while holding bulb with dominant hand.	
7. Aspirate irrigation solution, warmed to body temperature, into bulb syringe.	7. Aspirating through the catheter removes air and lubricates it for less traumatic insertion.
8. Irrigate wound. A. Insert tip of catheter or bulb syringe gently into wound; inject irrigation solution. B. Use sterile gauze pad in gloved hand to help direct flow of effluent. C. Direct flow of solution from cleanest to most contaminated for multiple wounds.	
9. Cleanse wound and skin; remove barrier drape, and dress wound.	

ACTION	RATIONALE

10. Assess and record:
   A. Condition of wound and skin.
   B. Amount and characteristics of drainage.	

WOUND CULTURES

Special Equipment

Aspiration technique:
    Syringe
    Large-bore needle
    Polyethylene tubing
    Small cork
    Sterile normal saline or iodophor solution
Swab technique:
    Aerobic culture tube
    Anaerobic culture tube
    Sterile normal saline or iodophor solution

Procedure

ACTION	RATIONALE
1. Remove surface debris and drainage with sterile normal saline or iodophor solution.	1. This removes surface contaminants that might alter culture results.
2. Milk wound gently.	2. This helps to obtain fresh drainage.

3. Select technique for obtaining wound culture.
   A. Aspiration technique:
      (1) Attach polyethylene tubing or large-bore needle to syringe.
      (2) Insert tubing or needle into wound and aspirate fresh drainage.
      (3) Evacuate air from syringe.
	
	A. This is the preferred technique for recovery of both aerobic and anaerobic organisms.
	
	(3) This facilitates recovery of anaerobic organisms.

ACTION	RATIONALE
(4) Cork needle, if using large-bore needle. If using polyethylene tubing, replace with a needle, expel air, and cork needle.	(4) Using cork rather than needle cap reduces risk of accidently stabbing oneself with the needle.

B. Swab technique:
  (1) Remove swab from aerobic culture tube and insert swab into wound.
  (2) Replace swab in tube, ensuring contact with transport media.
  (3) Repeat with anaerobic culture tube.

4. Transport specimens to laboratory immediately to facilitate recovery of fastidious organisms.

Precautions: General

1. Use solutions in unit-dose or small-capacity containers supplied to each individual patient.
2. Never use cotton balls, since loose fibers can act as foreign bodies.
3. Use unpowdered gloves, since powder particles can act as foreign bodies.
4. Avoid dislodging drains, drainage bags, or drainage suction tubing.

Related Care: General

1. Integrate the following concepts into wound care.
   A. Fluid collection, nonviable tissue, and drains diminish the ability of normal host defense mechanisms to rid a wound of organisms.
   B. An already infected wound can be invaded by other organisms and develop a secondary infection or superinfection. An infected wound can seed other sites and cause secondary infections.
   C. To reduce the risk of wound infection, a drain should exit the body through a separate stab wound rather than through the incision.
   D. Open drainage systems are a portal of entry for organisms from skin, dressings, and the air. Closed suction drainage systems utilizing small-diameter tubes greatly reduce the incidence of wound infection.
   E. Drainage bags should be used over open drains in the presence of heavy drainage to protect healthy skin or other nearby wounds.
   F. Montgomery straps should be used when frequent dressing changes or increased air circulation is needed. Straps should be periodically moved to new sites to prevent skin breakdown.

2. Ascertain whether plain gauze should be left dry or moistened with normal saline solution when dressing open wounds.
3. Enzyme or hydrophilic preparations may be prescribed for debridement of necrotic wounds (see "Wound Management: Decubiti").
4. Utilize wound precautions, as needed.

Complications

Primary, secondary, or superinfection of wound
Secondary infection in other sites
Secondary septicemia, with or without endotoxic shock
Wound dehiscence

Suppliers

Bard Hospital Division (wound drainage bags)
BBL, division of Becton Dickinson (Port-a-Cul—anaerobic culture tubes)
Flint Pharmaceutical (Travase—enzymatic ointment)
Heyer-Schulte (closed suction wound drains)
Hollister (wound drainage bags)
Marion Scientific Corporation (Cepti-Seal Culturette—aerobic culture tubes; Silvadene—antimicrobial cream)
Orthopaedic Equipment Company (Redi-vacette—closed suction wound drains)
Parke Davis and Company (Vi-Drape—adherent barrier drapes; Elase—enzymatic ointment)
Pharmacia Laboratories (Debrisan—hydrophilic preparation)
Schering Corporation (Garamycin—antimicrobial cream)
3M Company (Steri-Drape—adherent barrier drapes)
Winthrop Labs (Sulfamylon—antimicrobial cream)
Zimmer U.S.A. (Hemovac—closed suction wound drains)

REFERENCE

Taylor, V.: Meeting the challenge of fistulas and draining wounds. Nursing 80, *10*: 45 (June), 1980.

WOUND MANAGEMENT: DECUBITI

Sandra J. Pfaff, R.N., B.S.N.

Overview

There are a number of intrinsic and extrinsic factors that predispose to decubiti. Intrinsic (host) factors include diabetes, malnutrition, dehydration, coma, paralysis, incontinence, and fever. Extrinsic (iatrogenic) factors include immobilization (casts, traction) and sedation-induced insensitivity to pain.

Prevention of decubiti focuses on four basic nursing approaches: (1) recognition of high-risk patients (those with one or more predisposing factors); (2) monitoring for early signs of decubitus development; (3) nursing intervention, such as positioning, hygiene, and nutrition; and (4) patient protection, such as padding and the use of turning frames. Procedures for both the prevention and management of decubitus ulcers are presented. Objectives, precautions, related care, and complications are similar for both and are identified as "general."

Objectives: General

1. To prevent the development of decubiti through nursing management of the high risk patient.
2. To promote healing and prevent infection when a decubitus ulcer occurs.

PREVENTION OF DECUBITI

Special Equipment

> Karaya powder
> Adhesive foam padding
> Polyurethane foam padding

Procedure

ACTION	RATIONALE
1. Cleanse site with soap and water and dry thoroughly.	1. Sites to focus on are areas over bony prominences, areas experiencing undue or chronic pressure (intrinsic or extrinsic), and chronic reddened areas.

ACTION	RATIONALE
2. Gently massage site.	2. This stimulates circulation.
3. Sprinkle karaya powder liberally onto center of sticky side of adhesive foam padding.	
4. Apply adhesive foam padding to site and seal edges to skin.	
5. Cut a hole in polyurethane foam padding to fit it around adhesive foam padding.	
6. Apply to skin; add second layer if patient is very thin.	6. This prevents pressure on the site by distributing body weight more evenly around it.
7. Replace foam paddings: A. Immediately if they become wet, dislodged, or soiled. B. At least every 10 days.	7. This prevents discomfort and skin maceration.
8. Assess for skin turgor, erythema, and pain, and record findings.	

MANAGEMENT OF DECUBITI: KARAYA METHOD _____

Special Equipment

Karaya powder
Karaya ring
Polyurethane foam padding
Hydrogen peroxide solution

Sterile normal saline for irrigation
Iodophor solution
Irrigation equipment

Procedure

ACTION	RATIONALE
1. Irrigate decubitus with: A. Hydrogen peroxide. B. Then normal saline. C. Then iodophor solution.	A. This removes organic debris.
2. Cleanse surrounding skin with soap and water and dry thoroughly. Avoid removing karaya residue that adheres after irrigation.	

ACTION	RATIONALE
3. Massage area around decubitus gently.	3. This stimulates circulation.
4. Mold karaya ring to fit closely around edge of ulcer.	
5. Apply karaya powder. Use syringe to apply in hard to reach or very deep areas. A. Sprinkle karaya powder into decubitus. B. Allow it to absorb moisture in wound. C. Reapply until wound appears "dusty."	
6. Apply foam padding. A. Cut hole in polyurethane foam padding so it fits snugly around karaya ring. B. Apply to skin. C. Apply second layer, if needed, and extend 1 inch to 2 inches beyond perimeter of first layer for better pressure distribution.	C. This prevents pressure by distributing body weight more evenly.
7. Place plastic film from karaya ring over opening in ring.	7. This protects the wound from bed linens and ensures easy observation.
8. Add karaya powder every 8 to 9 hours to maintain dusty appearance.	
9. Irrigate and apply karaya powder daily.	
10. Change entire system: A. Immediately, if loose or soiled. B. At least every 10 days.	
11. Assess for infection; intervene as necessary.	
12. Assess and record: A. Size, depth, and condition of decubitus. B. Condition of surrounding skin. C. Amount and characteristics or drainage.	

MANAGEMENT OF DECUBITI: HYDROPHILIC BEAD METHOD _____

Special Equipment

Hydrophilic beads (dextranomer [Debrisan])
Wound cleansing solution
Irrigation solution
Sterile gauze pads
Tape
Sterile stretch gauze
Sterile gloves
Petroleum jelly
Sterile piston syringe
Sterile glycerin ⎫
Sterile bowl   ⎬ for irregular surfaces or hard-to-reach areas
Sterile tongue blades ⎭

Procedure

ACTION	RATIONALE
1. Cleanse wound area, using prescribed solution and standard technique.	1. This removes surface drainage and debris; it promotes circulation.
2. Irrigate wound and leave moist; dry surrounding skin.	2. Moisture facilitates cleansing action of hydrophilic beads.
3. Apply line of petroleum jelly around wound.	3. This contains beads within wound.
4. Pour beads into wound until layer is at least 3 mm. deep.	4. Bead action depends on its being at least this depth (or height in the case of shallow wounds).
5. Cover with sterile gauze pads, and secure with stretch gauze or tape.	5. The dressing should be tight enough to contain beads but not constrictive enough to interfere with blood flow. Stretch gauze may be preferable to tape to protect skin.
6. Mix 4 parts beads with 1 part sterile glycerin in a sterile bowl, using sterile tongue blade.	6. This is used for irregular surfaces or hard-to-reach areas.
7. Apply bead/glycerin paste to wound with sterile tongue blade, and apply dressing.	7. The layer should be at least 3 mm. in depth/height.

ACTION	RATIONALE
8. Change dressing at least daily, more often if drainage is moderate or heavy, or if beads change color.	8. When beads appear grayish yellow, they are fully saturated and no longer provide cleansing action. If not changed often enough, beads may form crust and adhere to wound.
9. Completely remove beads from wound at each dressing change by means of showering, irrigating with piston syringe, soaking (immersion or compresses), or mechanical cleansing.	

MANAGEMENT OF DECUBITI: ENZYME PREPARATION METHOD

Special Equipment

Enzyme preparation
Cleansing solution
Irrigation solution (sterile water or sterile saline, or hydrogen peroxide if fibrinolysin and desoxyribonuclease [Elase] ointment is being used)
Sterile gloves
Sterile tongue blades
Sterile dressings (nonadherent for Elase ointment; fine mesh gauze for Elase solution; gauze pads for sutilains [Travase] ointment)

Procedure

ACTION	RATIONALE
1. Cleanse wound area, using prescribed solution and standard technique.	1. This removes surface drainage and debris; promotes circulation.
2. Irrigate wound and leave moist; dry surrounding skin.	2. Antimicrobial cleansing solutions or ointments interfere with effectiveness of enzyme preparations.
3. Apply enzyme preparations in a thin layer, ensuring complete contact with all wound surfaces and extending ¼ to ½ inch beyond wound edge.	
4. Apply appropriate dressings.	

ACTION	RATIONALE

5. Repeat application and dressing change at recommended frequencies: Elase ointment at least daily, preferably 2 to 3 times/day; Elase solution every 6 to 8 hours; Travase 3 to 4 times/day.

Precautions: General

1. Use individual supplies for each patient.
2. If gloves are worn during care of extensive decubiti, use unpowdered gloves, since powder particles can act as foreign bodies.

Related Care: General

1. Integrate the following concepts into wound care.
   A. Nursing management centers on prevention of decubiti.
   B. Remote infection increases the risk of infection in decubiti and therefore requires early recognition and prompt intervention.
   C. Karaya is a vegetable gum that is slightly water soluble. It is effective for gentle debridement of ulcers and promotion of the development of granulation tissue.
   D. Enzyme preparations may be effective for debridement of necrotic tissue. Eschar must be removed prior to use of these preparations.
2. Support nutrition and hydration measures.
3. Turn or ambulate (or both) the patient routinely.
4. Use flotation beds, mattresses, or pads as necessary.

Complications: General

Infection
Extension of ulcer into muscle, which may require surgical intervention

Suppliers

Flint Pharmaceutical (Travase—enzyme preparation)
Parke Davis and Company (Elase—enzyme preparation)
Pharmacia Laboratories (Debrisan—hydrophilic beads)
E.R. Squibb and Sons (Stomahesive—adhesive foam padding)
3M Company (Reston—adhesive foam padding)

REFERENCES

Cameron, G.: Pressure sores—what to do when prevention fails. Nursing 79, 9:42 (Jan.), 1979.
Feustel, D.: Pressure sore prevention. Nursing 82, 12:78 (April), 1982.

WOUND MANAGEMENT: BURNS

Sandra J. Pfaff, R.N., B.S.N.

Overview

Physiologic abnormalities in burns alter normal healing processes. These include: (1) altered neutrophilic antibacterial activity, in which bacteria multiply and are protected from antibiotics while they are inside the burn neutrophils; (2) occluded vascular supply, which reduces the delivery of humoral and cellular defense mechanisms; (3) bacterial invasion by gram-positive organisms during the first 3 post-burn days, and by gram-negative organisms from beneath eschar by the fifth post-burn day; (4) edema, which neutralizes protective fatty acids; and (5) tissue necrosis, which enhances the growth of a bacterial population.

Medical therapy includes: (1) debridement by means of dressings or hydrotherapy; (2) surgical debridement with the application of heterografts; and (3) surgical debridement with the application of biologic dressings (cadaver skin, homografts, amniotic membrane homografts, porcine xenografts, or biosynthetic membranes).

Many critical care areas have a "resident" flora of multiply-resistant organisms. Prevention of patient colonization by these organisms is accomplished through rigid adherence to strict technique by all health care team members. Endogenous patient flora must be controlled to keep their total numbers below the infection threshold. Fluid and electrolyte losses through wounds must be adequately replenished.

Procedures for the management of open, intact second-degree, nonintact second-degree, and third-degree burns (also referred to as full-thickness burns) are presented. Because the objectives, precautions, related care, and complications are similar, they are presented only once, identified as "general."

Objectives: General

1. To promote healing of burns through wound care appropriate to the type of burn.
2. To prevent infection through inhibition of burn colonization by endogenous and exogenous flora.
3. To minimize contractures from burn scarring.

CARE OF FIRST-DEGREE BURNS _____

Procedure

ACTION	RATIONALE
1. Elevate and immobilize affected area.	1. This reduces pain and swelling.
2. Apply cold.	2. This provides comfort.
3. Keep area clean and dry; avoid application of ointments, creams, or lotions.	
4. Assess and record condition of burn and surrounding skin.	

CARE OF OPEN BURNS _____

Special Equipment

Sterile cotton swabs or sterile tongue blades
Iodophor solution
Antimicrobial cream
Bed cradle

Infrared lamp
Sterile gown
Sterile gloves
Mask

Procedure

ACTION	RATIONALE

1. Cleanse with iodophor and sterile water.
  A. Use all sterile supplies, gown, and gloves.
  B. Wear mask.
	A. This stimulates circulation and provides gentle debridement.

2. Apply antimicrobial cream (if prescribed by physician) in a thin layer with sterile cotton swab, sterile tongue blade, or sterile gloved hand.	
3. Use bed cradle to elevate top bed sheet.	3. This provides comfort and prevents adherence to burns.

ACTION	RATIONALE
4. Position infrared lamp above bed; position lamp carefully to prevent additional burning or pain to patient. If an infrared lamp in unavailable, adjust room temperature to prevent shivering due to decreased body temperature.	4. This helps to maintain body temperature.

5. Assess and record:
   A. Condition of blisters or eschar.
   B. Amount and characteristics of drainage.
   C. Signs of maceration.
   D. Pulse in affected extremities.
   E. Range of motion of affected extremities.

CARE OF INTACT SECOND-DEGREE BURNS (UNBROKEN BLISTERS)

Special Equipment

Sterile nonadherent surgical dressings
Stretch gauze
Iodophor solution
Sterile water

Procedure

ACTION	RATIONALE
1. Cleanse skin around burns with iodophor and sterile water; avoid any cleansing or manipulation of blisters.	
2. Apply sterile nonadherent pads *around* burns on bony prominences and pressure areas; secure with stretch gauze.	2. This protects blisters, relieves pressure, and enhances air circulation.
3. Assess and record condition of blisters and surrounding skin.	

CARE OF NONINTACT SECOND-DEGREE BURNS (BROKEN BLISTERS) _____

Special Equipment

Sterile, nonadherent surgical gauze roll
Sterile bulky gauze
Stretch gauze or net
Iodophor solution
Sterile water or sterile normal saline solution
Antimicrobial cream
Sterile gloves

Procedure

ACTION	RATIONALE
1. Cleanse with iodophor and sterile water or normal saline.	1. This stimulates circulation and provides gentle debridement.
2. Air-dry for 20 minutes.	
3. Apply antimicrobial cream, if prescribed by physician.	
4. Apply sterile, nonadherent surgical dressing.	
5. Apply bulky gauze dressings.	
6. Wrap with stretch gauze or net.	
7. Change dressings: A. Twice a day on deep wounds and on any wounds for which antimicrobial cream has been prescribed. B. Every 2 to 4 days on superficial wounds for which no antimicrobial cream has been prescribed.	
8. Assess and record: A. Condition of wound and surrounding skin. B. Presence of any odor. C. Amount and characteristics of drainage.	

CARE OF THIRD-DEGREE BURNS (FULL-THICKNESS BURNS

Special Equipment

Sterile nonadherent surgical gauze roll
Sterile bulky gauze
Stretch gauze or net
Antimicrobial cream
Bed cradle and heat lamp (if needed)
Iodophor solution
Sterile water or sterile normal saline solution
Sterile gloves
Mask

Procedure

ACTION	RATIONALE
1. Cleanse with iodophor and sterile water or normal saline.	1. This stimulates circulation and provides gentle debridement.
2. Air-dry for 20 minutes.	
3. Apply antimicrobial cream, if prescribed by physician.	
4. Apply sterile, nonadherent surgical dressing; use bed cradle and heat lamp, if needed.	4. The heat lamp helps to maintain body temperature.
5. Apply bulky gauze and stretch gauze *only* if large amounts of drainage are present.	
6. Change dressing as needed, depending on amount of drainage.	
7. Assess and record: A. Condition of wound, granulation tissue, and skin. B. Amount and characteristics of drainage. C. Pulse in affected extremities. D. Range of motion in affected extremities.	

Precautions: General

1. Use antimicrobial creams rather than ointments, since they are easier to apply and remove and are less occlusive.
2. Reduce the potential of cross-contamination from personnel and equipment. Personnel with an infection in *any* site should not care for burn patients. Masks should be worn when caring for second-degree burns with broken blisters or for third-degree burns.
3. Utilize a private room with positive air pressure. Cleaning should be done with wet cloths and mops and with minimal agitation of air currents. Burn care should be performed before or well after cleaning.

Related Care: General

1. Integrate the following concepts into wound care.
    A. Blisters on second-degree burns act as protective barriers for both fluid loss and the development of infection. They should not be cleansed or manipulated so that they are maintained intact as long as possible.
    B. Local application of moist compresses should be utilized, rather than hydrotherapy, if infection exists on another area of the body.
    C. Antimicrobial therapy should be instituted when the possibility of remote infection exists. Prophylaxis may be instituted if the blisters on second-degree burns break or after the eschar on third-degree burns is no longer intact.
    D. If used, dressings should be individualized according to the type, location, and depth of the wound. They should absorb fluid to prevent maceration, protect from trauma, and be comfortable. Nonadherent dressings are used for healing wounds; adherent dressings are used to debride infected wounds.
    E. Sterile bed linens and bed clothing should be used for nonintact second-degree burns and for third-degree burns.
    F. All patients should be assessed for remote infection and appropriate intervention taken.
    G. Change only bulky and stretch gauze on nonintact second-degree burns (blisters broken) if superficial wounds are clean and dry and no antimicrobial cream has been prescribed. Change dressings on superficial wounds more often if:
        (1) Any odor is detected.
        (2) Patient complains of discomfort.
        (3) Stretch gauze becomes soiled.
2. Integrate the following concepts into use of antimicrobial creams.
    A. Silver sulfadiazine cream (Silvadene) is the most frequently used agent for prophylaxis of burn wound infection. However, allergic reactions may occur, and patients should be monitored for leukopenia if this agent is used on extensive areas of the body.

B. Silver nitrate in 0.5% solution is often used on pediatric patients since it is painless. However, it does not penetrate eschar, is less effective against *Pseudomonas* species, and may leach sodium and chloride. Patient's electrolytes should be monitored and replaced as necessary.

C. Mafenide acetate cream (Sulfamylon) is able to penetrate eschar and has a broad antimicrobial spectrum. Because of pain upon application and metabolic side effects such as acidosis and decreased PCO_2, it is not frequently used for prophylaxis. Recent data indicate that its use for several days prior to grafting reduces local bacterial colony counts, thereby improving graft results.

D. Topical antimicrobials diffuse from wounds within 6 hours and therefore require reapplication at least every 12 hours.

3. Utilize barrier precautions, as necessary. These may include sterile gowns for personnel, and masks. Thorough handwashing with an antimicrobial agent prior to every patient contact is the most important barrier technique.

4. Maintain optimal fluid and electrolyte balances.

5. Monitor and assess the patient's nutritional status.

6. Utilize effective wound management of any infected wounds.

Complications: General

Infection, local or systemic
Dehydration
Hypothermia
Electrolyte imbalance

Suppliers

The Kendall Company (Telfa—nonadherent surgical dressings)
Marion Scientific Corporation (Silvadene—antimicrobial cream)
Schering Corporation (Garamycin—antimicrobial cream)
3M Company (Micropad—nonadherent surgical dressings)
Winthrop Labs (Sulfamylon—antimicrobial cream)

REFERENCES

Burke, J.F., Yannis, I.V., Quinby, W.C. Jr., et al.: Successful use of a physiologically acceptable artificial skin in the treatment of extensive burn injury. Ann Surg., *194*:413, 1981.

Herndon, D.N., and Kraft, E.R.: Temporary reduction of burn wound quantitative bacterial counts to less than 10^2 with subsequent 95% overall autograft survival. Surg. Forum, 33:61, 1982.

Macmillan, B.G.: Infection following burn injury. Surg. Clin. North Am. *60*:185, 1980.

INVASIVE SITE CARE
———— (VENOUS AND ARTERIAL) ————

Judith J. (Henderson) Boehm, R.N., M.S.N.

Overview

Effective site care for venous and arterial indwelling catheters is imperative to preserve the patient's skin integrity and to prevent any complications resulting from improper site care. The catheters referred to in these procedures may include:

1. Arterial
   A. Peripheral
   B. Left atrial
2. Venous
   A. Peripheral, steel needle and short catheter
   B. Central
   C. Pulmonary artery
   D. Right atrial

Whether these catheters are inserted by puncture, surgical cutdown, or transthoracically, the procedures for their care are quite similar. The precautions, related care, and complications apply to both short and long venous and arterial indwelling catheter site care and are identified as "general."

SHORT VENOUS AND ARTERIAL
INDWELLING CATHETER SITE CARE ——————————

Objectives

1. To decrease the incidence of phlebitis and infection at the catheter insertion site and catheter-related sepsis.
2. To assess the patient for phlebitis, infection, infiltration, and leakage of fluid at the catheter insertion site and catheter-related sepsis and, if present, to take appropriate nursing measures.
3. To preserve skin integrity at the insertion site.

Special Equipment

Sterile gloves
Sterile gauze pads and sterile solution (e.g.,
   normal saline)

Iodine and 70% alcohol, or iodophor solution
(for sensitive skin), or 70% alcohol (when
patient has allergy to iodine)
Povidone-iodine ointment
Adhesive tape

Procedure

ACTION	RATIONALE
1. Wash hands thoroughly.	
2. Expose site: A. Remove old dressings and tape from catheter insertion site. B. Leave one piece of tape in place to secure catheter.	
3. Don sterile gloves.	
4. Remove residual ointment or dried blood and secretions from site with sterile gauze pad or sterile solution (e.g., normal saline) as needed.	4. Dried blood and secretions can neutralize iodine's germicidal activity.
5. Assess insertion site for signs of inflammation, phlebitis, infection, infiltration, or leakage of fluid. A. If any of these is present, remove catheter. B. If infection at the site or sepsis is suspected, obtain appropriate cultures; see "Related Care" further on. C. Insert new catheter at another site with entirely new apparatus.	
6. Scrub skin around insertion site with iodine solution, using a circular motion from catheter outward to periphery. Allow the tincture to dry for 30 seconds, and then wash it off with 70% alcohol. If the patient has sensitive skin, an iodophor solution is used instead. It is allowed to dry in place and is not removed. If the patient has an allergy to iodine, scrub with 70% alcohol for at least 1 full minute.	6. Working from the cleanest area of the wound, the insertion site, to the less clean area, the periphery, prevents wound contamination and infection. Alcohol is used to decrease further the risk of burns from iodine. The iodophor solution's germicidal action is augmented by the sustained release of iodine.

ACTION	RATIONALE
7. Apply povidone-iodine ointment to insertion site and emerging catheter.	7. Iodine ointment is bactericidal, fungicidal, virucidal, and amebicidal. Some researchers suggest that the use of a polyantibiotic ointment may be more efficacious, especially for peripheral venous catheters.
8. Dress site and anchor needle or catheter. A. For a winged steel needle: 　(1) Apply short piece of ¼-inch adhesive tape across each wing parallel to needle. 　(2) Apply piece of ¼-inch tape across both wings, at right angle to needle (Fig. 7–2).	8. To-and-fro motion of the needle or catheter may facilitate entry of cutaneous microorganisms into the wound and increase risk of phlebitis by traumatizing the catheterized vessel.

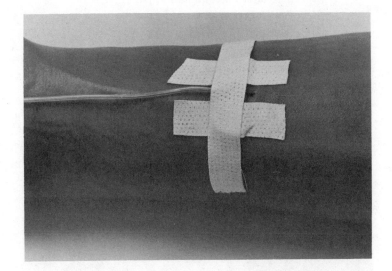

Figure 7-2.

(3) Place sterile gauze pad over insertion site and tape.	(3) Use of occlusive dressings remains optional, since there are no controlled investigative studies to warrant a definitive recommendation. An occlusive dressing is warranted at a site that could easily be contaminated.
(4) Make loop of intravenous tubing near to wings and tape it to skin; do not cross tubing over itself (Fig. 7–3).	(4) Compression of line may hinder flow.

ACTION   RATIONALE

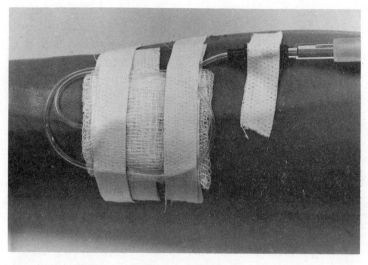

Figure 7-3.

B. For a short catheter:
   (1) Place small sterile gauze pad
       over insertion site, and tape.
   (2) Place piece of ¼-inch tape
       under hub of catheter,
       adhesive side up, crisscross it
       over hub, and secure it to
       dressing (Fig. 7–4).

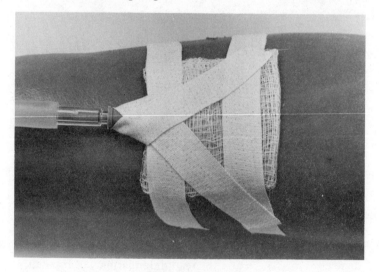

Figure 7-4.

   (3) Place piece of 1-inch tape
       across crisscrossed tape.
   (4) Place 1-inch strip of tape   (4) This helps to avoid discon-
       lengthwise over IV tubing   nection of the tubing and
       and hub. To allow for easy   hub.
       removal of the tape, fold tape
       onto itself, making a tab at
       distal end.

ACTION   RATIONALE

(5) Make loop of IV tubing and
     tape it to arm (Fig. 7–5).

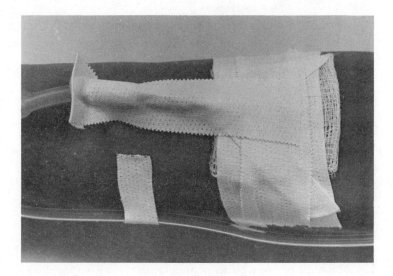

Figure 7-5.

9. Label new dressing with:
   A. Type, gauge, and length of needle
      or catheter in place.
   B. Date and time of insertion.
   C. Initials of person inserting device.
   D. Date of site care.

10. Record site care and catheter and skin
    integrity, as appropriate.

LONG VENOUS AND ARTERIAL INDWELLING CATHETER SITE CARE _____

Objectives

1. To decrease the incidence of phlebitis and infection at the catheter insertion site and catheter-related sepsis.
2. To assess the patient for phlebitis, infection, infiltration, and leakage of
   fluid at the catheter insertion site, and catheter-related sepsis and, if
   present, to take appropriate nursing measures.
3. To preserve skin integrity at the insertion site.

Special Equipment

Face mask
Sterile gloves
Sterile drapes
Fenestrated sterile gauze pads and sterile solution
   (e.g., normal saline)
Iodine and 70% alcohol, or iodophor solution
   (for sensitive skin), or 70% alcohol
   (when patient has allergy to iodine)
Povidone-iodine ointment
Tincture of benzoin
Adhesive tape

Procedure

ACTION	RATIONALE
1. Mask all persons in immediate area.	1. Optimum sterile technique is recommended, since many of these catheters remain in place longer than 48 hours.
2. Wash hands thoroughly.	
3. If catheter is in patient's arm or shoulder, abduct arm and have patient turn face away from site or place a mask over patient's face.	
4. Expose site: A. Remove old dressings and tape from catheter insertion site. B. Leave one piece of tape in place to secure catheter.	
5. Don sterile gloves.	
6. Place sterile drapes around exposed site.	
7. Remove residual ointment or dried blood and secretions from site with sterile gauze pad or sterile solution (e.g., normal saline) as needed.	7. Dried blood and secretions could neutralize iodine's germicidal activity.
8. Assess insertion site for signs of inflammation, phlebitis, infection, infiltration, or leakage of fluid. A. If present, remove catheter after consultation with physician.	

ACTION	RATIONALE
B. If infection at the site or sepsis is suspected, obtain appropriate cultures (see "Related Care" further on).	
C. When new catheter is inserted at another site, use entirely new apparatus.	
9. Scrub skin around insertion site, any sutures, and catheter with iodine solution, from catheter outward to periphery. Allow the tincture to dry for 30 seconds, and then wash it off with 70% alcohol. If the patient has sensitive skin, an iodophor solution is used instead. It is allowed to dry in place and is not to be removed. If the patient has an allergy to iodine, scrub with 70% alcohol for at least 1 full minute.	9. Working from the cleanest area of the wound, the insertion site, to the less clean area, the periphery, prevents wound contamination and infection. Alcohol is used to decrease further the risk of burns from iodine. The iodophor solution's germicidal action is augmented by the sustained release of iodine.
10. Apply povidone-iodine ointment to insertion site, emerging catheter, and sutures.	10. Iodine ointment is bactericidal, fungicidal, virucidal, and amebicidal.
11. Dress site and anchor catheter.	
A. For a central catheter:	
(1) Place fenestrated sterile gauze pad over insertion site, with catheter exiting in center (Fig. 7–6).	(1) Gauze under the catheter prevents it from pressing directly onto the skin.

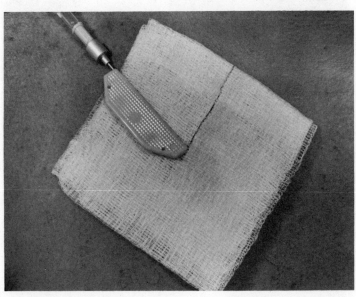

Figure 7-6.

ACTION	RATIONALE
(2) Place another sterile gauze pad over insertion site and catheter.	
(3) Apply tincture of benzoin to skin surrounding gauze; allow it to dry.	(3) Tincture of benzoin protects the skin and promotes adherence of the adhesive tape.
(4) Discard first layer of wide adhesive tape and apply fresh layer of tape over gauze, leaving connection of catheter to IV tubing exposed.	(4) Exposure of connection allows the IV tubing to be changed, if needed, without disturbing the dressing.
(5) Secure all edges of dressing with 1-inch tape.	
(6) Place 1-inch strip of tape lengthwise over IV tubing and connection. To allow for easy removal of the tape, fold tape onto itself, making a tab at the distal end.	(6) This avoids disconnection of the tubing and connection.
(7) Make loop of IV tubing and tape it on top of dressing (Fig. 7–7).	

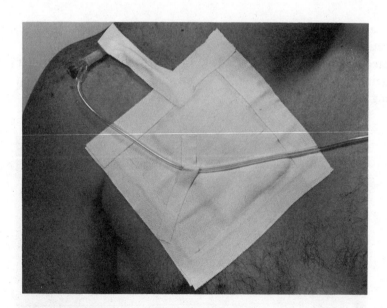

Figure 7-7.

B. For a right or left atrial line:
   (1) Place fenestrated sterile gauze pad over insertion site, with catheter exiting in center.

ACTION	RATIONALE
Suturing of line may not permit this step to be performed.	
(2) Place another sterile gauze pad over insertion site and line.	
(3) Discard first layer of wide adhesive tape and apply fresh layer of tape over gauze, cutting to center of tape.	(3) Cutting to center of the tape enables it to fit snugly around the catheter.
(4) Anchor exposed catheter to top of dressing or skin with tape.	

12. Label new dressing with:
    A. Gauge and length of catheter in place.
    B. Date and time of insertion.
    C. Date of site care.

13. Record site care and catheter and skin integrity, as appropriate.

Precautions: General

1. Maintain strict asepsis during site care, since contamination of the insertion site could progress to phlebitis or infection.
2. Do not leave short IV catheter in place longer than 72 hours, and preferably change at 48-hour intervals. If an IV catheter is not replaced after 72 hours, the nurse or physician should:
    A. Record in patient's medical record the rationale for leaving it in place longer than 72 hours.
    B. Ensure adherence to aseptic methods for the care of the line and site.
    C. Observe the site frequently for inflammation, phlebitis, infection, infiltration, and leakage of fluid, or any possibility of catheter-related sepsis.

Related Care: General

1. Perform site care once daily and when the dressing becomes contaminated.
2. Change IV tubing and solution at the same time site care is performed.
3. Remove hair from the site only if necessary to facilitate the placement or removal of adhesive tape. Remove hair with a depilatory or scissors, be-

cause razor shaving produces microabrasions of the skin, with resultant bacterial access and growth. The presence of hair bears little relation to the bacterial flora of skin, and methods used to clean the skin also suffice to clean hair.

4. Assess for signs of phlebitis plus purulent drainage if infection is suspected at the site. Collect any purulent material for culture and Gram stain. The catheter may then be cultured in the following manner.

   A. If the patient has no allergy to iodine, scrub the skin around the catheter with iodine and 70% alcohol, working from the catheter out to the periphery. Allow the iodine to dry for 30 seconds and then wash it off with 70% alcohol, working in a similar manner as above. Applying an antiseptic to the skin decreases the chance of contaminating the catheter with skin flora as it is removed.

   B. If the patient has an allergy to iodine, scrub the skin around the catheter with 70% alcohol solution for at least one full minute, working in a similar manner as above.

   C. Remove the catheter, applying pressure with dry sterile gauze to the artery or vein, as needed.

   D. Clip the tip of the catheter off with sterile scissors, letting it fall into appropriate tube for culture.

   E. Send specimens to the laboratory for culturing. A semiquantitative method of catheter culture is recommended.

5. Monitor the temperature of the patient regularly when a catheter is in place; an unexplained fever or chills may indicate catheter-related sepsis. If sepsis is present and thought to be related to infection from the catheter, blood may be drawn through the catheter. The catheter is then removed and cultured, as above.

6. Use taffeta, silk, or paper tape in place of adhesive tape to prevent skin irritation and allergic reaction as needed.

Complications: General

   Phlebitis
   Infection at insertion site
   Catheter-related sepsis
   Emboli
   Mechanical separation of lines
   Displacement or accidental removal of catheter
   Impairment of circulation

Suppliers

   Clinipad Corporation (general dressing change kits and central venous catheter care kits)

Concord Laboratories (TPN-CVP dressing change trays)
Shield Laboratories, Inc. (central venous catheter
   dressing change set)

REFERENCES

Maki, D.G., and Band, J.D.: A comparative study of polyantibiotic and iodophor ointments in prevention of vascular catheter-related infection. Am. J. Med., 70:739–744, 1981.

National Intravenous Therapy Association: Intravenous Nursing Standards of Practice. Belmont, MA, November, 1981.

Stratton, C.W.: Infection related to intravenous infusions. Heart Lung, 11:123–137, 1982.

8

THE
MUSCULOSKELETAL
SYSTEM

_____ CARE OF PERSONS IN TRACTION _____

Leona Mourod, R.N., M.S.N.

Overview

Multiple trauma is a frequent admitting diagnosis for patients to a critical care unit. With multisystem involvement, these patients require close monitoring of all body systems and expert handling of injured musculoskeletal tissues being treated with a form of skin or skeletal traction.

ESTABLISHMENT OF BALANCED SUSPENSION SKELETAL TRACTION TO THE FEMUR _____

Overview

Skeletal traction is used in fractures of the major long bones, which, because of spasms of large muscle masses, result in shortening, overriding, or displacement (or a combination of these) of the distal fragments. Skeletal traction permits use of greater amounts of weight for traction pull than could be applied to skin tissues without danger of damage or disruption. A Steinmann pin or a Kirschner wire may be used as the traction source, depending on the bone that was fractured, the severity of the fracture, and the amount of displacement. A Steinmann pin has a larger gauge than a Kirschner wire, requires larger entrance and exit openings in the skin and generates more heat during insertion through the bone, predisposing to the possibility of more bone cell loss. Because of its smaller gauge, a Kirschner wire necessitates smaller skin openings, causes less heat during insertion, and permits substantial strength for traction pull. The nursing care is the same when either the Steinmann pin or Kirschner wire is used for skeletal traction (Fig. 8–1).

Figure 8-1 *A*, Kirschner wire in a Kirschner bow or spreader. *B*, Steinmann diameter of pin compared to the wire pin. Note larger gauge.

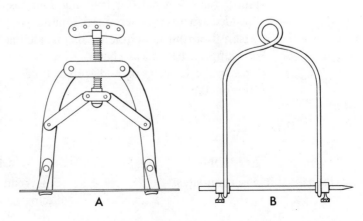

A   B

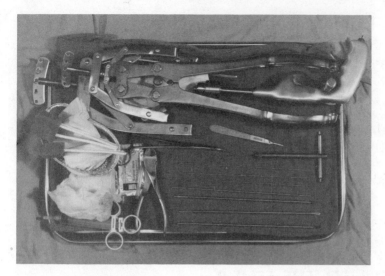

Figure 8-2 Sample Steinmann pin tray containing pins of varying sizes.

Objectives

1. To initiate weighted skeletal traction by use of a pin or wire through the proximal tibia.
2. To use balanced suspension to facilitate the skeletal traction and aid in patient care.

Special Equipment

Steinmann pin tray
or
Kirschner wire tray (Fig. 8–2)
Kirschner spreader bow
Scalpel handle and blades
Towels and drapes
Skin prep materials

Local anesthetic
Syringes and needles
Gloves
Gauze pads
Povidone-iodine or neomycin-based
  ointment

Additional Equipment

Electric or hand drill
Splint: may be a half- or full-ring Thomas, Harris, or other type,
  padded with felt-covered stockinette
Pierson (Pearson) attachment, also padded as above.
Foot support, padded as above
Ropes, pulleys, weights, and weight holders
Adhesive tape

Procedure

ACTION	RATIONALE
1. Prepare skin insertion sites.	1. This reduces the possibility of introducing bacteria into the pin tract.

ACTION	RATIONALE
2. Hold limb for skin prep, instillation of local anesthetic, and insertion of pin or wire.	2. This prevents additional trauma and provides stability for insertion.
3. Assist with application of spreader bow, application of splint, Pierson attachment, and foot support.	3. This facilitates establishing traction.
4. Assist with attaching ropes, pulleys, weights, and weight holders.	4. This provides safety to the patient while the traction is being established.
5. Assist with the elevation of the injured limbs in suspension and application of ropes, pulleys, and weights for countertraction.	5. This facilitates the traction pull and aids in patient comfort, reduces edema, and facilitates recovery and care.
6. Apply weights in exact amounts ordered for: A. Traction (may be 20 to 35 lbs.). B. Suspension (usually 6 to 8 lbs.). C. Countertraction (usually the same as for suspension).	C. Some countertraction comes from the patient's body; therefore the amount of weight may vary slightly from that used for suspension.
7. Assess patient's position and entire traction setup immediately; check all ropes, pulleys, knots, and weights for freedom of movement and security of knots (Fig. 8–3).	7. This assures proper position for safety and function and for optimal traction.

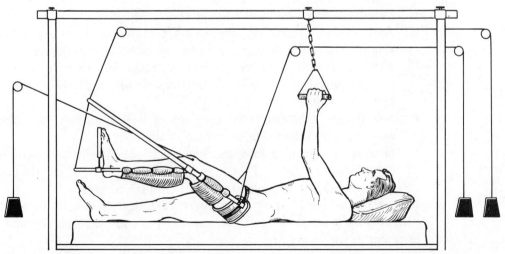

Figure 8-3 Skeletal traction to left lower extremity. Steinmann pin is placed in the proximal tibia to weights at the foot of bed. The splint and Pearson attachment are suspended by weights to the head of the bed. Countertraction begins at the top of the splint extending to weights at the head of the bed.

Precautions

1. Hold the injured limbs carefully during procedure to avoid undue motion or movement that could result in additional injury.
2. Never "lift" or release the weights once skeletal traction is initiated. The weights move freely over the ropes when the patient is moved up in bed. Check that nothing is preventing the free movement of the weights before moving a patient up in bed.
3. Observe the patient closely for development of compartment syndrome. A cardinal sign is *increasing pain on passive movement* (when digits are moved *for* the patient, not *by* the patient). Increasing pain on passive movement signifies anoxia within the muscle tissues. Compartment syndrome results from edema and continued arterial bleeding within a muscle held by its tight fascia. As the bleeding and edema progress, tissue pressure exceeds arterial pressure, preventing perfusion and oxygenation and leading to anoxia. Muscle cells may suffer irreversible damage if not adequately perfused for 6 hours. Surgical release of the tight fascia, called a fasciotomy, may be required to prevent such a complication. Neurovascular checks are performed to note perfusion of the tissues. In addition, intracompartmental pressure monitoring may be ordered (see "Intracompartmental Pressure Monitoring").

Related Care

1. Record the patient's responses and establishment of traction, including physician's name, time, site, type of traction, and amount of weight for traction, suspension, and countertraction.
2. Perform and record neurovascular assessments, comparing all findings with the opposite limb, incorporating each of the following components:
   A. Assess all peripheral pulses, including popliteal, anterior and posterior tibialis, and dorsalis pedis.
   B. Determine capillary refill time of at least two toes.
   C. Assess entire thigh, leg, and foot for presence of edema to assess venous return and amount of trauma or bleeding into tissues.
   D. Assess ability to move toes or foot to obtain data about motor function peripheral to injury site. Alert patient and staff not to bend the knee in traction.
   E. Ask patient to localize the presence of any numbness, tingling, or pain in injured tissues or elsewhere in the body.
   F. Note temperature of foot, leg, and thigh, specifically any significant temperature gradient. Foot may be slightly cooler but should not be cold or markedly different from calf or opposite foot.
3. If there is *no* head injury, administer narcotics judiciously during the patient's first days in skeletal traction to aid in muscle relaxation and adjustment to the injury and traction.

4. Maintain the patient in a low-Fowler back-lying position for most effective traction.

5. Provide information to the patient on how to use a trapeze and the "post" position to raise self. Post position involves placing the uninjured foot flat on the bed with the knee bent while grasping the trapeze and lifting the body off the bed. This position can be used during changing of linens, hygienic care, massage, or placing of a bed pan.

6. Monitor intake and output closely. Renal function may be initially decreased as a result of trauma and the stress response, but output should not be less than 30 to 50 cc/hour in adults.

7. Encourage oral intake of food and fluids if the patient's condition permits. Observe for paralytic ileus or peritoneal signs indicative of abdominal trauma. Initially, the patient may not be given anything by mouth until the extent of trauma is determined.

8. Measure thigh girth with tape measure and compare with uninjured thigh to determine if edema is increasing. Ice bags may be applied to decrease edema formation.

9. Observe patient for signs of increased restlessness, mental confusion, tachycardia, dyspnea, blood pressure changes, or development of petechial rash over upper area of chest and neck. These signs are indicative of *fat embolism,* which may be fatal. Immediate care is required to treat this complication: oxygen therapy, heparinization, IV therapy, antibiotics, and steroid administration. Fat embolization occurs most frequently in 24 to 72 hours after a long-bone fracture, but it can also occur later. Maintain watchfulness during the high incidence period and seek immediate medical care, particularly for increasing confusion, restlessness, dyspnea, tachycardia, and alterations in arterial blood gases.

10. Check laboratory data frequently for indications of hemoconcentration (increased hematocrit) or anemia (decreased hemoglobin), which could signify continuing bleeding or hemorrhage. Bleeding into cavities, including the chest, abdomen, capsule of the spleen, or muscle, may require emergency surgery to correct.

11. Perform pin care as ordered or needed. This care consists of using sterile applicators soaked in hydrogen peroxide to cleanse around pin entrance and exit sites, removing secretions gently to prevent additional trauma, rinsing with sterile saline, and applying a *thin* coating of an antibiotic ointment (either povidone-iodine or neomycin-bacitracin ointment). Pin care may be done as often as every 4 hours, if there is much drainage, or twice daily. Some physicians do not want special care given to the pin sites and request only cleansing during the bath time.

12. Assess all bony prominences regularly for signs of developing decubiti or pressure. Hygienic care, massage, position changes, bed foam pads, and elbow and heel protectors may all be needed to prevent decubiti.

13. Check entire traction setup regularly for intactness and proper functioning.

Complications

Hemorrhage	Volkmann's contracture
Compartment syndrome	Decubiti
Fat embolism	Renal calculi
Pulmonary embolism	Footdrop
Nonunion	Post-traumatic arthritis
Malunion	

REFERENCES

Carini, G. and Birmingham, J.: Traction Made Manageable. New York, McGraw-Hill, 1980, pp. 108–118.
Mourad, L.: Nursing Care of Adults with Orthopedic Conditions. New York, John Wiley, 1980, pp. 142–179.
The Traction Handbook. Warsaw, IN, Zimmer Co., 1975.

ESTABLISHMENT OF DUNLOP'S SKELETAL TRACTION TO THE HUMERUS _____

Overview

Dunlop's traction is used for treating fractures of the distal humerus when there is marked displacement, overriding, or comminution (multiple fragments). Usually a Kirschner wire is inserted in the distal humerus to which a spreader bow and weights are applied. The forearm is held vertically in Buck's extension traction to help maintain optimal traction to the humerus. Low props may be put under the wheels on the side of the bed of the injured arm to create a slight tilt for countertraction.

Dunlop's traction may also be done using only Buck's extension vertically and a sling near the elbow to pull the fractured bones into alignment (Fig. 8–4).

Objectives

1. To initiate Dunlop's skeletal traction to the humerus.
2. To maintain optimal traction position of the patient, injured arm, and forearm.

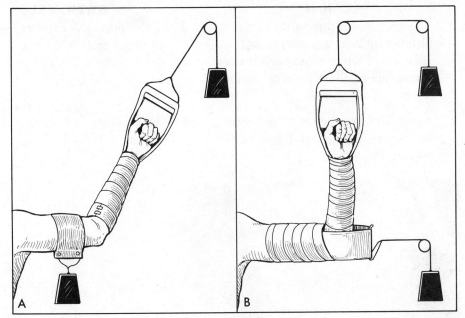

Figure 8-4 Dunlop's side arm traction. Position of the forearm varies according to the physician's preference and the patient's fracture.

Special Equipment

Kirschner wire tray with various lengths of wires
Scalpel handle and blades
Kirschner spreader bow
Towels and drapes
Syringes and needles
Skin prep materials
Local anesthetic
Gloves
Gauze pads
Povidone-iodine or neomycin-based ointment

Additional Equipment

Electric or hand drill
Ropes, pulleys, weights, and weight holders
Ace bandages
Moleskin or foam-backed adhesive strips
Hand support

Procedure

ACTION	RATIONALE
1. Assist with application of foam strips, Ace bandage, and initiation of Buck's extension to forearm.	1. This aids in maintaining the position of the forearm during insertion of wire.

ACTION	RATIONALE
2. Assist as needed during skin prep, infiltration of local anesthetic, and insertion of wire. Hold patient's arm firmly but gently to prevent additional injury.	2. This provides comfort and stability during insertion.
3. Assist with application of spreader bow, ropes, weights, and pulleys as needed (Fig. 8–5).	3. This facilitates initiation of traction.

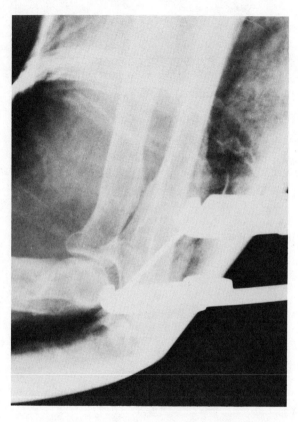

Figure 8-5 Skeletal Dunlop's traction. Pin is inserted through the distal humerus for this patient's particular fracture.

4. Assist with placement of lifts under wheels if needed for countertraction (Fig. 8–6).	4. This aids the function of the traction and helps patient maintain proper position for countertraction.

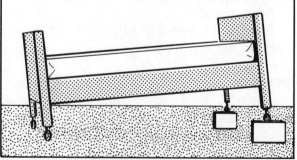

Figure 8-6 Angling bed using shock blocks to assist in maintaining patient's position while in Dunlop's traction. Side-to-side angling is the more common variation.

ACTION	RATIONALE
5. Check entire traction setup, skeletal and skin Buck's traction, ropes, pulleys, weights, and position of patient.	5. This provides baseline data.

Precautions

1. Do not release weights from Dunlop's skeletal traction to the arm. Only the skin Buck's extension can be removed from the forearm with written approval from the physician.
2. Observe for signs of circulatory compromise in arm and forearm, including complaints of increased numbness, or tingling, or increased pain on active or passive movement; changes in color; blanching; and temperature changes or edema of arm, forearm, or hand. Notify physician promptly of these changes or findings—they could signify compartment syndrome
3. Observe for increase in or presence of drainage at pin entry and exit sites. May indicate necrosis of bone cells or infection.

Related Care

1. Record patient's responses and establishment of traction, including physician's name, time, site, type of traction, and amount of weight to each type.
2. Perform and record neurovascular assessments, comparing all findings with the opposite limb. (See related care of "Establishment of Balanced Suspension Skeletal Traction to the Femur.")
3. Encourage the patient to exercise fingers every 4 hours to maintain movement and circulation.
4. Provide pin care (see related care of "Establishment of Balanced Suspension Skeletal Traction to the Femur").
5. Maintain back-lying, flat position at all times for most effective traction. Slight angling to either side permits hygienic care to back and buttocks and linen changes. Place side rail on side opposite traction in up position when care is completed.
6. Monitor laboratory data, intake and output, bowel functioning, appetite, pain patterns, mood and affect as indications of responses to trauma and imposed immobility.

Complications

Hemorrhage	Post-traumatic arthritis
Fat embolism	Wristdrop
Nonunion	Carpal tunnel syndrome
Malunion	Compartment syndrome

REFERENCES

Carini, G. and Birmingham, J.: Traction Made Manageable. New York, McGraw-Hill, 1980, pp, 152–164.
Mourad, L.: Nursing Care of Adults with Orthopedic Conditions. New York, John Wiley, pp. 158–159.

HOFFMANN EXTERNAL FIXATION TRACTION _____

Overview

External fixation devices may be used for various bone fractures, including those of the mandible, humerus, radius and ulna, pelvic bones, femur, and tibia and fibula (Figs. 8–7 and 8–8). Patients may be ambulatory while in these external devices, may be cared for in the home, and generally have more mobility and less disability. Multiple pins inserted transversely through the bones on either side of the fracture are held externally in the apparatus. The pins are inserted aseptically following skin preparation and infiltration of local anesthesia as in the other pin insertions mentioned previously for skeletal traction. Postinsertion care varies with the site and severity of trauma.

Precautions

1. Lift the extremity under the tissues in the Hoffmann apparatus, never by the apparatus itself, to avoid additional trauma to the affected tissues.

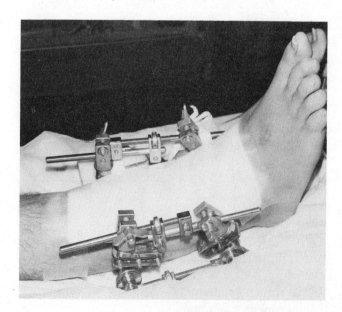

Figure 8-7 Hoffmann apparatus to tibia and fibula to maintain immobility while patient was being treated for osteomyelitis.

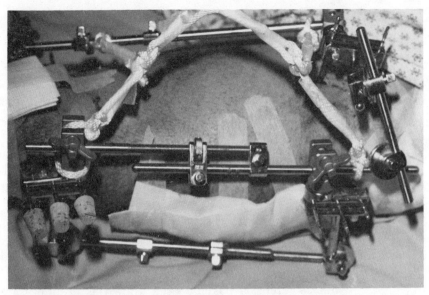

Figure 8-8 Hoffmann apparatus to the femur. Note corks placed to decrease trauma to patient and caregivers. Note also the cord used by the patient to assist with moving his leg while it was *simultaneously* being lifted from under the thigh and lower leg by the nursing personnel.

2. Encourage active muscle and joint exercises and movements within prescribed limitations and orders to prevent joint stiffness and muscle weakness in contiguous muscles and joints.

3. Check amount of weight bearing allowed for pelvic and lower-extremity fractures being treated with a Hoffmann external device. Weight bearing may be initially partial in one or both limbs with the patient using a walker or crutches as assistive supports, gradually progressing to full weight bearing. Instructions to patients regarding the amount of weight bearing should be explicit to avoid confusion or additional injury.

4. Explain techniques for use of crutches or a walker *before* the patient uses them so the patient knows how to use them and the amount of weight to be borne by the injured tissues.

Related Care

1. Complete meurovascular assessments for adequate tissue circulation and perfusion and sensory and motor functioning. (See related care of "Establishment of Balanced Suspension Skeletal Traction to the Femur") and record findings. As before, increasing pain on passive movement, increasing numbness and tingling, or color changes are signs of circulatory compromise and should be reported to the physician.

2. Provide pin care carefully and routinely because the multiple pin insertion and exit sites increase the possibility of infection. Systemic antibiotics may be administered initially to decrease the possibility of osteomyelitis because of the multiple skin/bone disruptions.

BUCK'S EXTENSION SKIN TRACTION TO A LOWER EXTREMITY

Overview

Buck's extension is a frequently used form of skin traction. It is used prior to surgical repair for fractures of the hip and subtrochanteric fractures of the femur. Postoperatively Buck's extension may be used to maintain the tissues in a desired position to assist muscles weakened by surgery, injury, or anesthesia. Additionally, Buck's extension may be used bilaterally for temporary traction to treat low back pain and degenerative conditions of the hips or knees.

As with all forms of skin traction, Buck's extension requires less weight than skeletal traction to the same area, is used for shorter periods, may be intermittently used, and may be removed for skin care and neurovascular assessments.

Buck's extension has also been known as running traction, as the traction "runs" over one pulley to the weights (Fig. 8–9).

Special Equipment

APPLICATION AND MAINTENANCE OF BUCK'S EXTENSION TO THE LEG

Skin-Trac boot, foam-backed adhesive strips, or moleskin strips
Elastic bandages
Spreader bar or foot plate
Ropes, pulleys, weights, and weight holders
Heel protectors (optional)
Cotton padding (optional)

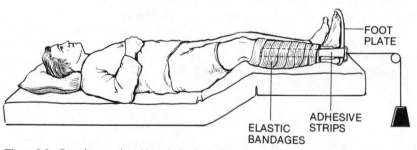

Figure 8-9 Running traction. Note similarity to Buck's extension.

Procedure

ACTION	RATIONALE
1. Assess all skin surfaces to be placed in traction for cleanliness, bruises, openings, or lesions that would prevent application over them.	1. This inspection should include running the hands around all surfaces to note their condition.

ACTION	RATIONALE
2. Shave the leg under the sites of adhesive application *only* if hirsute. Wash and dry gently and thoroughly after shaving. (Shaving is not needed with the Skin-Trac boot.)	2. This should be done carefully to avoid nicks or cuts. Long hair causes the adhesive strips to slide.
3. Apply the adhesive strips to the lateral aspects of the leg, beginning *below* the prominence of the lateral head of the fibula and extending down the leg.	3. This must be done carefully to avoid pressure where the peroneal nerve crosses over the head of the fibula. Peroneal nerve pressure results in footdrop.
4. Pad the ankle area to prevent placing adhesive directly over the malleoli.	4. This will help prevent skin pressure areas.
5. Cover the strips with the elastic bandages, beginning at the foot and extending *up* the leg to aid venous return. Wrap smoothly with pressure sufficient only to hold the adhesive strips in place	5. Wrapping in this manner follows venous return patterns and prevents developing of edema of the foot. Care should be taken to avoid undue tightness around the ankle and Achilles tendon. As above, applying the most distal straps first facilitates venous return.
or omit steps 4 and 5 and:	
Apply the Skin-Trac boot carefully under the foot and leg, gently lifting the leg and supporting it while placing the boot. Close the pressure-sensitive straps across the leg, moving up the leg until all are closed without undue tightness.	
6. Center the foot plate or spreader bar between the adhesive strips and attach to the strips evenly on each side.	6. This provides for even pull from each side.
7. Attach ropes to foot plate of adhesive strips or Skin-Trac boot and run over pulley.	7. This establishes traction route.
8. Attach weight holder with correct amount of weight to rope and lower gently to establish traction (Fig. 8–10).	8. This provides for "easing" into the full effect of the traction.
9. Adjust patient's position in bed to backlying in low Fowler.	9. This position helps maintain the traction optimally.
10. Assess the patient and check the entire setup thoroughly.	10. This assures patient safety and proper traction.

Precautions

1. Avoid use of a pillow under the leg in traction when the patient is in the back-lying position as this creates friction, causing resistance and lessening the traction effects.
2. Put side rails in up position for patient safety when no one is in attendance.
3. Check entire traction setup and freedom of movement of weights before moving patient up in bed.
4. Supply a trapeze so the patient can adjust own position to relieve pressure. Be sure to instruct the patient not to turn to the side without assistance.

Related Care

1. Record patient's responses and establishment of traction, including name of person applying traction (may be a physician, nurse, or orthopedic technician), time, site, type of traction, and amount of weight.
2. Monitor patient's position, responses, and neurovascular findings hourly at first, then at times ordered by physician.
3. Remove the Skin-Trac boot or elastic bandages for skin care and check at least daily, preferably twice daily. Removal should follow institutional policies and specific orders from physician.
4. Maintain a back-lying low-Fowler position for the majority of time in traction. The patient may be turned to the uninjured side for back care and position changes if needed. Either the lowermost leg or a pillow may be placed to support the leg in traction while the patient is on the side.
5. Continue hourly neurovascular assessments carefully for the first 24 hours, lengthening time between checks as patient's condition or orders permit.

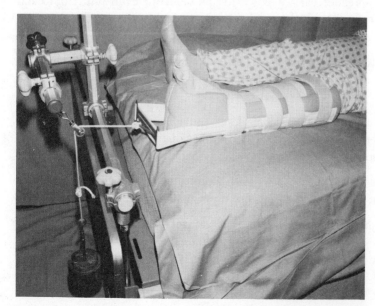

Figure 8-10 Buck's extension to the leg using Skin-Trac Boot. Note elastic hose under boot used to decrease venous stasis.

Complications

Thrombophlebitis	Achilles tendon shortening
Footdrop	Tarsal tunnel syndrome

REFERENCES

Brunner, N. A.: Orthopedic Nursing. A Programmed Approach. St. Louis, C.V. Mosby, 1979.

Carini, G. and Birmingham, J.: Traction Made Manageable. New York, McGraw-Hill, 1980. pp. 86–87.

Mourad, L. Nursing Care of Adults with Orthopedic Conditions. New York, John Wiley, 1980, pp. 110–115.

INTRACOMPARTMENTAL PRESSURE _ MONITORING: WICK OR SLIT CATHETER _

Rae Nadine Smith, R.N., M.S.N.

Overview

Intracompartmental pressure monitoring is an invasive procedure used to determine intramuscular and interstitial pressures to aid in diagnosis and management of compartment syndrome.

Compartment syndrome occurs when the pressure within a closed space confined by bone and unyielding fascia (osseofascial compartment) increases to the point at which it interfers with the perfusion of the muscle and nerves within the involved compartment. This may be caused by an increase in the volume of the compartment or a decrease in the size of the compartment.

The degree of functional loss depends on how long surgical decompression is delayed. Irreversible changes may occur as early as 4 hours after injury if near-total tissue devascularization is present.

Compartment syndrome has been reported in the four compartments of the leg (most common), the forearm, arm, shoulder, thigh, and buttocks. Some clinical studies have reported no significant differences in physical findings in patients with high and low compartment pressure. Intracompartmental monitoring provides an objective, quantitative technique with minimal risk for aiding in the diagnosis of compartment syndrome.

While there are several monitoring techniques, the Wick catheter (Myocath) or Slit catheter technique is the currently preferred method. It provides continuous, direct measurement of interstitial fluid pressure and is suitable for both acute and chronic (intermittent) compartment syndromes. The system is simple, reliable, inexpensive, commercially available, and disposable and provides accurate, objective data.

Compartmental pressure may be monitored continuously or intermittently for up to 48 hours with periodic checks for catheter patency. Normal intracompartmental pressure ranges from 0 to 8 mm. Hg. In a recumbent person the average compartment pressure is 4 mm. Hg. Pain and paresthesias first appear when pressure reaches approximately 20 to 30 mm. Hg. Intracompartmental pressure of 30 mm. Hg. or more is an indication for decompression, since intracompartmental pressure above 30 mm. Hg. can produce irreversible changes.

Objectives

1. To monitor one or more intracompartmental pressures continuously or intermittently with one catheter insertion per compartment.
2. To assist in the early diagnosis and treatment of compartment syndrome.
3. To avoid unnecessary surgery.
4. To prevent neuromuscular deficits.

Special Equipment

Slit catheter or Wick catheter monitoring kit
(Figs. 8–11 and 8–12)

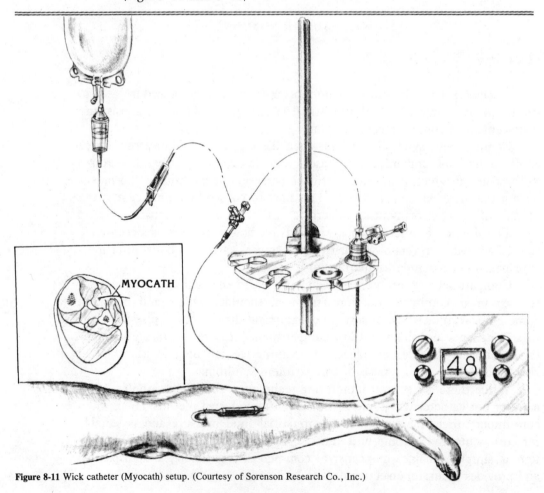

MYOCATH

Figure 8-11 Wick catheter (Myocath) setup. (Courtesy of Sorenson Research Co., Inc.)

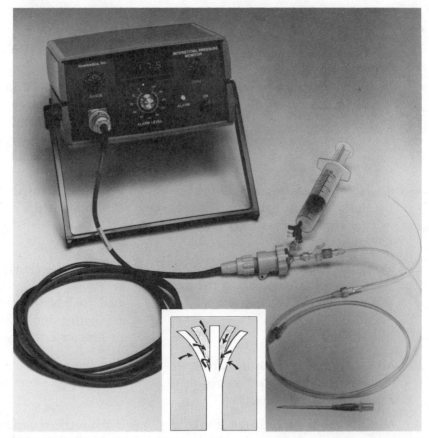

Figure 8-12   Slit catheter setup. Slit tip on catheter consists of 5 petals that allow a patent fluid path and prevent occlusion with material or tissue. (Photo courtesy of Howmedica, Inc.)

Razor
Sterile gauze pads or prep sponges
Povidone-iodine prep solution
Alcohol 70%
Sterile gloves, mask
Suture
Tape
IV pole
Transducer
Transducer mount
Pressure monitor (scope and amplifier)
Normal saline (0.9% sodium chloride) IV solution
Local anesthetic (optional)
Sodium heparin for IV flush soltution (optional)
   If monitoring kit is not used, assemble the following sterile components:
      IV administration set-up or 30 ml. syringe
      Slit or Wick catheter
      Approximately 48 inches of male-female connector pressure tubing
      Three-way stopcock
      1-ml. syringe
      Disposable transducer dome

Procedure

ACTION	RATIONALE
1. Prepare a flush solution.	
A. IV normal saline is recommended.	A. Although IV solution such as lactated Ringer's is satisfactory for pressure monitoring, normal saline is the preferred solution from the standpoint of infection control.
B. Heparin may be added to the flush solution: 1 unit/ml. or 2 units/ml. are frequently used dilutions.	B. This is used when clotting is anticipated.
2. Set up the transducer and monitor, placing a venting stopcock on the top or venting port of the transducer.	2. Since physiologic pressures are relative to atmospheric pressure, transducers used for invasive physiologic pressure monitoring must be vented to room air for correct balancing procedures.
3. Attach a length of pressure tubing, 48 inches or less, to the side port or monitoring port of the transducer.	3. This limits damping artifacts that may give false pressure readings.
4. Advance the Wick catheter, if it is being used, until the wick just appears in the orifice.	4. If the catheter is advanced beyond the heel of the needle bevel, there is danger of shearing or damaging the catheter.
5. Mark the conduit, with a ball point pen, at the base of the groove where the conduit joins the needle hub.	5. Marking allows determination of Wick insertion into the compartment.
6. Retract the catheter tip carefully until the wick cannot be seen.	6. This facilitates insertion and prevents tissue from entering the needle.
7. Connect the following to the side port of the stopcock:	7. Both gravity filling, via an IV administration set from an IV bag, and syringe filling are acceptable filling techniques.
A. IV administration flush line *or*	
B. 30-ml. filled syringe.	B. Smaller syringes exert more pressure, which could damage the transducer if the stopcock were incorrectly positioned, or dislodge the wick from the Wick catheter.

ACTION	RATIONALE
8. Open the venting stopcock on the transducer dome to air and permit the flush solution to fill the tubing and transducer dome.	8. Any air bubbles between the transducer diaphragm and the Slit or Wick catheter will result in false low or high pressure measurements.
9. Close the venting stopcock when no air bubbles remain.	
10. Turn the stopcock on the catheter to slowly flush the catheter. A drop of solution should be seen at the tip of the Slit catheter.	10. Rapid flushing may introduce air into the system or fail to remove all air. When air free, the catheter is ready for insertion into the muscle compartment.
11. Prepare the insertion site.	11. This reduces the risk of infection.
12. Provide for local anesthetic if appropriate.	12. Some patients do not require local anesthetic since their injury may have induced anesthesia.
13. Secure the catheter inserted into the affected muscle compartment by means of suture or tape or both (Fig. 8–13).	

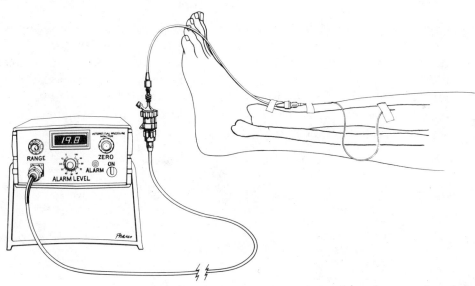

Figure 8-13   Tape and suture are used to secure the catheter.

| 14. Turn the stopcock off toward the patient. Level the open port of the venting stopcock at the level of the tip of the intracompartmental catheter (Fig. 8–14). | 14. For every inch of discrepancy between the port of the venting stopcock and the tip of the intramuscular catheter, there will be a measurement error of approximately 2 mm. Hg. due to the effect of hydrostatic pressure. |

ACTION   RATIONALE

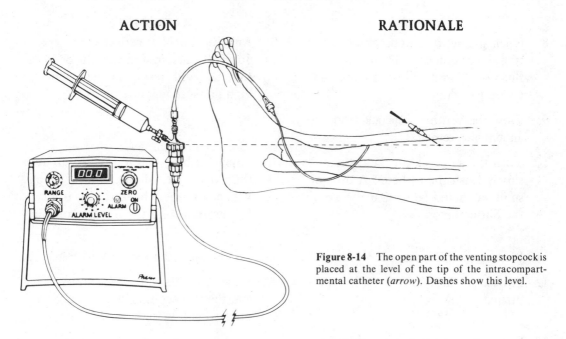

Figure 8-14   The open part of the venting stopcock is placed at the level of the tip of the intracompartmental catheter (*arrow*). Dashes show this level.

15. Balance and calibrate the monitoring system (see "Hemodynamic Monitoring, Single Pressure Transducer System").

16. Check the response of the system by palpating the area over the catheter tip and observing the scope for small, temporary elevations in the pressure pattern. A similar check may be made by having the patient flex-extend the appropriate distal joint (Fig. 8–15). Sys-

15. False high or false low pressures result when monitoring equipment is improperly set up, balanced, and calibrated.

16. A normal pressure response consists of a rapid rise of compartmental pressure with contraction, and a rapid fall to normal, without interstitial pressure summation on repetitive contractions. Patients with symptoms of compartment syndrome demonstrate a rapid

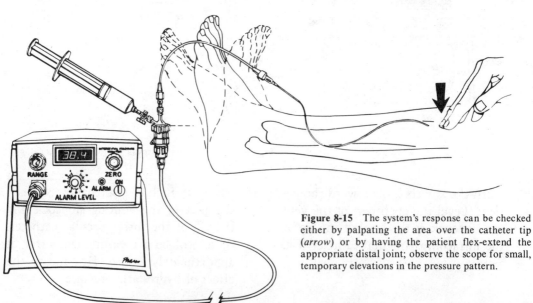

Figure 8-15   The system's response can be checked either by palpating the area over the catheter tip (*arrow*) or by having the patient flex-extend the appropriate distal joint; observe the scope for small, temporary elevations in the pressure pattern.

ACTION	RATIONALE
tem response should be checked routinely at least every 6 hours.	rise of compartmental pressure with contraction, with summation of baseline pressures, and the onset of pain at 15 to 20 mm. Hg. There is a slow fall to baseline after the cessation of contractions.

17. Record the pressure from each catheter.

18. Flush the catheter by slow infusion through it of 0.1 ml. or flush solution if the system is unresponsive to palpation or flexion-extension exercises.

18. This removes tissue or other material occluding the tip of the catheter. Catheters require flushing approximately every 6 hours to keep the wick or petals moist enough to communicate pressure via the fluid column to the transducer.

Precautions

1. Maintain sterile technique throughout the monitoring procedure.
2. Attempt to correct any bleeding abnormalities prior to catheter insertion.
3. Eliminate all potential causes of measurement errors, such as air and incorrect balancing and calibration procedures prior to treating a patient for an increase in intramuscular or interstitial pressures.
4. Avoid using excessive syringe pressures to reduce risk to the transdcuer and certain types of catheters.
5. Avoid advancing the Wick catheter past the needle bevel as it cannot be withdrawn without risk of damaging the catheter.
6. Position stopcocks correctly to obtain correct measurements and avoid equipment damage, particularly to the transducer.
7. Dispose of all intracompartmental catheters following use.

Related Care

1. Read and observe the setup and instruction procedures included with the compartment-monitoring catheters and related equipment.
2. Check the response of the system periodically. If the response is unsatisfactory, the catheter should be flushed with 0.1 ml. normal saline. If the response remains unsatisfactory, the catheter should be removed.
3. Check to see that the wick of the Wick catheter is removed when the catheter is removed. If the wick detaches from the catheter, remaining in the tissue, remove it by pulling the monofilament safety line attached to the wick.
4. Remove the catheter after 48 hours to reduce the risk of infection.

5. Obtain blood and urine samples for myoglobin levels, usually during the first 24 hours after injury.
6. Assess the patient frequently for sensory and motor function, the presence of distal pulses, and tenseness of the involved compartment.
7. Notify the physician of pressure increases or clinical signs and symptoms of compartment syndrome. Decompression procedures are usually initiated for intracompartmental pressure above 30 mm. Hg.

Complications

Infection
Equipment malfunctions
User error

Suppliers

Howmedica, Inc. (Slit catheter)
Sorenson Research Company, Inc. (Wick catheter—Myocath)

REFERENCES

Crossland, S. and Deyerle, W.: Compartmental syndrome. Nursing 80, *10*:51–53 (Dec.), 1980.
Gelberman, R.H., et al.: Compartment syndromes of the forearm: Diagnosis and treatment. Clin. Orthop., *161*:252–261, 1981.
Koman, L.A., et al.: Wick catheter in evaluating and treating compartment syndromes. South. Med. J., *73*:303–309, 1981.
Kuska, B.M.: Acute onset of compartment syndrome. J. Emerg. Nurs., *8*:75–79 (March/April), 1982.
Matsen, F.A.: Compartmental syndromes. Hosp. Prac., *15*:113–117 (Feb.), 1980.
Mubarek, S.J., et al.: Acute compartment syndrome: Diagnosis and treatment with the aid of the Wick catheter. J. Bone Joint Surg., *62*:1091–1095 (Dec.), 1978.
Saffle, J.R., et al.: Intramuscular pressure in the burned arm: Measurement and response to escharotomy. Am J. Surg., *140*:825–831, 1980.

9

NUTRITIONAL
SUPPORT

TOTAL PARENTERAL NUTRITION

Rita Colley, R.N., B.A.

Overview

Administration of total nutrition by vein has evolved into a specialty with its own nomenclature—total parenteral nutrition (TPN), hyperalimentation, or intravenous hyperalimentation (IVH). The object of TPN is to provide sufficient nutrients by vein to achieve anabolism and to promote weight gain, when necessary.

The solutions are made with hypertonic glucose, amino acids, electrolytes, minerals, vitamins, and trace elements. Intravenous lipid emulsions are also needed to prevent essential fatty acid deficiency or supply calories or both. (IV lipids are administered separately; see "Lipid Therapy—Administration of Intravenous Lipids.")

Indications for TPN are varied and include inflammatory bowel disease, draining fistulas, hypermetabolic demands, often from major trauma, inadequate gastrointestinal (GI) tract as a consequence of malabsorption, and short-bowel syndrome. TPN is also used as adjunctive therapy with some cancer treatments. The common factor that should always be present in a patient before this therapy is instituted is the inability of the GI tract to function in a manner that allows achievement of anabolism. This point is made because the therapy is not without risk, and use of the GI tract (for feeding) is easier, safer, and more economical.

The solutions must be prepared in the pharmacy under a laminar airflow (LAF) unit. Using a closed transfer method and in-line filtration during admixture, the pharmacist is able to provide the highest degree of quality control. Extreme preoccupation with asepsis is necessary, because sepsis is the most dreaded complication of TPN therapy; yet, it may almost always be avoided when proper technique is used in every aspect of the therapy.

The solutions should be refrigerated until use; ordinarily they should be used within 24 hours of preparation time. The expiration date and time should be placed on the solution container label, along with all other necessary identifying information.

Although it is desirable to have total admixture done in the pharmacy under a LAF unit, some institutions find it necessary to add to the solutions after they have been obtained from the pharmacy. It is prudent to delegate this responsibility only to a qualified IV nurse therapist. Admixture would then be done by the IV nurse therapist in a specifically designated place in the clinical area. Compatibility of any additive with the basic TPN mixture should be authorized by the pharmacy department. Integrity of the solution container must always be preserved, during and after placement of additional additives.

INSERTION OF A SUBCLAVIAN TOTAL PARENTERAL NUTRITION CATHETER (ASSISTING WITH) _____

Overview

The usual intracatheter for TPN infusion is 8 to 12 inches long and is made of polyurethane, polyvinylchloride (PVC), or siliconized rubber. There are many brands available, and choice is dependent upon the physician and institutional availability. The advantages of siliconized rubber over PVC intracatheters have been reported. Many physicians now theorize that this less reactive catheter will not irritate the vein wall as easily as PVC catheters seem to do. It has also been reported that siliconized rubber catheters have far less fibrin sheath formation on them; theoretically this reduces the possibility of bacterial seeding upon the catheter. Because siliconized rubber is more flexible than PVC, it must be secured to the skin with great care to avoid kinking of the catheter.

Placement of a catheter for infusion of TPN solution is a sterile procedure, usually performed in the patient's room. Before infusion begins, the patient should be clean, with all wound dressings freshly changed to decrease the chance of contamination. The patient's blood volume should be or have been restored to normal so that adequate venous pressure exists. This prevents the physician from attempting to puncture the collapsed vein of a dehydrated hypovolemic patient. Clotting factors should also be normalized to avoid prolonged bleeding during or after placement.

Objective

To monitor and support the patient during insertion of a TPN catheter, assisting at crucial moments.

Special Equipment

This consists of a sterile catheter placement kit, containing:
Four sterile drapes
Three towel clips
Ten sterile gauze pads

Two 3-ml. syringes
One silk suture with atraumatic straight needle
Two hemostats
One pair scissors
One 10-ml. vial 1% lidocaine
Povidone-iodine ointment
One subclavian intracatheter
One gown
Two pairs sterile gloves
Two masks
One bottle acetone ⎫
One bottle 1% tincture of iodine ⎬ new, unopened bottles
One bottle 70% isopropyl alcohol ⎭
One can tincture of benzoin
One 6-inch × 8-inch sterile adhesive-backed drape
One roll 1-inch plastic nonallergenic tape
One 500-ml. bottle 5% dextrose in water for IV infusion
One adult drip IV tubing
One towel (to be used as a towel roll)

Procedure

ACTION	RATIONALE
1. Wash hands with surgical scrub solution and rinse.	
2. Prepare site for catheter insertion by washing and shaving area of catheter insertion. It is preferable to shave the area the night before catheter insertion in case surface abrasions occur in the skin.	2. This is done to eliminate pain during adhesive removal at future dressing changes, as well as to facilitate aseptic technique.
3. Place catheter insertion implements on clean, alcohol-scrubbed bedside table. Prime IV tubing and prepare flow control device if one is being used.	
4. Place patient in supine position with towel roll (12-inches long and 3-inches in diameter) along thoracic vertebrae (Fig. 9–1).	4. The towel roll elevates the clavicle, facilitating location of the subclavian vein and separating it from the apex of the lung.

ACTION   RATIONALE

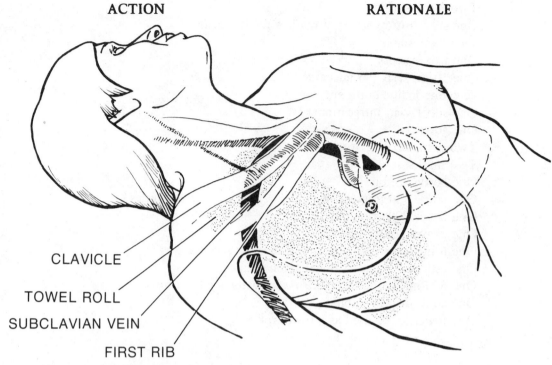

CLAVICLE

TOWEL ROLL

SUBCLAVIAN VEIN

FIRST RIB

Figure 9-1 Positioning of patient for subclavian catheter insertion.

5. Place bed in Trendelenburg position at approximately 45 degrees. If the patient has difficulty tolerating this position, do not implement it until the procedure actually begins.

5. This position aids in filling the subclavian veins.

6. Instruct patient to turn head away from insertion site.

7. Mask all persons in immediate area, except patient. (Gowning and gloving is required for the person performing the invasive procedure.)

7. The patient's face will be draped and does not require a mask.

8. Assist in surgical preparation of skin and surgical draping.
    A. Prep is similar to dressing change scrub: acetone, iodine, and alcohol.
    B. Do not cover eyes or nose with drape.

    B. This panics some patients.

9. Ensure patient comfort.
    A. Explain that area will sting as it is infiltrated with local anesthetic (similar to a bee sting), that the stinging will subside, and that medication will be given time to take effect.

ACTION	RATIONALE
B. Hold patient's hand— enormous comfort and security are usually provided by this simple gesture. C. Make sure anesthetic is given time to take effect.	
10. Inform patient that there will be a feeling of pressure as catheter needle penetrates skin.	10. This should not be extremely painful or anxiety provoking if the patient is prepared.
11. Instruct patient to perform Valsalva maneuver after venous blood has been aspirated into syringe and before syringe is disconnected to allow catheter introduction. A. Compress abdomen if patient is unable to perform Valsalva maneuver. B. Effect Valsalva maneuver in intubated patient by maintaining inspiratory phase of Ambu bag (effective approximately 3 to 5 seconds after inspiration is initiated).	11. The Valsalva maneuver must be maintained until the intracatheter is threaded to the needle hub, occluding it. Failure to do this invites air embolism. Remember to tell the patient when it is all right to breathe again!
12. Encourage a single suture at insertion site and placement of catheter straight down on chest as intracatheter is sutured (Fig. 9–2).	12. This allows cleaning of the catheter beneath it (during dressing changes) and prevents kinking.

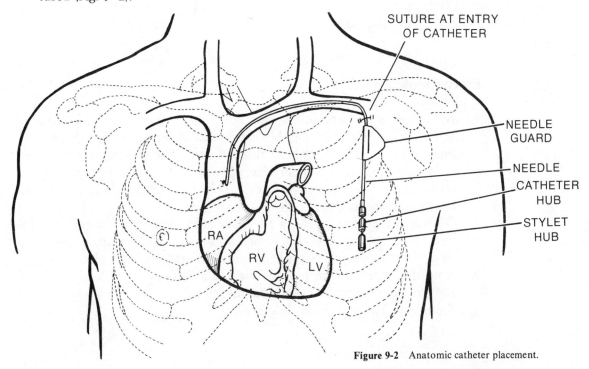

SUTURE AT ENTRY OF CATHETER

NEEDLE GUARD

NEEDLE
CATHETER HUB

STYLET HUB

RA

RV   LV

Figure 9-2   Anatomic catheter placement.

ACTION	RATIONALE
13. Instruct patient to perform Valsalva maneuver as catheter hub plug is removed and isotonic IV infusion is hooked up. A. Set rate at 20 cc/hour. B. Maintain this rate until catheter tip location is verified by x-ray.	13. This is done so that the catheter is not open to the air unnecessarily.
14. Lower IV bottle below heart level to observe venous backflow of blood into tubing.	14. This helps to verify venous placement of the catheter; it is also the reason a filter has not yet been connected— it could clog with venous blood.
15. Bring patient out of Trendelenburg position.	
16. Remove surgical drapes and towel roll.	
17. Apply dressing (see "Total Parenteral Nutrition Subclavian Catheter Site Care").	
18. Prepare patient for chest x-ray.	
19. Initiate the first bottle of TPN upon verification of catheter tip location by x-ray (Fig. 9–2). Correct catheter tip location is the mid-superior vena cava or the innominate vein. The right atrium is the only acceptable location for soft flexible cannulas, and only when authorized by hospital policy.	

Precautions

1. *Never* use the catheter for anything other than TPN—e.g., central venous pressure monitoring, blood withdrawal, bolus or piggy back infusions should not be permitted through the TPN catheter. It is an inviolate system. However, in emergency situations the TPN catheter is often used for central venous access. The catheter should not be reused for TPN in these cases.
2. Observe the patient carefully for signs and symptoms of respiratory distress (e.g., dyspnea, decreased breath sounds, chest pain, cyanosis or shock) and a slowly growing hematoma following catheter placement.
3. Note that some cardiac patients may be asked only to hold their breath and not to perform the Valsalva maneuver to avoid precipitating dysrhythmia. This is a medical decision.

Related Care

1. Clean the tracheostomy wound of tracheostomy patients prior to catheter insertion and cover with povidone-iodine sponges as part of the surgical preparation. A sterile, adhesive, waterproof plastic drape or transparent semipermeable membrane dressing should be placed between the tracheostomy tube and the insertion area as an additional barrier. The catheter insertion site should be located as far away from the tracheostomy as possible.

2. Place the catheter on the side with a thoracostomy tube, if applicable, because the tube often prevents pleural space complications during catheterization.

3. Place the catheter on the side opposite the planned surgical incision if patients are preoperative for head, neck, or thoracic surgery.

4. Monitor TPN solution administration; a flow control device should be used — preferably a pump.

5. Maintain catheter asepsis. The patient should have routine temperatures taken frequently, and any elevation should be reported. There seems to be no single febrile pattern associated with TPN sepsis; it can be manifested by a low-grade temperature, either constant or intermittent, by daily temperature spikes, or by a dramatic elevation accompanied by clinical signs of septicemia. Glucose intolerance is often an early warning of catheter related sepsis in the TPN patient. If this develops suddenly for an unexplained reason, catheter sepsis should be suspected. If a TPN patient has a single dramatic temperature spike the total IV system (down to the catheter hub) should be removed and cultured, including the solution from the solution container and from the IV tubing, both proximal and distal to the filter, if one is used. Any TPN patient with a fever should have a complete history and physical examination, and thorough culturing, followed by serologic diagnostic monitoring. If the fever remains inexplicable, the catheter should be removed and cultured (see "Culturing a Total Parenteral Nutrition Subclavian Venous Catheter"). If blood cultures are positive and recurrent, or if the patient is in septic shock, the catheter should also be removed.

6. Note that a commercially available prepackaged catheter placement kit may be substituted for the equipment described.

7. Note that a different procedure, involving placement of the catheter over a guidewire, may be done. The basic procedure varies little, but care is taken to use a soft, flexible, atraumatic wire to avoid vein wall trauma or perforation.

Complications

Sepsis	Lymphatic leak
Pneumothorax	Air embolism
Hemothorax	Catheter embolism

Hydrothorax
Extravasation
Nerve damage

Myocardial irritability
Myocardial perforation
Thrombosis

REFERENCE

Grant, J.P.: Subclavian catheter insertion and complications. *In* Grant, J.P. (ed.): Handbook of Total Parenteral Nurtition, Philadelphia, W.B. Saunders, 1980, pp. 47–69.

MONITORING DAILY INFUSION OF TOTAL PARENTERAL NUTRITION THERAPY

Objectives

1. To provide nutrients by vein to achieve anabolism and promote weight gain.
2. To deliver TPN in a manner that avoids untoward metabolic complications.

Procedure

ACTION	RATIONALE
1. Begin initial infusion at a slow rate (approximately 60 to 80 ml./hour).	1. This allows pancreatic insulin production to increase and helps to avoid glucose intolerance.
2. Increase infusion in slow increments (approximately 25 ml./hour/day).	2. This also allows pancreatic insulin production to increase and helps to avoid glucose intolerance.
3. Time-tape the TPN solution container; infuse via flow-control device (preferably a pump), and frequently check accuracy of volume delivered.	3. This prevents fluid overload and glucose overdose.
4. Weigh patient daily, at same time with same clothing.	
5. Keep accurate record of intake and output.	5. Calorie count and fluid balance are calculations necessary to determine correct prescription of TPN solution and additional fluids, if needed.

ACTION	RATIONALE
6. Measure urinary sugar and acetone levels every 6 hours.	6. This indicates glucose tolerance.
A. If sugar is 2+ or greater report glycosuria.	A. This requires serum glucose measurement and treatment.
B. Use Tes-tape if patient is receiving cephalosporins, large doses of aspirin, or vitamin C.	B. Clinitest tablets may yield a false positive result.
7. Decrease infusion in slow increments—i.e., "wean" the solution.	7. This helps to prevent hypoglycemic shock by allowing serum insulin level to naturally decline.

Precautions

1. Be alert for the signs and symptoms of hypoglycemia, hyperglycemia, hyperosmolar coma, electrolyte imbalance, dehydration, and deficiency states of vitamins, essential fatty acids, and trace elements.
2. Monitor serum laboratory values closely and frequently. When the patient's condition is stabilized, the frequency of intervals will decrease.

Complication

Altered fluid administration

REFERENCES

Colley, R.: Total parenteral nutrition in 1981. *In* Wesdorp, R.I.C., and Soeters, P.B. (eds.): Clinical Nutrition '81, New York, Churchill Livingstone, 1982, pp. 331–338.

Kennedy, G.: Monitoring the parenteral nutrition patient. *In* Jeejeebhoy, K.N. (ed.): Total Parenteral Nutrition in the Hospital and at Home. Boca Raton, CRC Press, 1983, pp. 57–60.

TOTAL PARENTERAL NUTRITION SUBCLAVIAN CATHETER SITE CARE _____

Overview

The subclavian catheter dressing should be changed every 48 hours or three times a week on Monday, Wednesday, and Friday. The actual prepping of the skin should be done with gentle but abrasive action to ensure removal of all debris and adhesive residue. The entire catheter should also be cleansed. This involves some motion of the catheter so that the underside (including the needle guard and needle, when present) is thoroughly cleansed. Because many TPN patients are malnourished, their skin is particularly sensitive and therefore solutions, dressing materials, and tapes should be selected appropriately.

The dressing should always be maintained so that it is aseptic, dry, and air occlusive. If the dressing becomes loose or wet it should be considered contaminated and changed immediately.

Objectives

1. To keep the catheter stable, secure, free of debris, and aseptic, thereby minimizing the potential for mechanical and septic complications.
2. To preserve skin integrity at the insertion site.

Special Equipment

This consists of the sterile subclavian dressing change kit, containing:
Three aluminum cups
One disposable clamp
Scissors
Ten sterile gauze pads
Povidone-iodine ointment
Two pairs sterile gloves
One 6-inch × 8-inch adhesive-backed sterile drape
One bottle acetone ⎫
One bottle 1% tincture of iodine ⎬ new, unopened bottles
One bottle 70% isopropyl alcohol ⎭
One can tincture of benzoin aerosol
One new roll 1-inch adhesive tape

Procedure

ACTION	RATIONALE
1. Wash hands with surgical scrub solution and rinse.	
2. Mask all persons in immediate area. Do not mask patient if this causes respiratory difficulty; instead, have patient turn head away from catheter site.	2. This protects the catheter from nasopharyngeal organisms. The mask also protects the patient from the disturbing odors of some of the prep solutions and the benzoin.

ACTION	RATIONALE
3. Place patient in supine or semi-Fowler's position and remove pillow(s).	
4. Clear off bedside table, cleanse with isopropyl alcohol, and allow it to dry thoroughly.	4. This promotes asepsis.
5. Wash hands again with surgical scrub solution and rinse.	
6. Prepare subclavian dressing change kit (Fig. 9–3) in a sterile fashion; fill three cups with acetone, iodine, and alcohol.	

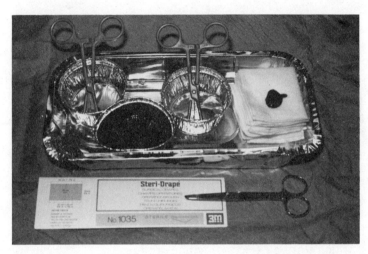

Figure 9-3 Subclavian dressing change kit.

ACTION	RATIONALE
7. Squeeze povidone-iodine ointment onto double-thickness gauze pad.	
8. Remove old dressing. A. Stabilize catheter to avoid dislodging it.	
B. Pull skin away from tape (rather than tape away from skin).	B. There is less trauma.
C. If gauze sponges do not adhere to dressing over insertion sites (therefore coming off with it) put on sterile gloves, remove sponges, and then change gloves.	
9. Don sterile gloves; trim gauze with ointment to a 2-inch × 2-inch size; place this outside aluminum cups but well within borders of sterile field.	9. This keeps the ointment and sponges away from solutions and therefore dry.

ACTION	RATIONALE
10. Observe catheter insertion site for erythema, edema, drainage, or crusting. Culture and report to physician, if appropriate.	
11. Defat catheter insertion site and surrounding skin. A. Use an acetone-prepared gauze pad. B. Always begin at insertion site and prep in wider-to-wider concentric circles. C. Prep only out to border of dressing. The necessary number of gauze sponges varies and is determined by their being clean after prepping. D. Avoid acetone prep of catheter if manufacturer warns against this.	11. Defatting removes debris that could harbor organisms and clears the surface for the iodine. B. This is the "clean-to-dirty method." D. Acetone may degrade some catheters.
12. Prep skin with iodine solution in same manner as above. A. Use a 2-minute scrub. B. Allow iodine to air dry. C. Concentrate half the time on the insertion site.	12. Iodine is antibacterial and antifungal.
13. Prep skin with isopropyl alcohol solution until all traces of iodine are removed; allow alcohol to evaporate fully.	13. Iodine left on the skin may burn it. Traces of wet alcohol may combine with the povidone-iodine ointment and burn the skin.
14. Apply povidone-iodine ointment on double-thickness gauze to catheter insertion site.	
15. Remove sterile gloves.	
16. Spray surrounding skin with tincture of benzoin; allow benzoin to dry until sticky.	16. Wet benzoin can cause poor adhesion of dressing and skin irritation.
17. Cover catheter with sterile, adhesive-backed drape. A. Place drape halfway down catheter hub to create approximately a 1-inch border around gauze.	17. This placement at the catheter hub allows access to it later for IV tubing change.

ACTION	RATIONALE
B. Make sure the patient's arm is abducted so that dressing will not bind.	B. If dressing binds it could prevent range of motion.
C. Do not touch adhesive back of drape.	C. This will contaminate it.

18. Apply tape to lateral and upper edge of drape.

19. Make a ½-inch slit in tape to be applied to lower border of drape; place this slit piece of tape up under catheter hub and then seal lower border.

    19. This insures occlusion at the catheter hub.

20. Place a piece of tape along lower border, over (and halfway down) catheter hub (Fig. 9–4).

    20. This helps to stabilize the catheter hub.

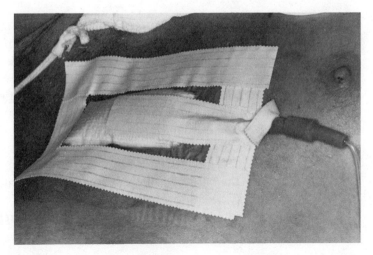

Figure 9-4 Subclavian dressing.

21. Secure all IV tubing and catheter hub junctions with tape.

    21. This prevents accidental tubing separation.

22. Anchor filter (or IV tubing if a filter is not used) to drape on patient's skin.

    22. This prevents catheter dislodgment by focusing inadvertent tension here rather than on the insertion site.

23. Label dressing with date and initials. Write on the basic dressing and not on the anchoring tape, which may be removed.

Precautions

1. Substitute alcohol as a defatting agent if the patient or catheter is sensitive to acetone.

2. Use povidone-iodine solution if the patient is sensitive to iodine. If

povidone-iodone is nonirritating (this is almost always the case) leave it on the skin—i.e., do not remove it with alcohol. Povidone-iodine solution is long lasting and effective even after drying. Also, its removal by alcohol could create a strong tincture of iodine, which is very irritating to the skin.

3. Substitute one of the adhesive sprays used in ileostomy care (e.g., Hollister adhesive) if tincture of benzoin irritates the skin.

4. Substitute a sterile, cloth, adhesive-backed tape or try a transparent semipermeable membrane dressing if the sterile plastic, adhesive-backed drape irritates the skin. A transparent semipermeable membrane dressing is also waterproof, but it allows moisture vapor beneath it to escape while still affording sterile protection from the environment. If a transparent semipermeable membrane dressing is used, do not surround the upper and lateral edges of the dressing with tape—i.e., only the bottom edge should have tape on it.

Related Care

1. Protect the basic dressing with additional tape if the type of tape used to secure the IV tubing–catheter hub junction and to anchor the filter (or tubing) to the dressing tears the dressing (likely with the plastic drape or the transparent semipermeable membrane dressing).

2. Waterproof a cloth dressing (Fig. 9–5) for patients:
   A. With tracheostomy or with draining wounds.
   B. In high humidity areas.
   C. With oxygen apparatus that beads moisture.
   D. With nasogastric tubes.

3. Note that use of a prepackaged, commercially available dressing change kit may be substituted in this procedure.

4. Substitute a liquid benzoin or other skin prep if the aerosol bothers the patient.

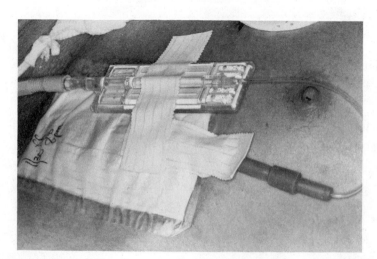

Figure 9-5 Waterproofed cloth dressing.

5. The frequency of dressing change may be other than specified, depending on hospital policy.

Complication

Sepsis (if dressing not maintained properly)

REFERENCES

Colley, R.: Total parenteral nutrition—nursing approach. *In* Plumer, A.L.: Principles in Practice of I.V. Therapy, 2nd ed. Boston, Little, Brown, 1975, pp. 185–213.
Ryan, J.A., Abel, R.M., Abbott, W.M., Hopkins, C.C., Chesney, T.M., Colley, R., Phillips, K., and Fischer, J.E.: Catheter complications in total parenteral nutrition. A prospective study of 200 patients. N. Engl. J. Med., *290*:757–761, 1974.

TOTAL PARENTERAL NUTRITION SUBCLAVIAN CATHETER INTRAVENOUS TUBING AND FILTER CHANGE

Overview

IV tubing for TPN is changed every 24 hours. This is a reasonable standard of care and follows the recommendations of the Centers for Disease Control in Atlanta. More frequent tubing changes should be unnecessary and may even increase the risk of bacterial contamination because they involve multiple daily manipulations of the catheter hub–IV tubing junction. It is crucial that the actual procedure be done aseptically and that air embolism precautions be taken.

Tubing and filter change should be timed to coincide with the change of the IV solution container. This minimizes the number of times the closed system is manipulated. If a filter is used, the choice should be determined by patient and institutional need. The best selection of a filter would be one that is of 0.2-micron porosity and is air eliminating. A 0.2-micron filter will trap both particulate matter and all bacterial and fungal organisms. These filters also have the capacity to eliminate air and to maintain a normal gravity flow rate for 24 hours, even with hypertonic solutions.

This procedure is written for positive pressure infusion. Make sure that the pounds per square inch pressure tolerance of the filter is not exceeded by the infusion pump.

Objectives

1. To change the IV tubing and final filter in an aseptic, efficient manner.
2. To minimize the potential risk for microemboli.

Special Equipment

TPN infusion container
IV tubing
0.2-micron filter
Aseptic hemostat
Sterile needle
Aseptic tape

Procedure

ACTION	RATIONALE
1. Wash hands with surgical scrub solution and rinse.	
2. Make sure TPN solution is as prescribed by physician; check expiration date of solution.	
3. Inspect solution against a strong light for cloudiness, turbidity, or particulate matter; also inspect solution container for cracks (in a bottle) or minute punctures (in a bag).	3. This could indicate solution contamination, in which case its use is contraindicated.
4. Be certain that solution container is waterproof and airtight.	4. This guarantees asepsis.
5. Remove protective covering from IV solution container.	
6. Clamp off IV tubing.	
7. Remove protective covering from IV tubing.	
8. Spike IV solution container.	
9. Invert solution container, fill drip chamber, and prime IV tubing; purge tubing of all air, including air usually trapped in side-arm injection sites.	

ACTION	RATIONALE
10. Insert IV tubing into filter housing and prime filter. Follow manufacturer's specific instructions for priming a filter; all filters differ slightly.	10. Correct filling of the filter is essential to its proper operation.
11. Shut off IV solution and cover end of filter tubing with a sterile needle; label IV tubing drip chamber and filter housing with date.	11. Dating the tubing and filter helps insure that they will be changed on time.
12. Place a tape marked in hourly increments on new TPN solution container. It should be checked every 30 minutes.	12. The time-tape allows for easy visualization of flow accuracy.
13. Place patient in supine position.	13. This helps to prevent air embolism.
14. Remove tape anchoring filter to the dressing and tape securing catheter hub–filter tubing junction; stabilize dressing with one hand.	14. This guards against catheter dislodgment.
15. Turn off patient's TPN infusion pump.	
16. Remove used tubing from infusion pump and establish gravity flow.	
17. Quickly insert new tubing into infusion pump and reprogram as necessary.	
18. Instruct patient to perform Valsalva maneuver before used filter tubing is removed from catheter hub.	
19. Turn off TPN infusion.	
20. Replace used filter tubing with new filter tubing while patient performs Valsalva maneuver. A. Grasp catheter hub with clean hemostat. B. Lift hub slightly up off chest wall. C. Rotate old filter tubing out gently and twist new tubing in.	20. Successful performance of the Valsalva maneuver creates a positive venous pressure that may cause backflow of blood through the catheter. B. Lifting the hub off the chest avoids contamination. C. Most catheter junctions have a Luer slip fit that requires this. If a Luer-Lok junction is used, secure the lock.

ACTION	RATIONALE
21. Turn TPN infusion on; instruct patient to breathe normally again.	
22. Tape all tubing junctions and tubing-hub junction.	22. This provides additional protection against accidental tubing separation.

Precautions

1. Integrate air embolism precautions into the procedure.
2. Integrate aseptic technique into the procedure.
3. Note that to avoid precipitation of dysrhythmias, some cardiac patients may be asked only to hold their breath and not to perform the Valsalva maneuver. This is a medical decision.

Related Care

Option: Paint all IV tubing junctions with an antimicrobial solution before disconnecting them. Although this has not been required in the above procedure, it may be a desirable addition in some cases.

Complications

Sepsis
Emboli

REFERENCES

Colley, R., and Wilson, J.: Hyperalimentation: A plus for nitrogen balance. *In* Hamilton, H. (ed.): Monitoring Fluid and Electrolytes Precisely. Horsham, PA, Intermed Communications, 1978, pp. 183–188.

REMOVAL OF A SUBCLAVIAN TOTAL PARENTERAL NUTRITION CATHETER

Overview

Removal of a subclavian catheter is a routine nursing procedure in some institutions; in others, this practice is restricted to a physician. This procedure is written for those nurses who are authorized to remove subclavian catheters.

Objectives

1. To remove the subclavian catheter in a safe, aseptic manner.
2. To assess skin integrity at site, post-TPN catheter removal.

Special Equipment

Sterile gauze pads
Povidone-iodine ointment
Isopropyl alcohol
Plastic tape (new clean roll)
Sterile scissors

Sterile forceps
Sterile gloves
Sterile hemostat
Sterile towel
Sterile bowl

Procedure

ACTION	RATIONALE
1. Review patient's record for catheter placement note; check for description of internal venous cutdown or subcutaneous tunnel exit.	1. If either condition exists, the nurse should not remove the catheter.
2. Shut off intravenous infusion.	
3. Wash hands with surgical scrub solution and rinse.	
4. Open sterile towel to create sterile field and place sterile equipment on it.	
5. Fill sterile bowl with alcohol.	
6. Squeeze povidone-iodine ointment onto sterile sponge.	
7. Place patient in a supine position without a pillow.	7. This helps to prevent air embolism.
8. Expose catheter insertion site.	
9. Don sterile gloves.	
10. Prep catheter insertion site and surrounding skin with alcohol; allow alcohol to dry. Prep in same manner as described in "Total Parenteral Nutrition Subclavian Catheter Site Care."	

ACTION	RATIONALE
11. Remove suture at insertion site, using scissors and forceps. If suture is difficult to cut, a pediatric suture set may be easier to use.	
12. Remove catheter. A. Grasp catheter at distal end with sterile forceps and *withdraw slowly*. B. Have patient perform Valsalva maneuver as catheter is withdrawn. C. Do not force catheter removal: if it is difficult to remove: (1) Stop. (2) Tape catheter in place. (3) Notify physician immediately.	
13. After catheter is removed: A. Apply povidone-iodine to insertion site *immediately* while sterile forceps hold catheter. B. Observe catheter for correct length and normal tip.	A. Occlusion of this site maintains asepsis and prevents air embolism if tract formation exists. B. Expected catheter length varies according to catheter inserted, and should have been noted in the patient's record at the time of catheter insertion.
14. Apply dressing. A. Secure dressing with plastic tape. B. Layer tape to make a totally occlusive seal.	
15. Observe dressing for active bleeding, hematoma formation, or edema. If bleeding occurs: A. Apply direct pressure. B. Notify physician immediately.	
16. Label dressing with date and time applied and with notice to leave it on, occlusive, for 72 hours.	
17. Record length of removed catheter in patient's record.	
18. Activate nursing care plan to reassess insertion site in 72 hours. It should be closed; if not, apply a new occlusive dressing immediately.	

Precautions

1. Integrate air embolism precautions into the procedure.
2. Initiate suspected catheter embolism precautions immediately if a portion is missing from the removed catheter: Place patient in left lateral Trendelenburg position and notify physician.
3. Note that to avoid precipitation of dysrhythmias, some cardiac patients may be asked only to hold their breath and not to perform the Valsalva maneuver. This is a medical decision.

Related Care

Culture the catheter if sepsis is suspected. See "Culturing a Total Parenteral Nutrition Subclavian Venous Catheter."

Complications

Catheter embolism
Exudate or fibrin sheath on internal portion of
    catheter (indicating possibility of infection).

CULTURING A TOTAL PARENTERAL NUTRITION SUBCLAVIAN VENOUS CATHETER _____

Objective

To culture the catheter tip in the most effective manner when catheter-related sepsis is suspected.

Special Equipment

See equipment list for "Removal of a Subclavian
    Total Parenteral Nutrition Catheter," plus:
        Sterile culture tube
        Sterile scissors
        Sterile wound culture tube

Procedure

ACTION	RATIONALE
1. Follow procedure for "Removal of a Subclavian Total Parenteral Nutrition Catheter," steps 1 through 12.	
2. After catheter has been withdrawn and is still being kept up and away from skin, proceed with following steps.	

NOTE:

The following steps must be done **swiftly** *as the patient continues to perform the Valsalva maneuver. Failure to maintain this maneuver increases the danger of air embolism. Concern with this persists until the occlusive dressing is covering the catheter exit site.*

3. Milk wound, attempting to express pus, after catheter removal.	3. Pus could indicate suppurative thrombophlebitis—a very serious complication requiring immediate physician diagnosis and treatment.
4. Culture any pus expressed, using sterile wound culture tube.	
5. Note any redness, edema, warmth, or palpable hardness at or near wound.	5. This could indicate phlebitis, thrombosis, or sepsis.
6. Apply povidone-iodine ointment gauze to insertion site immediately while holding catheter with sterile forceps.	6. Occlusion of this site maintains asepsis and prevents air embolism if tract formation exists.
7. Observe catheter for correct length and normal tip.	7. Expected catheter length varies according to catheter inserted, and should have been noted in the patient's record at the time of catheter insertion.
8. Culture catheter tip.	
A. Take second pair of sterile scissors and cut catheter several millimeters inside former skin surface portion.	
B. Drop catheter tip segment into sterile culture tube and re-cover tube.	
9. Apply dressing.	
A. Secure dressing with plastic tape.	
B. Layer tape to make a totally occlusive seal.	

ACTION	RATIONALE
10. Observe dressing for active bleeding, hematoma formation, or edema. If bleeding occurs: A. Apply direct pressure. B. Notify physician immediately.	
11. Label dressing with date and time applied and with notice to leave it on, occlusive, for 72 hours.	
12. Record length of removed catheter in patient's record.	
13. Activate nursing care plan to reassess insertion site in 72 hours. It should be closed; if not, apply a new occlusive dressing immediately.	
14. Hand-carry catheter culture to laboratory immediately after dressing application.	14. This prevents the specimen from drying out.
15. Request that the laboratory perform a semiquantitative culture.	15. This method involves the use of a sheep blood agar plate (see Maki references, below).

Precautions

1. Integrate air embolism precautions into the procedure.
2. Initiate suspected catheter embolism precautions immediately if a portion is missing from the removed catheter: Place patient in left lateral Trendelenburg position and notify physician.
3. Note that to avoid precipitation of dysrhythmias, some cardiac patients may be asked only to hold their breath and not to perform the Valsalva maneuver. This is a medical decision.

Related Care

1. Complete fever work-up to determine its cause.
2. Culture additional segment of catheter (skin interface segment), if ordered. This requires additional sterile scissors to avoid cross-contamination.

Complications

Catheter embolism
Exudate or fibrin sheath on internal portion of catheter (indicating possibility of infection.)

REFERENCES

Maki, D.G., Jarrett, F., and Sarafin, H.W.: A semiquantitative culture method for identification of catheter-related-infection in the burn patient. J. Surg. Res., *22*:513–520, 1977.

Maki, D.G., Weise, C.E., and Sarafin, H.W.: A semiquantitative culture method for identifying intravenous-catheter-related infection. N. Engl. J. Med., *296*:1305–1309, 1977.

TOTAL PARENTERAL NUTRITION HICKMAN CATHETER SITE CARE

Overview

The last few years have seen a marked increase in the use of long (approximately 90 cm.) silicone catheters that are generically referred to as "right atrial catheters". The catheters most frequently used are the Hickman and Broviac brands. The two catheters are similar but have different internal diameters and capacities. The Broviac catheter has an internal lumen of 1.0 mm. and a volume of approximately 1.0 ml.; the Hickman catheter has an internal lumen of 1.6 mm. and a volume of approximately 2.0 ml. The catheter is trimmed to the desirable length prior to placement. Placement of the catheter is done in the operating room, either by surgical cutdown or percutaneously. The cephalic or jugular vein is catheterized, and the silicone catheter is advanced via a long subcutaneous tunnel into the superior vena cava or the right atrium (Fig. 9–6). A Dacron mesh cuff surrounds the catheter in the subcutaneous exit tunnel approximately 30 cm. from the

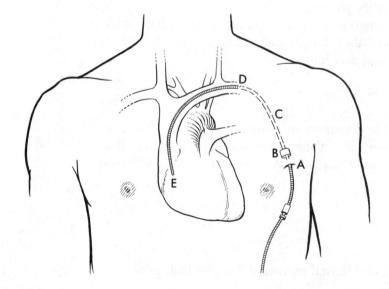

Figure 9-6 Hickman catheter. Silicone rubber catheter tunneled subcutaneously and positioned in right atrium. *A*, incision site; *B*, Dacron cuff; *C*, subcutaneous tunnel; *D*, insertion into subclavian vein; *E*, right atrium.

catheter hub. Eventual fibrous tissue infiltration of this cuff is thought to stabilize the catheter. The long subcutaneous exit is thought to minimize infection of the intravascular system by locating the distal portion of the catheter far from the venous entrance. These catheters were originally designed for home total parenteral nutrition patients but are being used increasingly for patients who require long-term venous access in multiple therapies. The following content focuses on the Hickman catheter.

Objectives

1. To keep the catheter stable, secure, free of debris, and aseptic, thereby minimizing the potential for mechanical and septic complications.
2. To preserve skin integrity at the insertion site.

Special Equipment

This consists of the sterile Hickman dressing change kit containing:
 Two aluminum cups
 One disposable clamp
 Scissors
 Eight sterile gauze pads
 Povidone-iodine ointment
 Two pairs sterile gloves
 One 4-inch × 4-inch adhesive-backed sterile drape
 One bottle povidone-iodine solution ⎫ new unopened bottles
 One bottle 70% isopropyl alcohol ⎭
 One can tincture of benzoin aerosol
 One new roll 1-inch tape

Procedure

ACTION	RATIONALE
1. Wash hands with surgical scrub solution and rinse.	
2. Mask all persons in immediate area. Do not mask patient if this causes respiratory difficulty; instead, have patient turn head away from catheter site.	2. This protects the catheter from nasopharyngeal organisms. The mask also protects the patient from the disturbing odors of some of the prep solutions and the benzoin.
3. Clear off bedside table, cleanse with isopropyl alcohol, and allow it to dry thoroughly.	3. This promotes asepsis.

ACTION	RATIONALE
4. Wash hands again with surgical scrub solution and rinse.	
5. Prepare Hickman dressing change kit in a sterile fashion; fill two cups with isopropyl alcohol and povidone-iodine solution.	
6. Squeeze povidone-iodine ointment onto double-thickness gauze pad.	

7. Remove old dressing.
  A. Stabilize the catheter to avoid dislodging it.
  B. Pull skin away from tape (rather than tape away from skin).
  C. If gauze sponges over insertion site do not adhere to dressing (therefore coming off with it) put on sterile gloves, remove sponges, and then change gloves.
	B. There is less trauma.

8. Don sterile gloves; trim gauze with ointment to a 2-inch × 2-inch size; place this away from aluminum cups but well within borders of sterile field.	8. This keeps the ointment and sponges away from solutions and, therefore, dry.

9. Observe catheter exit site for erythema, edema, drainage, or crusting. Culture and report to physician, if appropriate. Defat catheter insertion site and surrounding skin.
  A. Use an alcohol-prepared gauze pad.
  B. Prep in wider-to-wider concentric circles.
  C. Prep only out to border of dressing. The necessary number of gauze sponges varies and is determined by their being clean after prepping.
	9. Defatting removes debris that could harbor organisms and clears the surface for the iodine.
	
	B. This is the "clean-to-dirty method."

10. Prep skin with povidone-iodine solution in same manner as above.
  A. Use a 2-minute scrub.
  B. Allow povidone-iodine to air dry.
  C. Concentrate half the time on the insertion site.
	10. Povidone-iodine is antibacterial and antifungal.

ACTION	RATIONALE
D. Prep catheter, usually under dressing as well.	
11. Apply povidone-iodine ointment on double-thickness gauze to catheter insertion site.	
12. Remove sterile gloves.	
13. Spray surrounding skin with tincture of benzoin; allow benzoin to dry until sticky.	13. Wet benzoin can cause poor adhesion of dressing and skin irritation.
14. Cover catheter with sterile, plastic, adhesive-backed drape. A. Create approximately a 2-inch border around gauze. B. Do not touch adhesive back of drape.	B. This will contaminate it.
15. Apply tape to lateral and upper edges of drape.	
16. Make a ½-inch slit in tape to be applied to lower border of drape; place this slit piece of tape up under catheter hub and then seal lower border.	16. Slit ensures occlusive seal.
17. Securely anchor external portion of catheter to drape.	17. This prevents catheter dislodgment by focusing inadvertent tension here rather than on the insertion site.

Precautions

1. Avoid the use of acetone or tincture of iodine with the Broviac and Hickman catheters; the manufacturers discourage it.
2. Substitute one of the adhesive sprays used in ileostomy care, e.g., Hollister adhesive, if tincture of benzoin irritates the skin.
3. Substitute a sterile, transparent, waterproof, semipermeable membrane dressing if waterproofing is necessary or if the original dressing irritates the skin.

Related Care

1. Protect the basic dressing with additional tape if the type of tape used to secure the IV tubing–catheter hub junction and to anchor the filter (or

tubing) to the dressing will tear the dressing (likely with transparent dressings).

2. Waterproof a cloth dressing (see Fig. 9–5) with a plastic drape in patients:
   A. With tracheostomy or with draining wounds.
   B. In high-humidity areas.
   C. With oxygen apparatus that beads moisture.
   D. With nasogastric tubes.
3. Use of a prepackaged, commercially available dressing change kit may be substituted in this procedure.
4. Substitute a liquid benzoin or other skin prep if the aerosol bothers the patient.
5. The frequency of dressing change may be other than specified, depending on hospital policy.

Complication

Sepsis

REFERENCES

Duval, A., and Hennessy, K.: Care of the Broviac catheter. N.I.T.A., 6:40–42, 1983.
Wilson, J.: Right atrial catheters (Broviac and Hickman): Indications, insertion, maintenance and protocol for home care. N.I.T.A., 6:23–37, 1983.

TOTAL PARENTERAL NUTRITION
INTRAVENOUS TUBING AND FILTER CHANGE
FOR A HICKMAN CATHETER

Overview

When a Hickman catheter is disconnected from a continuous infusion, backflow of blood in the catheter should be avoided to maintain catheter patency. This is done through a special maneuver that involves clamping the catheter while positive pressure still exists; immediately following this action the positive pressure is discontinued. This procedure is written for a positive pressure infusion; the catheter has a long and flexible portion outside of the body that is easily subject to kinking, and infusion is best maintained via an infusion pump.

Objectives

1. To change the IV tubing and final filter in an aseptic, efficient manner.
2. To minimize the potential risk for microemboli.
3. To minimize backflow of blood into the catheter and subsequent clotting.

Special Equipment

TPN infusion container
IV tubing
0.2-micron filter
Sterile needle
Aseptic tape

Procedure

ACTION	RATIONALE
1. Wash hands with surgical scrub solution and rinse.	
2. Make sure TPN solution is as prescribed by physician; check expiration date of solution.	
3. Inspect solution against a strong light for cloudiness, turbidity, or particulate matter; also inspect solution container for cracks (in a bottle) or minute punctures (in a bag).	3. This could indicate solution contamination, in which case its use is contraindicated.
4. Be certain that solution container is waterproof and airtight.	4. This guarantees asepsis.
5. Remove protective covering from IV solution container.	
6. Clamp off IV tubing.	
7. Remove protective covering from IV tubing.	
8. Spike IV solution container.	
9. Invert solution container, fill drip chamber, and prime IV tubing; purge tubing of all air, including air usually trapped in side-arm injection sites.	

ACTION	RATIONALE
10. Insert IV tubing into filter housing and prime filter. Follow manufacturer's specific instructions for priming a filter; all filters differ slightly.	10. Correct filling of the filter is essential to its proper operation.
11. Shut off IV solution and cover end of filter tubing with a sterile needle; label IV tubing drip chamber and filter housing with date.	11. Dating the tubing and filter helps insure that they will be changed on time.
12. Place a tape marked in hourly increments on new TPN solution container. It should be checked every 30 minutes.	12. The time-tape allows for easy visualization of flow accuracy.
13. Remove tape anchoring catheter to the dressing and tape securing catheter hub–filter tubing junction; stabilize dressing with one hand.	13. This guards against catheter dislodgment.
14. Clamp Hickman catheter with atraumatic clamp and *immediately* shut off infusion pump.	14. This avoids backflow of blood into catheter and subsequent clotting.
15. Remove used tubing from infusion pump.	
16. Quickly insert new tubing into infusion pump and reprogram as necessary.	16. The infusion should be interrupted as briefly as possible. Establish a brief period of gravity flow if necessary.
17. Remove used filter tubing from catheter hub; keep catheter hub sterile.	
18. Replace used filter tubing with new filter tubing. A. Remove sterile protective needle from new tubing. B. Insert new tubing and secure Luer-Lok junction.	B. Luer-Lok fittings are almost always used with Hickman catheters. They are strongly advocated to prevent accidental separation of tubing.
19. Turn on infusion pump and simultaneously unclamp Hickman catheter.	19. This avoids backflow of blood into catheter and pressure on catheter.
20. Retape tubing and hub junction.	20. This provides additional protection against accidental separation of tubing.

Precautions

1. Implement air embolism precautions in this procedure.
2. Integrate aseptic technique into the procedure.
3. Clamp and unclamp rapidly, as specified, to avoid subjecting the clamped catheter to positive pressure.

Related Care

1. Option: Paint all IV tubing junctions with an antimicrobial solution before disconnecting them. Although this has not been required in the above procedure, it may be a desirable addition in some cases.
2. Change the tubing every 24 hours.

Complications

Sepsis
Air embolism

REFERENCES

Guidelines for prevention of intravascular infections, Centers for Disease Control. N.I.T.A., 5:39–46, 1982.
Total parenteral nutrition (T.P.N.) nursing standards of practice. N.I.T.A., 1:77–80, 1982.
Wilson, J.: Right atrial catheters (Broviac and Hickman): Indications, insertion, maintenance and protocol for home care. N.I.T.A., 6:23–27, 1983.

HEPARINIZATION OF A TOTAL PARENTERAL NUTRITION HICKMAN CATHETER

Overview

When patients receive intermittent infusion of total parenteral nutrition, it will be necessary to place a heparin lock between infusions. Heparinization preserves catheter patency. A single standard indicating volume or strength of heparin flush solution for this procedure does not exist. Concentrations of heparin/saline flush solution typically range from 10 units/ml. to 1000 units/ml., and volume varies from 2 to 3 ml. to 6 to 8 ml. per flush procedure. Although a standard is also lacking for frequency of heparinization, once a day should be sufficient. Intermittent total parenteral nutrition is often called cyclic feeding. It may be prescribed for metabolic reasons (to imitate circadian rhythm) or in preparation for home total parenteral nutrition.

Objective

To maintain patency of the Hickman catheter between IV infusions.

Special Equipment

Prefilled heparin syringe
Sterile Luer-Lok hard plastic cap
Atraumatic catheter clamp

Procedure

ACTION	RATIONALE
1. Wash hands with surgical scrub solution and rinse.	
2. Open Luer-Lok cap package, preserving sterility of cap.	
3. Untape tubing/hub junction.	
4. Clamp Hickman catheter with atraumatic clamp and *immediately* shut off infusion pump.	4. This avoids backflow of blood into catheter, and subsequent clotting.
5. Remove used filter tubing from catheter hub; keep fluid pathway of catheter hub sterile.	
6. Connect heparin syringe (without needle) securely to catheter after purging syringe of air.	6. A Luer-Lok fitting on the syringe is preferable to preserve the integrity of the connection.
7. Apply gentle pressure to syringe plunger and *immediately* release catheter clamp.	7. This avoids backflow of blood into catheter and subsequent clotting.
8. Inject prescribed volume of heparin/saline flush.	
9. After prescribed volume has been injected, and *before the syringe is empty*, reclamp the catheter while pressure to syringe plunger is maintained.	9. This avoids backflow of blood into catheter and subsequent clotting.
10. *Immediately* release pressure on syringe plunger.	10. This avoids pressure on catheter.

ACTION	RATIONALE
11. Disconnect syringe from catheter, keeping fluid pathway of exposed hub sterile.	
12. Carefully remove sterile, hard plastic Luer-Lok cap from package and connect to the catheter.	
13. Secure Luer-Lok junction and retape.	13. This prevents accidental separation of tubing.

Precautions

1.   Implement air embolism precautions in this procedure.
2.   Integrate aseptic technique into the procedure.
3.   Clamp and unclamp rapidly, as specified, to avoid subjecting the clamped catheter to positive pressure.
4.   Keep the Hickman catheter clamped when the infusion is not occurring. (This is an optional safeguard.)
5.   Note that the dose of heparin administered should not interfere with the patient's clotting factors.
6.   Note that the volume of the heparin/saline flush administered should always exceed the capacity of the catheter being heparin locked.

Related Care

1.   Option: Use soft latex injection cap in place of the hard plastic cap. This should also be a Luer-Lok fitting.
2.   If heparinization is administered through a latex soft cap, use a needle that is shorter than the cap to avoid accidental perforation of the catheter.
3.   Option: Paint all IV tubing junctions with an antimicrobial solution before disconnecting them. Although this has not been required in the above procedure, it may be a desirable addition in some cases.

Complication

Catheter clotting

REFERENCE

Wilson, J.: Right atrial catheters (Broviac and Hickman): Indications, insertion, maintenance and protocol for home care. N.I.T.A., 6:23–27, 1983.

LIPID EMULSION THERAPY

Rita Colley, R.N., B.A.

ADMINISTRATION OF INTRAVENOUS LIPID EMULSIONS

Overview

There are presently three brands of intravenous lipid emulsion commercially available in the United States—Intralipid injection (Cutter) and Travamulsion injection (Travenol) are soybean emulsions and Liposyn injection (Abbott) is a safflower emulsion. Lipid emulsions are isotonic, ranging from 280 mOsm./liter to 340 mOsm./liter, depending on the concentration of the emulsion. All of the emulsions contain similar emulsifying agents and additives: the main difference is in the triglyceride source of Liposyn injection.

Lipid emulsions are available in 10% and 20% concentrations; a 10% emulsion contains 1.1 calorie/ml. and a 20% emulsion contains 2.0 calories/ml. Because the emulsions are isotonic, they may be administered peripherally.

There are two main indications for administering IV lipids: (1) to prevent or treat essential fatty acid deficiency and (2) to obtain the high caloric yield of fat. Essential fatty acid deficiency is a state that may be more common than formerly believed. Some typical symptoms are thrombocytopenia, thinning hair, dry or scaled skin, and liver function abnormalities. Chemical confirmation of this deficiency state is possible by determining the triene/tetraene ratio.

Infusion of IV lipid emulsions requires some specific guidelines. Lipid emulsions are administered simultaneously with a parenteral nutrition solution but are usually infused as a solo IV or through a **Y**-connection system close to the catheters. Additives to the lipid emulsion are usually not advocated. However, a new method of lipid administration has recently been introduced; that involves admixture of the lipid emulsion with a solution containing amino acids, dextrose, electrolytes, vitamins, and trace elements. If this method of total parenteral nutrition is utilized, the manufacturer's specific recommendations for additive compatibilities should be followed.

Objective

To administer intravenous fat in a safe, efficient manner, with full awareness of possible complications.

Special Equipment

IV lipid emulsion

Procedure

ACTION	RATIONALE
1. Before infusing:	
A. Inspect emulsion for frothiness, separation, or oily appearance.	A. These could indicate a cracked bottle of emulsion; administration would then be contraindicated.
B. If cold, allow emulsion to come to room temperature; this takes only a few minutes.	B. Cold emulsion causes pain and could produce blanching of the skin.
2. Prime IV tubing administration set provided with lipid emulsion and connect in usual fashion.	
3. Infuse IV lipid emulsion as a separate infusion or as a **Y**-type infusion connected to catheter hub.	3. This prevents mixing with other solutions, which might cause emulsion instability.
4. Follow manufacturer's recommendations for rate and dose. Initial rates are very slow. Maximum rates are limited both by flow rate and by total dose.	4. This allows time to notice adverse reactions and avoids overdosage.

Precautions

1. Do not filter IV lipid emulsion; it would clog the filter and might crack the bottle of emulsion.
2. Place only specified allowable additives in the lipid emulsion. This practice is severely restricted when the lipid emulsion is administered separately from the TPN solution.
3. Observe the patient carefully during the first 15 to 30 minutes of infusion; note any adverse reactions that might occur and report to physician immediately.
4. Do not interrupt IV lipid emulsion infusion or reuse an opened bottle, since IV lipid emulsion could become contaminated.
5. Do not administer lipid emulsion to a person with a known disturbance of normal fat metabolism, e.g., pathologic hyperlipemia, lipoid nephrosis, or acute pancreatitis if accompanied by hyperlipemia.
6. Use caution and closely monitor patients with severe liver damage, blood coagulation disorders, anemia, pulmonary disease, or conditions that predispose the patient to fat embolism.

Related Care

1. Review the *current* package insert regarding product information before administration of this drug.

2. Assess serum opacity 4 to 6 hours after terminating infusion. Serum will appear cloudy or opaque if the lipids have not cleared the bloodstream.
3. Store the lipid emulsion at a temperature of 25° C. (77° F.) or less.
4. Routinely monitor the patient's ability to tolerate lipid emulsion (liver function tests, cholesterol, triglycerides, plasma-free fatty acids, and blood coagulation studies).

Complications

Thermogenic reaction	Altered hemodynamic state
Blood dyscrasias	Flank pain
Dyspnea	Anaphylaxis
Hyperlipemia	Headache
Cyanosis	Sleepiness
Flushing	Nausea
Dizziness	Vomiting
Hyperthermia	Sweating
Transient increases in liver enzymes	Chest pain

Suppliers

Abbott Laboratories (Liposyn injection 10% and 20%)
Travenol Laboratories, Inc. (Travamulsion injection 10% and 20%)
Vitrum of Sweden (Intralipid injection 10% and 20% distributed in the United States by Cutter Laboratories, Inc.)

REFERENCES

Englert, D.: Rational use of fat emulsions. Nutri. Sup. Serv. 2(9):35–40, 1982.
Tsallis, G.: Products for parenteral nutrition. *In* Jeejeebhoy, K.N. (ed.): Total Parenteral Nutrition in the Hospital and at Home. Boca Raton, CRC Press, 1983, pp. 133–135.

ENTERAL NUTRITION VIA
——— AN ENTERAL FEEDING TUBE ———

Rita Colley, R.N., B.A.

Overview

The focus of this section is enteral nutrition via narrow-bore nasogastric or transpyloric tubes that are introduced through the nares. Attention is given to proper administration techniques for continuous and intermittent enteral feedings. A variety of enteral feeding tubes are available; most are soft and flexible, of narrow bore to avoid pharyngeal and esophageal irritation, and usually made of silicone or polyurethane. The decision to place a tube through the pyloric sphincter is often made to avoid the potentially lethal complication of feeding aspiration. However, it is often impossible to obtain confirmation of transpyloric tube location via conventional methods, and care must be taken to obtain x-ray confirmation of such tubes before feeding is initiated.

CONTINUOUS ENTERAL TUBE FEEDING ADMINISTRATION ————————————————

Objective

To provide a safe method of continuous enteral nutrition to those patients unable to ingest food normally.

Special Equipment

Feeding tube in place
Enteral feeding solution
Enteral feeding administration set and solution container
  (often preattached)
60-ml. aspirating syringe
Feeding tube clamp
Sterile water for irrigation
Stethoscope

Procedure

ACTION	RATIONALE
1. Obtain enteral feeding and warm to room temperature as necessary.	1. Extremely cold feeding may cause cramping.
2. Fill feeding solution container and, if not preattached, connect to administration set.	
3. Prime administration set tubing (this is not necessary if the tubing is already in use.)	
4. Change enteral feeding administration set every 24 hours.	4. This is an infection control principle.
5. Change enteral feeding solution container every 8 hours.	5. This is an infection control principle.
6. Keep head of bed elevated at least at a 30-degree angle at all times.	6. This discourages pulmonary aspiration of enteral feeding or gastric contents.
7. Aspirate gastric contents every 4 hours, using aspirating syringe. *NOTE:* Aspiration of transpyloric tubes is not done; check for x-ray confirmation of tube location and stability of tube fixation.	7. This confirms tube placement in the stomach and indicates the volume of gastric residual. Consistent length of tube remaining outside of body helps to indicate that the tube position is unchanged.
8. Return gastric aspirate to stomach.	
9. Continue feeding if gastric aspirate is less than 100 ml.	9. Gastric residual of 100 ml. is an insignificant amount.
10. Discontinue feeding and notify physician if gastric aspirate is more than 100 ml. Also, assess the patient for abdominal distention.	10. Gastric retention may be significant.
11. Inject 20 cc. of air and listen with stethoscope for rush of air over stomach if gastric aspirate is unavailable.	11. This confirms gastric placement of feeding tube.
12. Confirm bowel sounds with stethoscope. If bowel sounds are absent, discontinue feeding and notify physician.	12. Ileus may exist.
13. Clamp feeding tube and change administration set if tubing change is occurring.	

ACTION	RATIONALE
14. Infuse enteral feeding as prescribed, maintaining consistency of rate.	14. This avoids glucose intolerance and gastrointestinal intolerance.
15. Instill 30 ml. of water every 4 hours, whenever feeding is discontinued, or if clogging of tubing is suspected.	15. This maintains tube patency.

Precautions

1. Use an enteral feeding pump to avoid tube kinking and subsequent clogging and to maintain prescribed consistency of rate.
2. Make sure gag reflex is present in patients receiving gastric feedings to avoid pulmonary aspiration.
3. Observe the patient carefully for signs of gastrointestinal intolerance to the enteral feeding, e.g., nausea, vomiting, distention, cramping, hyperactive bowel sounds.

Related Care

1. Maintain nasal and oral hygiene with particular emphasis on avoiding pressure points from the tube. Change the tape and apply new tape so that stress does not cause skin or mucosal irritation.
2. Do not initiate enteral feeding at full strength or volume; usually both are increased separately and gradually to allow development of patient tolerance.
3. Monitor metabolic parameters to determine glucose tolerance and electrolyte requirements.
4. Monitor intake and output to determine fluid balance and requirements.
5. Mix enteral feeding solutions well, with blender if necessary, to maintain patency of administration set tubing and feeding tube.
6. Use liquid medication to maintain patency of administration set tubing and feeding tube.

INTERMITTENT ENTERAL TUBE FEEDING ADMINISTRATION _____

Objective

To provide a safe method of intermittent enteral nutrition to those patients unable to ingest food normally.

Special Equipment

Feeding tube in place
Enteral feeding solution
Enteral feeding administration set and solution container (often preattached)
60-ml. aspirating syringe
Sterile water for irrigation
Stethoscope
Feeding tube clamp
Gauze sponge
Elastic band

Procedure

ACTION	RATIONALE
1. Obtain enteral feeding and warm to room temperature as necessary.	1. Extremely cold feeding may cause cramping.
2. Elevate head of bed to at least a 30° angle.	2. This discourages pulmonary aspiration of enteral feeding or gastric contents.
3. Unclamp feeding tube and aspirate gastric contents every 4 hours, using aspirating syringe. Do this before feeding. *NOTE:* Aspiration of transpyloric tubes is not done; check for x-ray confirmation of tube location and stability of tube fixation.	3. This confirms tube placement in the stomach and indicates volume of gastric residual. Consistent length of tube remaining outside of body helps to indicate tube position is unchanged.
4. Return gastric aspirate to stomach.	
5. Begin feedings if gastric aspirate is less than 100 ml.	5. Gastric residual of less than 100 ml. is an insignificant amount.
6. Check with physician before feeding if gastric aspirate is more than 100 ml. Also assess for abdominal distention.	6. Gastric retention may be significant.
7. Inject 20 cc. of air and listen with stethoscope for rush of air over stomach if gastric aspirate is unobtainable.	7. This confirms gastric placement of feeding tube.
8. Confirm bowel sounds with stethoscope. If bowel sounds are absent, discontinue feeding and notify physician.	8. Ileus may be present.

ACTION	RATIONALE
9. Pinch feeding tube closed, disconnect syringe from feeding tube, and reconnect barrel of syringe without plunger. Fill barrel with feeding solution.	
10. Unpinch feeding tube.	
11. Continuously administer prescribed volume of feeding, allowing it to run in slowly by gravity.	11. If feeding is viscous it may need to be diluted.
12. Administer prescribed volume of water into tube after feeding is completed. Instill at least 30 ml. of water.	12. This maintains tube patency.
13. Clamp feeding tube, remove syringe, and cover exposed tip with gauze pad secured by elastic band.	
14. Keep syringe clean and change it every 24 hours.	14. This is an infection-control principle.
15. Maintain head of bed elevation for at least 30 to 60 minutes.	

Precautions

1. Make sure gag reflex is present in patients receiving gastric feedings to avoid pulmonary aspiration.
2. Observe the patient carefully for signs of gastrointestinal intolerance to the enteral feeding, e.g., nausea, vomiting, distention, cramping, hyperactive bowel sounds.

Related Care

1. Maintain nasal and oral hygiene with particular emphasis on avoiding pressure points from the tube. Change the tape frequently, and apply new tape so that stress does not cause skin or mucosal irritation.
2. Do not initiate enteral feeding at full strength or volume; usually both are increased separately and gradually to allow development of patient tolerance.
3. Monitor metabolic parameters to determine glucose tolerance and electrolyte requirements.
4. Monitor intake and output to determine fluid balance and requirements.
5. Mix enteral feeding solutions well, with blender if necessary, to maintain patency of administration set tubing and feeding tube.

6. Use liquid medication to maintain patency of administration set tubing and feeding tube.

Complications: General

Tube malposition
Pulmonary aspiration
Gastrointestinal intolerance
Glucose intolerance
Fluid and electrolyte imbalance
Contaminated enteral feeding
Irritation of skin or mucosa by tube or tape
Hyperosmolar load
Tube obstruction

REFERENCES

DelRio, D., Williams, K., and Esvelt, B.: Handbook of Enteral Nutrition, A practical Guide to Tube Feeding. El Segundo, Calif., Medical Specifics Publishing, 1982.
Enteral nutrition, continuous feeding. *In* Massachusetts General Hospital Manual of Nursing Procedures, 2nd ed., pp. 90–91, Boston, Little, Brown, 1980.
Konstantinides, N.N., and Shronts, E.: Tube feeding, managing the basics. Am. J. Nurs., *83*(9):1312–1320.
Matarese, L.: Standardized enteral nutritional support. Nutri. Sup. Serv., *3*(8):27–30, 1983.

10

SAFETY

INFECTION SURVEILLANCE IN
THE CRITICAL CARE UNIT _____

Elaine Larson, R.N., Ph.D., F.A.A.N.

Overview

Infection control measures in the critical care unit can effectively reduce the incidence of nosocomial infections. The impact of measures instituted must be evaluated continually in conjunction and cooperation with the total hospital infection surveillance program.

A formal infection control and surveillance program should ideally be developed by an Infection Control Practitioner (ICP). In addition, a nurse with expertise and interest in infection control should be designated as a liaison between the unit and other hospital departments, especially between infection control committee members and personnel concerned with surveillance. Responsibilities of the ICP or nurse designated by the infection control committee include the steps presented in the procedure below.

Objectives

1. To identify endemic and epidemic organisms that are present in the critical care unit.
2. To be informed of infection rates in the unit.
3. To evaluate the effectiveness of infection control measures instituted and practiced in the unit.

Procedure

ACTION	RATIONALE
1. Review monthly infection reports from hospital infection control officer.	1. A monthly review helps to note trends in infection within the unit and rapidly identify the presence of epidemic or endemic strains in the unit.
2. Establish, review, and maintain unit infection control policies in collaboration with hospital infection control committee. The hospital infection control committee should review these policies and procedures annually.	2. This ensures the updating and conformance of policies and procedures with accepted standards of practice and aids in compliance with the standards of the Joint Commission on Accreditation of Hospitals.
3. Review and interpret critical care unit policies and collected data with personnel in unit.	
4. Assist with defining unit infection control needs.	

ACTION	RATIONALE
5. Interpret infection control needs and communicate them to appropriate departments and personnel.	
6. Coordinate efforts to evaluate effectiveness of unit infection control practices.	
7. Use environmental sampling judiciously and sparingly. This includes cultures of such fomites as walls, floors, irrigating fluids, electrodes, and sinks. Valid reasons for environmental sampling are to: A. Search for fomites of a specific organism that is causing nosocomial infection problems. B. Document necessity for improved cleaning procedures. C. Increase personnel sensitivity and awareness of potential role of environment in infection control.	7. Results are difficult to interpret and do not necessarily reflect direct risk to patients.
8. Minimize air sampling, as it is of limited use. Use only to: A. Establish quantity of airborne organisms in case of unit crowding. B. Identify types of airborne organisms in case of an epidemic situation (Fig. 10–1).	8. Results are difficult to interpret; airborne contamination plays a relatively small part in most nosocomial organisms.

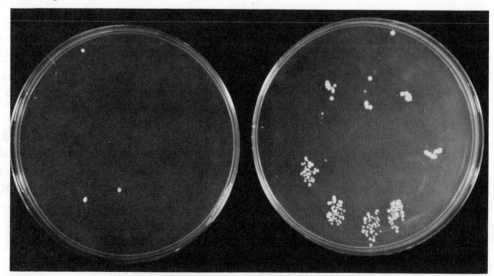

Figure 10-1 The transmission of organisms via air and hands. The culture plate on the left shows bacterial growth after an hour's air sampling using the Mattson-Garvin slit air sampler. There are three colonies of skin flora present. The culture plate on the right shows bacterial growth from an ICU employee's fingers. The organisms are too numerous to count. Both samples were taken in a six-bed medical-surgical ICU during the same time period. Plates were incubated at 37° C. for 48 hours.

ACTION	RATIONALE
9. Establish critical care unit standing policies for routine patient culturing when clinical symptoms of infection occur: A. Respiratory: when purulent, bloody, or foul tracheal secretions are present. B. Wound or skin: when purulence, redness, or induration is present with or without insertion of catheters, tubes, etc. C. Urinary: when urine is foul smelling or cloudy.	
10. Integrate microbiologic culture reports of patients into nursing assessment and care. A. Teach personnel the normal flora of body sites, symptoms of infection, and common opportunistic and more virulent pathogens. B. Note antimicrobial susceptibility patterns of organisms reported. Notify physician if patient is receiving an antimicrobial to which the organism(s) present is resistant.	10. This aids personnel in becoming informed of organisms present in the unit. A. This enables personnel to interpret culture results adequately. B. An antimicrobial agent will be ineffective if organism(s) present are resistant; inadequate or inappropriate antimicrobial usage encourages the growth of resistant strains.

Precautions

These are an integral part of the procedure.

Related Care

1. Review and revise policies annually, utilizing appropriate resources.
2. Involve support services in development of protocols regarding environmental and equipment cleaning, and encourage compliance by incorporating infection control practices into personnel performance evaluation.
3. Identify problems that might be appropriate for quality assurance study.

Complications

Late detection of infection sources, agents, and infections
Infection

REFERENCES

Hargiss, C., and Larson, E.: How to collect specimens and evaluate results. Am. J. Nurs., *81*:2166, 1981.

Roderick, M.A.: Infection Control in Critical Care. Rockville, Aspen Systems Corporation, 1982.

Simmons, B.P.: Guideline for hospital environmental control. *In* Guidelines for the Prevention and Control of Nosocomial Infections. Atlanta, Centers for Disease Control, 1981.

U.S. Dept. of Health and Human Services: Management Skills for Infection Control Nurses. Atlanta, Centers for Disease Control, 1982.

INFECTION CONTROL IN THE
CRITICAL CARE UNIT

Elaine Larson, R.N., Ph.D., F.A.A.N.

Overview

Approximately one in four patients in critical care units acquires noso-comial organisms if the stay is more than 3 days, with the risk increasing as the stay is prolonged. Because personnel are the key to infection control, all control measures implemented must place major emphasis on the role of the multidisciplinary health care team.

Procedures for three elements of infection control—personnel, equipment, and environment—are presented.

Objectives

1. To minimize the risk of infection to the critically ill patient by:
   A. Meticulous hand washing and personal hygiene of personnel.
   B. Appropriate sterilization, cleaning, and monitoring of equipment that contacts the patient.
   C. Instituting, maintaining, and monitoring housekeeping procedures, especially those related to floors, sinks, storage, and utility rooms.
2. To prevent patient-to-patient spread of organisms by means of personnel, fomites, contact, or air.
3. To segregate patients of potential hazard to others by:
   A. Establishing and maintaining isolation policies for the unit.
   B. Practicing satisfactory containment technique.

INFECTION CONTROL MEASURES: PERSONNEL

Procedure

ACTION	RATIONALE

1. Establish hand washing policies and dress code for unit.
   A. Educate all new employees concerning these policies.
   B. Provide intermittent (biannual) reeducation of personnel.
	1. Hands of personnel have been demonstrated to be the primary mode of transmission for nosocomial infections.

ACTION	RATIONALE

2. Provide adequate hand washing facilities.
   A. If a soap dispenser is not used, use soap rack with adequate drainage and small bars; dispensers and soap racks must be cleaned routinely.
   B. Check sinks for splashing; if splashing occurs:
      (1) Lower water pressures, or
      (2) Erect splash guards, or
      (3) Insert faucet filters; however, they must be cleaned every month.

A. Contaminated dispensers have been associated with nosocomial infections. Soap, especially in a pool of liquid, may support the growth of microbes.
B. Splashing will contaminate clothing.

(3) Filters can harbor organisms.

3. Provide an acceptable hand washing agent; most soaps or antiseptics are acceptable.
   A. Choose an agent, using the following criteria:
      (1) Effectiveness against organisms most commonly found in unit.
      (2) Cost effectiveness.
      (3) Having least undesirable side effects (skin drying, burning).
   B. Agents include:
      (1) Hexachlorophene. This may be preferable if staphylococci are a problem.

      (2) Iodophors. These are preferable if gram-negative organisms (e.g., *Escherichia coli, Serratia, Klebsiella, Pseudomonas*) are a problem.
      (3) 70% alcohol. Its use should be limited to those occasions when hand washing facilities are poor or unavailable.
      (4) Other agents:
         (a) Bar soaps adequately remove transient organisms but are not adequate if the patients are known to be infected.

3. Although some antiseptics are more active against certain organisms, technique and frequency of hand washing are as important as the agent used.

(1) Hexachlorophene is effective only against gram-positive organisms; its effectiveness is increased with duration of use.
(2) Iodophors are effective against gram-negative and gram-positive organisms, fungi, and some viruses.
(3) 70% alcohol will adequately disinfect skin in 15 to 20 seconds but is very drying.

ACTION	RATIONALE

(b) Chlorhexidine (Hibiclens) is effective against both gram-negative and gram-positive organisms; its residual effectiveness lasts up to 6 hours (in the absence of recontamination).

(c) Aqueous benzalkonium chloride (Zephiran) is *not* an acceptable skin cleanser.

4. Employ effective hand washing technique.
   A. Lather and rub with friction for at least 15 seconds under a stream of warm water.
   B. Rinse and dry with a paper towel.
   C. Turn off faucet with another paper towel.

   D. Wash hands before each patient contact.
   E. Remove all rings other than plain bands.
   F. Remove cracked or chipped nail polish.

4. Hand washing is the most effective infection control measure available.

   C. Organisms are spread from a contaminated faucet through a wet towel.

   E. Organisms are difficult to remove from crevices.

5. Prevent skin drying and dermatitis of hands.
   A. Alternate agents or use bar soap if a hand washing agent is too drying.
   B. Wear gloves, especially during high-risk procedures such as catheterization and wound care.
   C. Use hand creams with caution.
      (1) Use small containers with "squirt" lids (*not* lids that will unscrew).
      (2) Discard when empty, or clean thoroughly and refill routinely.
      (3) Avoid hand cream application immediately after hand washing while in critical care

5. Dry, cracked skin harbors more organisms.

   C. Hand creams are easily contaminated and are a known cause of nosocomial infections.

      (3) This decreases the chance of causing infections due to contaminated hand cream and

ACTION	RATIONALE
unit; apply while off duty (coffee or lunch breaks, times away from direct patient care).	may reduce the residual effect of antiseptics.

6. Protect patients from organisms spread on clothing and hair.
   A. Wear scrub attire or other washable clothing not worn outside the hospital, and which is changed daily. A clean gown or lab coat must be worn when leaving unit.
   B. Wear hair pulled back or covered.
   C. Have visitors wash their hands well before entering and when leaving the unit.
   D. Have visitors don clean gown when entering critical care unit; when they leave unit, gown is discarded.

6. Clothing and hair are demonstrated fomites of infection.

7. Minimize traffic in unit (especially during sterile or invasive procedures).

7. Increased movement increases bacterial movement in the air.

8. Ensure that entry into unit is through a "clean" area (not through a dirty utility room, for example).

9. Require participation of all unit personnel in hospital employee health program.
   A. Keep records of immunization, chest x-rays, or tuberculin tests up to date.
   B. If renal dialysis or transplant patients are cared for in unit, adopt policies for hepatitis surveillance of personnel and patients.

10. Exclude personnel and visitors with bacterial infections from the unit; these include common cold, influenza, hepatitis, herpes, and infections due to *Staphylococcus aureus* or beta-hemolytic streptococcus.

ACTION	RATIONALE
11. Maintain an infection control orientation and education program for all personnel in consultation with and supervised by Infection Control Practitioner (see "Infection Surveillance in the Critical Care Unit").	11. This helps to increase staff awarenesss regarding their responsibility in infection control.

INFECTION CONTROL MEASURES: ENVIRONMENT

Procedure

ACTION	RATIONALE
1. Ensure, as much as possible, that the critical care unit is ventilated adequately.	1. Certain organisms (staphylococci, pneumococci, tubercle bacilli, and others) are known to be airborne.
A. Air should be exchanged at least 12 times each hour.	A. This removes airborne organisms, preventing a cumulative build-up.
B. If window fans or air conditioners are used, have filters changed routinely (at least twice a year)	B. Contaminated fans can be sources of nosocomial microbial acquisition, especially for certain soil organisms such as *Legionella pneumophila*.
C. Avoid open windows in critical care unit.	C. Contaminated outside air can increase the risk of infection to patients during invasive procedures. In addition, insects may enter.
D. In rooms with regulated air flow ("isolation" rooms), keep door closed, and fans off.	D. Regulated air flow is ineffective when outside air is allowed to enter or inside air is allowed to exit.
E. Avoid shaking of linen and violent curtain pulling.	E. Organisms become airborne.
2. Collaborate with housekeeping personnel in setting up critical care unit procedures, especially regarding:	2. This decreases the possibility of nosocomial infections acquired through contact with contaminated surfaces.
A. Mopping technique with schedule, i.e., every 8 hours and whenever necessary.	
B. Terminal cleaning after patient leaves unit.	

ACTION	RATIONALE
C. Cleaning surfaces and patient areas. All surfaces should be cleaned daily and *immediately* after contamination with blood or other body fluids.	C. Because of increased risk of infections such as hepatitis, all body fluids should be treated as contaminated.
D. Cleaning of sinks.	
E. Cleaning agents.	
F. Methods for evaluating cleaning effectiveness.	
3. Segregate clean and dirty areas; place linens and other clean supplies in least trafficked, most protected areas.	
4. Prohibit from admission, when possible, patients with influenza and viral upper respiratory infections, especially during epidemic seasons.	4. Such conditions are highly contagious and may cause severe pulmonary complications in the debilitated patient whose defense systems are impaired.
5. For infected patients requiring intensive care, use hospital standards outlined and accepted for isolation techniques.	5. Effective isolation techniques cannot be carried out in curtained cubicles.
A. Single-room isolation with adequate hand-washing facilities must be provided.	
B. Segregate immediately patients harboring organisms with unusual resistance to antimicrobial agents (especially multiresistant gram-negative bacteria such as *Serratia marcescens* and methicillin-resistant staphylococci).	B. Epidemics with such organisms have been increasingly reported in critical care units. Multiresistant organisms are difficult to treat.

INFECTION CONTROL MEASURES: EQUIPMENT _____

Procedure

ACTION	RATIONALE
1. Incorporate infection control principles into all patient care activities associated with infection risk.	1. This decreases risk to patients, visitors, and staff.
A. Procedures of particular concern include:	
(1) Insertion of intravascular needles and catheters.	(1) These have been demonstrated to be the major causes of nosocomial infections.

ACTION

(2) Use of respiratory therapy equipment.

(3) Insertion and care of urinary catheters.

(4) Use of thermometers.

(5) Care of intubated patients.

(6) Wound care.

(7) Total parenteral nutrition (hyperalimentation).

B. Carefully assess need for invasive techniques.

C. Help maintain strict asepsis when such procedures are performed in unit.

D. Evaluate written procedures of these activites to ensure that they delineate infection control measures.

2. Establish and maintain a cleaning schedule for emergency equipment, including defibrillator, pacemakers, and intubation and resuscitation equipment.

RATIONALE

Precaution

Hexachlorophene has been demonstrated to cause neurologic toxicity in infants and in adults after massive exposure of mucous membranes.

REFERENCES

Bond, G.B.: Serratia—an endemic hospital resident. Am. J. Nurs., *81*:2183, 1981.

Cross, A.S., and Roup, B.: Role of respiratory assistance devices in endemic nosocomial pneumonia. Am. J. Med., *76*:681–695, 1981.

Hargiss, C., and Larson, E.: Guidelines for prevention of hospital-acquired infection. Am. J. Nurs., *81*:2175, 1981.

Infection control: Putting principles into practice. Am. J. Nurs., *81*:2165–2186, 1981.

Larson, E.: Persistent carriage of gram-negative bacteria on hands. Am. J. Infect. Control, *9*:112, 1981.

Pantelick, E.B.: Anaerobic Infections: Some Practical Considerations for the Nurse. Upjohn, 1979.

Preston, G.A., Larson, E.L., and Stamm, W.E.: The effect of private isolation rooms on patient care practices, colonization and infection in an intensive care unit. Am. J. Med., *70*:641–643, 1981.

Roderick, M.A.: Infection Control in Critical Care. Rockville, Aspen Systems, 1983.

ELECTRICAL SAFETY

ELECTRICAL SAFETY FOR PATIENTS AND MEDICAL DEVICE OPERATORS

Kit Stahler-Miller, R.N., M.S.N.

Overview

A simple analogy can be made between electricity and the cardiovascular system. Electricity and blood can be envisioned as having distribution and return systems. Current (amps) corresponds with blood flow, and voltage (volts) with blood pressure. Although voltage is the driving force that causes current to flow, the physiologic effects from an electric shock are caused by current.

Conductors are materials through which electricity easily flows. Examples are all metals (copper is the most widely used) and ionic fluids. Insulators are materials that are highly resistant to the flow of electrical current. Although a perfect insulator does not exist, effective examples include glass, rubber, and intact dry skin. Skin insulation or resistance is undesirably decreased when skin is wet or compromised by a needle, catheter, or wound. Electrolyte gels are used to decrease skin resistance so that voltages generated internally can be detected externally through the intact skin.

Grounding is the most important principle in electrical safety. A ground is a low-resistance electrical pathway to the earth. Its purpose is to limit or carry away undesirable leakage (stray) current from the metal cabinet of electrically operated devices. Electrical current will follow the path of least resistance to seek ground. However, this route may not be the intended circuit. A patient or an equipment operator may be the link in an inadvertent pathway to ground. Remember to ground *equipment*, not the patient.

Electricity has both positive and negative physiologic effects. Positive or therapeutic effects occur from its controlled use, as in nerve stimulation, electroshock therapy, defibrillation, cardioversion, and cardiac pacing. Negative or hazardous effects occur from contact with devices that have stray currents on their metal chassis. Perceptible shock sensation resulting from contact with current 1 ma. or greater is termed macroshock. The current diffuses through the body in such a way that little of it passes through the heart. Physiologic effects are dependent on both the magnitude of the current and its path through the body. Effects range from a tingling sensation to ventricular fibrillation, organ damage, severe thermal burns, cardiac arrest, and death (Table 10–1).

Microshock is an imperceptible hazard that may result in ventricular fibrillation when current less than 1 ma. is delivered directly into the heart by a conducting pathway; thus, patients with a central conductive catheter are susceptible. Wire catheters directly into or in proximity to the heart include temporary pacemaker lead wires, esophageal and tracheal electrodes, and thermistor probes. Other central catheters containing conductive fluids include venous and arterial lines attached to transducers and cardiac output apparatus. Minute leakage current levels of only tens of millionths of an ampere can induce ventricular fibrillation (Table 10–1). It is important to note that peripheral intravascular catheters or completely implanted permanent pacemakers do not carry a risk of microshock.

The recent explosion of health care technology has vastly increased the knowledge, capability, and sophistication of patient care and has further increased the potential of electrical shock for patients and personnel. Therefore, operators of complex electronic equipment should understand the accompanying electrical hazards and initiate appropriate measures to safeguard patients, themselves, and others. The combination of practical and theoretic knowledge associated with this milieu should be part of the nurse's knowledge base. Overall responsibility of the critical care nurse includes an understanding of the following:

1. Why the device is being used, what it does, and its clinical function.
2. The basic operating principles and mechanics of the device—how it works and how it is applied.
3. The device's unique problems and hazards, appropriate precautions necessary to avoid adverse effects, and how to recognize its failures.
4. Psychologic relationships among the patient, equipment, and operator that may create insecurity, fear, or overdependence.
5. One's own limitations, especially of how and when to request help, training, or service assistance.

Objectives

1. To provide an electrically safe environment through application of basic electrical principles and associated precautions.
2. To identify nursing responsibilities associated with the safe and effective use of equipment.
3. To utilize clinical engineering in an effective equipment control program to conduct periodic testing, maintenance, calibration, equipment pre-use inspection, plus consultation during equipment procurement, and staff education.

Procedure

ACTION	RATIONALE
1. Use electrically operated equipment that has been inspected for safety within the last 6 months. The tag on the device should indicate the date of the last inspection.	1. This helps to avoid using hazardous equipment that is malfunctioning or deteriorating. Equipment can still operate with unobservable defective ground connections.

TABLE 10-1.   Physiologic Effects of 60 Hz current (1-second Duration) on the Body

PATH	AVERAGE CURRENT	EFFECT		COMMENT
Current through body trunk*	10 amp (A)	Severe burns, physical injury, respiratory paralysis, and possible death		Physical injury (e.g., nerve damage, blood coagulation, deep muscle necrosis).
	1 A	Sustained myocardial depolarization; entire heart tetanized	Danger of respiratory arrest at CNS level	Normal rhythm returns if current removed in time; otherwise, death.
	100 milliamps (ma)†	Danger of ventricular fibrillation; localized myocardial desynchronization		Usually does not revert to normal rhythm when current removed; thus external defibrillation essential to tetanize and resynchronize the rhythm.
				These lower intensities are more dangerous than tetanizing currents because of local desynchronization.
				Approximate current flowing in a 100-watt bulb.
	50 ma	Major muscle massess involved in electrical excitation	Tetanization of respiratory muscles	Physical injury (e.g., fractures, contusions, lacerations).
		Pain, possibly fainting, exhaustion, physical injury		Spasmodic skeletal muscle contractions and involvement of intercostal or diaphragmatic muscles may lead to exhaustion, respiratory failure, and death.
	20 ma	"Can't let go"; muscle contraction forces the hand closed	Responses localized at the points of entry and exit	Injury from violent muscle spasm or from throwing oneself free. This "secondary accident" is perhaps the most frequent form of injury in a 120-volt electrical accident.
	10 ma	Threshold of pain		Commonly accepted upper limit of safe current.
	5 ma			Main danger is startle and involuntary reaction (e.g., dropping/spilling things; pulling out IV).
	1 ma ‡	Threshold of sensation		Nearly 50 times the amount necessary to cause ventricular fibrillation if the current flows directly into the heart.

PATH	AVERAGE CURRENT	EFFECT	COMMENT
Current directly through heart	180 micro amps (μa)	Ventricular fibrillation	Current required to intentionally fibrillate adult human hearts during open heart surgery.
	100 μa	Ventricular fibrillation	Current required to achieve ventricular fibrillation in dogs.
	20 μa	Premature ventricular contractions	
		Ventricular tachycardia	
	10 μa		Accepted maximum level of leakage current as observed by most manufacturers of medical devices.

1 A = 1.0 (1)

1 ma = .001 (1 x 10^{-3})

1 μa = .000001 (1 x 10^{-6})

*Current flowing from arm to arm through the chest with large areas of the hands touching conductive surfaces.

†Conventional abbreviation. Note: MA is the abbreviation on several models of pacemakers (both letters capitalized).

‡ The threshold of sensation is much lower for light contact, smaller electrodes, or on contact with parts of the body more sensitive than the palms.

ACTION	RATIONALE
2. Send dropped equipment to the biomedical engineering department before reuse.	2. This is done to test for damaged components and to assure safety. Equipment may look intact but be damaged.
3. Inspect equipment for electrical hazards such as: A. Cracked or frayed line cords and cables. B. Inadequate strain relief (see "Electrical Terms, Strain Relief"). C. Broken or defective connectors, knobs, and switches. D. Damaged or absence of U.L. listed three-prong plugs, identified by a green dot (Fig. 10–2). (see "Electrical Terms, Plug Caps").	3. This is done to identify, remove from service, label, and report hazardous equipment.

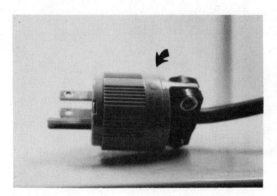

Figure 10-2 Hospital grade plug. Arrow points to green dot.

4. Ensure that all equipment is plugged into properly grounded receptacles (wall outlets) that are tested at least annually to ensure adequate ground connections.	4. This protects the patient from hazards associated with leakage (stray or faulty) current.
5. Report all outlets that do not firmly hold a plug.	5. This decreases the possibility of an electrical hazard. A plug that is loose in an outlet indicates a need to replace the outlet.
6. Avoid plugging in multiple devices that draw high current (e.g., ventilator, radiant warmer) in a single duplex receptacle.	6. This eliminates the possibility of overloading the circuit, drawing too much current, and creating a hazard.

ACTION	RATIONALE
7. Number the faceplate of the receptacle with the number of the corresponding circuit breaker. Number the legend on the breaker door to correspond with the numbers on the faceplate.	7. This speeds identifying which circuit breaker has tripped.
8. Isolate the patient from ground. A. Use equipment with isolated patient inputs (monitors with isolated front ends). B. If the patient is in an electric bed, make sure the bed is either double-insulated or equipped with an isolation transformer.	8. This prevents the patient from acting as an inadvertent pathway to the ground by effectively separating the patient from the power distribution system.
9. Remove discontinued and unused electrically operated equipment from the bedside.	9. This decreases the possibility of accidental damage or failure resulting in electrical hazards.
10. Prohibit the use of patient-owned ungrounded electrical equipment, including chargers or converters for battery-operated devices (e.g., televisions, radios, tape recorders, razors, toothbrushes, hair dryers).	10. The possibility of a person plugging a rechargeable battery-operated unit into the wall is an unwarranted risk. This eliminates the risk of introducing unsafe equipment into the patient's environment.
11. Turn equipment to "off" position before unplugging.	11. This prevents arcing (sparks) that may cause fires or secondary startle-reaction injuries.
12. Maintain relative humidity of 50% to 60% in clinical areas.	12. This will minimize generation of electrostatic charges and reduce the possibility of injury to patient and staff (from a startle reaction) or damage to equipment.
13. Remove plug from wall outlet by grasping plug rather than line cord; pull steadily and straight out.	13. This prevents unobservable and potentially dangerous damage to the line cord and plug.
14. Ensure that there are meaningful and ongoing continuing education sessions provided jointly by staff development and clinical engineering departments.	14. This promotes a continuing awareness of the safe use of complex electrical equipment in the clinical environment.

Precautions

1. Avoid:
   A. Use of equipment that fails inspection.
   B. Use of extension cords.
   C. Use of cheater adapters.
   D. Use of equipment that shocks, sparks, or smokes.
   E. Ungrounded equipment in the patient's environment.
   F. Use of patient-owned appliances in the patient's environment.
   G. Simultaneous contact with the patient and equipment housing.
   H. Storage and spillage of liquids on electrical equipment.
   I. Dangling or kinking patient cables and power cords.
   J. Draping power cords on pipes or plumbing or laying them on a wet surface.
2. Do not depend upon equipment failure to warn of hazardous currents.
3. Identify and remove equipment causing 60 hertz (cycle) interference on cardiac monitors.
4. Also see "Electrical Safety Precautions for Patients with Direct Conduction Pathways to the Myocardium."

Related Care

1. Periodically inspect staff-owned equipment that is used in the hospital as if it were hospital-owned (e.g., radios, coffee makers, clocks).
2. Maintain a log of records provided by clinical engineering department regarding preventive maintenance, electrical safety checks, and maintenance performed.

Complications

Macroshock: startle reactions, neurologic dysfunction, burns, and ventricular fibrillation
Microshock: ventricular fibrillation

Electrical Terms

Alternating current (AC). An electrical current that reverses its direction of flow periodically. In the United States, AC current cycles or reverses exactly 60 times a second; 60 cycles per second and 60 hertz (Hz.) are synonymous. Related terms are power cord, line cord, wall current, interference.

Ampere (amp). A unit of electrical current; the number of electrons passing a given point per second. Fuses and circuit breakers help protect against potentially hazardous current overload.

Chassis. The metal housing, casing, frame, or cabinet of electrical devices.

Circuit A closed electrical pathway. The current flows from the power source to the device and back to the power source or ground. Electricity does not flow through an open system. That is why birds can sit on bare high-voltage power lines and not get shocked.

Direct current (DC). An electrical current that flows through a circuit in one direction. It is produced by a battery (chemical reaction). Battery-operated devices include defibrillators, monitors, oxygen analyzers, and pacemakers.

Fuse. A protective disposable switch that opens and stops the flow of electricity whenever the electrical current is too high. Every fuse has a rating for how much current it can tolerate. When this is exceeded (e.g., from a short circuit, defective component, or a device or devices drawing large currents from the same line), the circuit overheats and the soft metal connection inside the fuse melts and breaks the current pathway. Replacement of the fuse restores the continuous circuit. A circuit breaker is similar but does not have to be replaced; it is manually reset.

Ground. A low resistance electrical pathway to the earth. The ground wire connects the chassis to the earth. Equipment should be grounded, NOT the patient. Related terms are three-pronged plug; safety, green, or ground wire.

Ground fault. When the ground wire is not intact. The device will continue to operate BUT a valuable protective mechanism will be lost. A device called a ground fault circuit interrupter (GFCI) built into the receptacle will discontinue the power when this occurs. However, GFCI's are not recommended where critical life support equipment is used. It is better to lose a ground than to automatically shut down the equipment. GFCI's are typically used in electrically sensitive areas such as dialysis and hydrotherapy units where water is prevalent. (See "Hemodialysis, Overview—Electrical Power.")

Insulator. A material highly resistant to the flow of electricity. There are no perfect insulators.

Leakage current. Current that has strayed from its usual pathway and is seeking ground. Source: AC. Related terms are chassis fault and damaged or poorly designed equipment.

Plug caps (commonly called plugs)
   Standard two-bladed. A pair of flat blades for connecting the lead

wire ("hot" wire that carries the current or power to the device or "load") and the return wire ("neutral" wire that returns the current to the power source).

Standard three-pronged. A pair of flat blades to connect the lead and return wires, plus a ground pin that is connected through the green wire in the line cord. The **U**-shaped or round pin is longer than the flat blades. Therefore it is the first connection made and the last one broken when plugging-in or unplugging equipment.

Newer models of hospital-grade molded plug. U.L. listed as hospital grade. Sturdier construction provides adequate strain relief (Fig. 10–3).

Short circuit. An accidental electrical connection between a hot wire within the instrument and the instrument case. A short circuit can occur through mechanical damage or insulation breakdown. A fluid spill into monitoring equipment will cause the insulation to be bypassed and result in contact between the hot and neutral or ground wires. The excessive current generally causes arcing and sparks, which in turn cause the circuit breaker or fuse to open, thus disrupting power to the instrument.

Strain relief. Anchoring of the line cord's insulating jacket to the chassis of an electrical device. It is designed to minimize stresses such as tug-

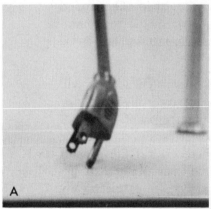

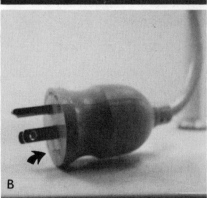

Figure 10-3 *A,* Older molded plug. Note the limited strain relief where the cord enters the plug compared with Figures 10-2 and 10-3*B*. *B,* Newer molded hospital grade plug. Arrow points to green dot on the face of the plug.

ging, bending, and pulling on the conducting wires of the line cord. Inadequate strain relief may cause damage to the conductors, resulting in serious shock hazards.

Voltage. Electrical pressure or potential, the driving force that causes current to flow.

Watt. The electrical measure of power.

REFERENCES

Cooper, K.L.: Electrical safety: The electrically sensitive ICU patient. Focus on Health Devices. AACN, 9:17–19, 1983.

Electrical safety. Health Devices. 3:ES3–23, 1974, pp. 239–261.

Kinney, M.R., Packa, D.R., Branyon, M.E., and Miers, L.J.: Care of the cardiac patient. *In* Andreoli, K.G., Fowkes, V.K., Zipes, D.P., and Wallace, A.G. (eds.): Comprehensive Cardiac Care: A Text for Nurses, Physicians, and Other Health Professionals, 5th ed. St. Louis, CV Mosby, 1983, pp. 474–477.

Mersh, J. Hemodynamic pressure monitoring. *In* Hudak, C.M., Lohar, T.H., and Gallo, B.M. (eds.): Critical Care Nursing, 3rd ed. Philadelphia, J.B. Lippincott, 1982, pp. 172–173.

Poulton, R.J.: Monitoring critically ill patients in the hyperbaric environment. Med. Instrum., 5(2): 81–84, 1981.

Warren, J.: Provisions for electrical safety. *In* Kenner, C.V., Guzzetta, C.E., and Dorsey, B.M. (eds.): Critical Care Nursing: Body-Mind-Spirit. Boston, Little, Brown, 1981, pp. 67–71.

ELECTRICAL SAFETY PRECAUTIONS FOR PATIENTS WITH DIRECT CONDUCTION PATHWAYS TO THE MYOCARDIUM

Betty W. Norris, R.N., M.S.N.

Objective

To establish minimum essential precautions that reduce electrical hazards to patients with direct cardiac conductors.

Procedure

ACTION	RATIONALE
1. Wear rubber gloves when working with conductive pathways to the myocardium.	1. Temporary pacemaker catheters and saline-filled central venous, pulmonary artery, and left atrial catheters provide low resistance current pathways to the myocardium.

ACTION	RATIONALE
2. Avoid contact with conductive ends of catheters while touching electrical equipment or metal parts of bed.	2. Minute alternating current levels can induce ventricular fibrillation.
3. Use only properly grounded equipment in vicinity of these patients.	3. This reduces the risk of leakage current that may be conducted directly to the myocardium.
4. Ensure that defibrillation equipment is immediately available.	4. There is a potential risk for stimulating the myocardium in the vulnerable period of the cardiac cycle, which could produce ventricular fibrillation.
5. Provide continuous dysrhythmia monitoring of patients with direct cardiac conductors.	5. This permits observation and determination of dysrhythmias and their appropriate treatment.
6. Use a 5% dextrose in water infusion for fluid-filled catheters inserted to or in the myocardium.	
7. Provide special attention to the following for temporary transvenous pacemaker catheters.	
A. Use battery-powered rather than line-operated devices when being connected to pacemaker terminal.	A. This reduces the possibility of transmitting leakage current.
B. Check for strong electrical fields; these are usually evidenced by erratic deflection of sense/pace indicator needle to left.	B. This may interfere with demand function.
C. Protect pacemaker, catheter, and connections from moisture.	C. Moisture or fluid may cause malfunction of the pacemaker.

Precautions

1. Maintain constant alertness for potential risk sources.
2. Minimize electrical equipment in use.
3. Also see precautions for "Electrical Safety for Patients and Medical Device Operators."

Related Care

1. Ensure that inspection and preventive maintenance programs are performed.
2. Maintain a log of pacemaker battery usage.

3. Also see related care for "Electrical Safety for Patients and Medical Device Operators."

Complications

Macroshock: startle reactions, neurologic dysfunction, burns, and ventricular fibrillation
Microshock: ventricular fibrillation

REFERENCES

The Heart and Electrical Hazards: Directions in Cardiovascular Medicine. Somerville, N.J., Hoechst Pharmaceutical. Book 9: Vol. 3, 1973.
External Pacemaker. Minneapolis, Medtronics.

RADIATION SAFETY

Ellen Frances Lenihan, R.N., M.S.

Overview

The number of diagnostic procedures dependent on images and the measurement of radioactive isotopes and x-rays has increased considerably over the past few years. There are several fundamental principles of roentgenology and nuclear medicine that will enable the knowledgeable nurse in the critical care unit to protect herself or himself against undue radiation exposure.

Diagnostic roentgenology is based on the differential absorption of x-rays by the various tissues in the body. This absorption will increase or decrease, depending on three elements. First, the atomic number of the material being radiated affects absorption. As the atomic number increases, absorption increases. Lead, which has a high atomic number, absorbs x-rays well. Likewise, bone, the components of which have a higher atomic number than most body tissue, will absorb more x-ray than other parts of the body. Density is the second element affecting absorption. Air, which is low in density, does not absorb x-rays as well as fluid. Finally, as thickness increases, absorption increases. The x-rays that are not absorbed by tissues will pass through the body, forming an image on photographic film.

Diagnostic nuclear medicine procedures consist of administering a drug containing a radioactive tracer to the patient. This radiopharmaceutical localizes in an organ or a system. The gamma rays emitted by the radioisotope within the patient can be detected externally by scanners, cameras, or probes. In vitro procedures entail adding the radiopharmaceutical to the patient's blood, urine, or fecal material to determine the amount of a specific substance present.

The basic difference between roentgenology and nuclear medicine procedures, relative to radiation safety, is that the source of radiation in x-rays is the vacuum tube within the x-ray machine while the source in nuclear medicine procedures is the patient. For this reason, nuclear medicine images are sometimes referred to as emission images, while x-ray images are sometimes referred to as transmission images.

Several factors affect the amount of radiation an individual will receive on exposure, and each factor must be taken into consideration when one is caring for a patient undergoing a procedure involving radioactive material.

The *amount* of radioactivity present is the first factor that should be considered. It varies according to the specific radioactive material utilized and the dose being administered.

The second factor is the *distance* of the individual from the radiation source. Distance protects in two ways: absorption and scattering by air and attenuation by geometry (i.e. the shape and form that make up the distance). The intensity of a radiation field is inversely proportional to the distance between the source and the observer.

The *time* spent in actual contact with the source of radiation is the third factor affecting the amount of radiation exposure. Exposure to radiation over a year should not exceed 0.5 rad or 500 millirads. It is regulation that a person receive no more than 2 millirads a day. The amount of radiation present and the distance from the source are variables that affect allowable exposure time. It is important to stress that radiation is cumulative.

The fourth factor is the degree of *shielding* utilized. Shielding is chosen according to the type of radiation: alpha, beta, or gamma. The effective distance between a source and a worker can be increased by using an absorbing shield between them, thus allowing one to work closer to the source with negligible increase in risk. The exact attenuation nature of shielding depends on the nature of the radiation.

Several methods are utilized in measurement of the amount of radiation a worker has been exposed to. The two most frequently seen in the clinical area are the pocket dosimeter and the film badge. The pocket dosimeter is usually calibrated in roentgens or subunits of it. Essentially it is a charge-measuring electroscope. The film badge measures beta, gamma, and x-radiation exposures. It consists of a plastic holder that contains a wrapped piece of radiation-sensitive film. When the film is developed, it compares the worker's exposure film to standard film that has been exposed to various calibrated radiation doses. The worker's total exposure can then be determined. All persons involved in caring for the patient(s) should have their own film badge or pocket dosimeter. It is usually worn for a one-month period. It should be worn at the waist at all times while in the clinical area; the worker, however, should not wear the badge home.

RADIOPHARMACEUTICAL RADIATION SAFETY PRECAUTIONS _____

Objectives

1. To identify nursing responsibility related to safe care of the patient undergoing a nuclear medicine procedure.
2. To provide a safe environment for the nurse and patient after completion of the procedure.

Procedure

ACTION	RATIONALE
1. Wear the film badge at waist level.	1. The amounts of radioactive substances contained in diagnostic doses of radiopharmaceuticals are very small.

ACTION	RATIONALE
	Lead shields are therefore not necessary. The amount of radiation exposure must be recorded, however, and the film badge should be placed at the position closest to the patient.
2. Wear rubber gloves when disposing of urine during the first 24 hours following a nuclear medicine procedure.	2. Technetium (half-life 6 hours) is excreted via the kidneys. The half-life of thallium is 73 hours and of gallium, 78 hours.
3. Wash hands before and after removing the gloves.	3. The chance of internal contamination is avoided.
4. Provide soap and water for patient to wash his hands thoroughly after he handles his urine.	4. This avoids undue internal contamination for the patient.

Precautions

1. If pregnant, curtail *immediate contact* with a patient for 24 hours after the patient has undergone a nuclear medicine procedure.
2. Wear only the assigned film badge.

Nuclear Medicine Terms

Blood-pooling scanning. A nuclear medicine procedure utilizing technetium-99m human serum albumin for differentiation between diffuse left ventricular hypokinesis and a potentially large aneurysm and assessing the severity of right ventricular dysfunction.

Decay, radioactive. Spontaneous emission of charged particles from an unstable nucleus.

Dose. The radiation delivered to a specified region.

Half-life, biologic. The time required for the body to eliminate, through biologic processes, one half of a given amount of a radioactive substance that has been introduced into it.

Half-life, effective. The reduced half-life due to the combination of physical decay and biologic elimination.

Half-life, physical. The time required for the radioactive material to be reduced to 50% of its initial activity by natural radioactive decay.

Infarct scintigraphy. A nuclear medicine procedure that utilizes technetium-99m pyrophosphate, an infarct-avid radiopharmaceutical used in the diagnosis of acute myocardial infarction.

Irradiate. To subject to the action of x-ray or other rays from a radioactive substance for diagnostic or therapeutic purposes.

Isotope. An element that has the same chemical properties and same atomic number as another, but a different atomic weight, and in the case of radioisotopes, different radioactive behavior.

Lung profusion scan. A nuclear medicine procedure that delineates areas in which pulmonary arterial circulation is deficient. It is useful in patients with suspected pulmonary embolism.

Myocardial perfusion imaging. A nuclear medicine procedure using thallous chloride, an analogue of potassium, effective in evaluating regional myocardial perfusion.

RAD. The unit of measurement of the absorbed dose of radiation.

Radioactivity. The property of emitting rays or particles of matter as a result of nuclear disintegration. The rays can pass through various substances opaque to light rays and produce certain chemical and electrical effects.

Radiopharmaceutical. A drug that has been tagged with a radioactive element.

Renal scan. A nuclear medicine scan that provides visualization of the urinary tract. It is useful in detecting renal infarction and renal atherosclerosis or trauma and in monitoring rejection of a transplanted kidney.

Scan. A scintigram. The developed film of a nuclear medicine diagnostic procedure.

Tracer (radioactive). A radioactive isotope, capable of being incorporated into compounds, which when introduced into the body "tags" a specific portion of the molecule so that its course may be traced.

REFERENCES

Chandra, R.: Introductory Physics of Nuclear Medicine. Philadelphia, Lea & Febiger, 1982.
Kinney, E., et al.: Nuclear Cardiology. Philadelphia Med. *75*:57–61, 1979.

PORTABLE X-RAY RADIATION SAFETY PRECAUTIONS

Objectives

1. To provide a safe environment for the nurse while the patient is undergoing a portable x-ray procedure in the clinical unit.
2. To insure the safety of other patients in the clinical area.

Procedure

ACTION	RATIONALE
1. Provide safe distance for other patients in the vicinity during x-ray. If necessary, separate with a lead shield.	1. This will prevent undue radiation exposure.
2. Stand behind camera while the x-ray is being taken.	2. The source of radiation is the vacuum tube. An appropriate distance must be maintained to avoid undue radiation exposure.
3. Wear lead-lined apron if you must stay with patient during the x-ray.	3. Lead has a high atomic number and will absorb the x-rays.
4. Wear the film badge on your collar while wearing the lead apron.	4. The lead apron will cover the waist and RADS will not be recorded.

Precautions

1. If pregnant, do not stay with patient while x-rays are being completed.
2. See precautions for Nuclear Medicine Procedures.

Radiology Terms

Radiation dose rate. The amount of radiation delivered per unit time.

RAD. The unit of measurement of the absorbed dose of radiation.

Roentgen rays. Forms of electromagnetic energy that travel at the speed of light but have considerably shorter wave lengths. This property enables the radiation to penetrate organs and tissues according to density and thickness.

See "Nuclear Medicine Terms."

REFERENCES

Harvey, A. M., et al.: The Principles and Practice of Medicine, 20th ed. New York, Appleton-Century-Crofts, 1980.
Thompson, T.: Primer of Clinical Radiology, 2nd ed. Boston, Little, Brown, and Company, 1980.

11

ORGAN
DONATION

ORGAN DONATION

Peggy J. Reiley, R.N., M.S.

Overview

In the past few years, registries have been established to keep statistics on all organ transplants. Kidney transplants have constituted the largest number, followed in frequency by heart, liver, lung, and pancreas transplants. In addition, corneas, bone, and skin are transplanted frequently.

Critical care nurses play a vital role in facilitating organ donation by recognizing potential organ donors. This section will deal mainly with kidney donation, since it is the organ transplanted most often. Although the donation of tissues such as eyes, skin, and bone will not be presented in detail, reference will be made when appropriate.

Since 1970 all 50 states have adopted a form of the Uniform Anatomical

'Renew a life 30'   UNIFORM DONOR CARD

Please fill out and carry this card with you at all times.

of _____

(Print or type name of donor)

In the hope that I may help others, I hereby make this anatomical gift, if medically acceptable, to take effect upon my death. The words and marks below indicate my desires.

For the purpose of transplantation, therapy, medical research or education, I give:

(U)____Any Needed Organs or Parts

(KE)___Kidneys and Eyes Only

(K)____Kidneys Only

(E)____Eyes Only

Limitations or special wishes, if any:_____

_____

Figure 11-1 Both sides of a Uniform Donor Card.

Signed by the donor and the following two witnesses in the presence of each other:

DATE SIGNED   DATE OF BIRTH OF DONOR

STREET

CITY   STATE

SIGNATURE OF DONOR

WITNESS

WITNESS

This is a legal document under the Uniform Anatomical Gift Act or similar laws.

Gift Act. This act legally provides anyone above the age of 18 with the right to indicate willingness to become an organ donor at the time of death. This intent is made known in the form of a signed document, witnessed by two people. This is called a uniform donor card (Fig. 11–1). In many states laws have been passed whereby the intent to become an organ donor can be indicated on the driver's license. The Uniform Anatomical Gift Act also authorizes the next of kin to donate useful organs.

RECOGNIZING POTENTIAL ORGAN DONORS _____

Objective

To facilitate organ donation by recognizing potential donors and respecting medicolegal parameters.

Procedure

ACTION	RATIONALE
1. Legal evaluation: A. Ascertain if written permission has been obtained for donation of organs by potential donor or next of kin. (1) Determine if donor has signed a uniform donor card with signature of two witnesses, all of whom were over the age of 18 when the signing took place. (2) Establish next of kin priority for authorization as follows: (a) Spouse (b) Adult son or daughter (c) Either parent (d) Adult brother or sister (3) Utilize hospital-approved form or form provided by the organ bank. B. Ascertain if Medical Examiner's permission has been obtained for use of organs, when appropriate.	A. To remove tissues or organs, appropriate permission must be obtained. B. The Medical Examiner's permission for the donation of organs is necessary if death occurs within 24 hours of admission to the hos-

ACTION	RATIONALE
	pital; as the result of an accident, a homicide, or suicide, or any other unnatural cause; or following a critical event in the hospital.
2. Medical evaluation: A. Note age of potential donor.	A. There are upper age limits for organ donation. In most instances the maximum age for kidney donation is 65 years; donation of tissue such as bone also has age limits. However, age does not usually interfere with eye donation.
B. Assess health history for any pre-existing disease processes of potential donor, particularly history of: (1) Renal disease (2) Hypertension (3) Diabetes mellitus (4) Malignant disease (5) Hepatitis	B. The existence of any of these disease processes may interfere with the donation of kidneys (with the exception of a primary brain tumor in the case of malignant disease).
C. Assess for presence of infection or infectious process of potential donor; if sepsis is suspected, obtain cultures.	C. Known infection or septicemia interferes with all types of organ donation owing to potential for transmitting the infectious process to the recipient of the graft.
D. Confirm renal status of potential kidney donor by having following laboratory tests performed: (1) BUN (2) Creatinine (3) Urinalysis (4) SMA 6 (5) Blood type (6) Urine and blood culture	
E. Confirm neurologic status of potential kidney donor, ascertaining pronouncement of death according to standard medical practice.	E. When pronounced dead on the basis of neurologic evidence, the donor can be taken to the operating room for organ removal.
F. Assist in control of warm ischemia. (1) Maximum amount of time that kidneys can withstand warm ischemia (absence of	F. Cardiopulmonary support continues during this time despite pronouncement of death to prevent warm ischemia of the donor organ.

ACTION	RATIONALE
blood flow in a warm body) and still function successfully when transplanted is 60 minutes.	
(2) Neurologic death is not necessary for tissue donations such as eyes, skin, or bone. These tissues can withstand a much longer warm ischemia time.	

3. Alert organ bank or transplant center in local area when medical and legal evaluation is accomplished and patient is recognized as a potential donor.

Precautions

1. Evaluate the patient's legal status as a potential organ donor: When a driver's license is coded to indicate that a person is an organ donor, this is not sufficient data to remove the organs legally; the signature of the donor and of two witnesses, or the signature of the next of kin, is required legally.
2. Declaration of brain death is made according to standard medical practice. More than half of the states have adopted legislation recognizing brain death. In states in which there is no such legislation, the concept has already been upheld when specific cases have been presented to the courts.

Related Care

Contact the transplant center or organ bank in the local area regarding organ protocols, information, or questions.

Complications

Medical
Legal

REFERENCES

AMA 1980 Interim Meeting Report: Organ donation and transplantation. J. Tenn. Med. Assoc., 74:7 507–515, 1981.

Davis, F.D.: Current strategies in the procurement of cadaveric kidneys for transplantation. Nurs. Clin. North Am., *16*:565–571, 1981.

Romeo, K.C., and Abbott, N.K.: Facilitating organ donation. J. Emerg.Nurs., 4:35–36, (July–Aug.), 1978.

Stuart, F.P., Veith, F.J., and Cranford, R.E.: Brain death laws and patterns of consent to remove organs for transplantation from cadavers in the United States and 28 other countries. Transplantation, *31:*238–244 (Apr.), 1981.

FACILITATING ORGAN DONATION _____

Objectives

1. To support the person/family who is considering organ donation.
2. To ensure that the organ for donation is in optimum physiologic condition to maintain homeostasis and perfusion of the kidneys.
3. To protect the organ against potential infectious processes.

Procedure

ACTION	RATIONALE
1. Provide psychologic support to the family and, when appropriate, the patient when discussing organ donation. A. Approach of the individuals is best done by someone they know and trust. B. Maintain sensitivity to and concern for the family's grief. C. Ascertain if family understands the concept of brain death and the hopelessness of the donor's condition. D. Explain to the family that organs will be removed in the operating room; there will be no visible evidence that organs have been removed; there will be no charge to them for organ removal. E. Support the family or patient or both in their decision regarding donation.	1. Accurate knowledge about transplantation will aid in supporting the family or patient or both.
2. Maintain strict sterile technique: be alert to sources of contamination such as vascular invasive techniques, catheter, tracheotomy, or wounds.	2. Development of an infectious process could, in many instances, eliminate the possibility of the patient's being an acceptable organ donor.

ACTION	RATIONALE
3. Maintain an hourly urinary output with a minimum volume of 50 to 100 ml. with the use of IV therapy. Suggested therapy includes 5% dextrose in Ringer's lactate alternating with 5% dextrose in water. Titrate at a rate equal to the last hour's urine output plus 50 ml. Maintain electrolyte balance in standard fashion.	3. Urinary output of 50 ml. or more is a good indication that the kidneys are being well perfused.
4. Maintain systolic blood pressure at a level that will provide a urinary output of 50 ml. or more. Generally this will be maintained when the blood pressure is approximately 100 mm. Hg.	4. Prolonged hypotension will result in decreased urinary output and subsequent poor renal perfusion.
5. If, after vigorous hydration, adequate perfusion cannot be maintained, consider use of these vasopressors, in order of perference: A. Dopamine (Intropin) B. Isoproterenol (Isuprel) C. Metaraminol bitartrate (Aramine) D. Levarterenol bitartrate (Levophed)	5. Intropin and Isuprel, although they are vasoconstrictors, do not decrease renal blood flow, whereas Aramine and Levophed have this effect.
6. Consider using mannitol or furosemide (Lasix) if an adequate output of 50 to 100 ml./hour or more cannot be maintained despite sufficient volume replacement and adequate blood pressure.	6. An adequate urinary output is necessary to provide protection against acute tubular necrosis in the transplanted kidney.
7. Utilize a wetting solution and tape eyelids closed if the patient is an eye donor.	7. This protects the corneas from drying and being abraded.
8. Maintain body temperature between 97° and 102° F.	8. This prevents possible damage to the kidneys from hyperthermia or hypothermia.
9. Avoid the use of nephrotoxic drugs if possible.	9. This prevents possible damage to the kidneys.
10. Utilize vasopressin (Pitressin) 5 to 10 units IV or subcutaneously every 2 to 4 hours.	10. This prevents acute tubular necrosis from dehydration.

Precautions

If adequate renal perfusion cannot be maintained, a rise in the levels of BUN and creatinine may make the patient an unacceptable donor.

Related Care

1. Consult the transplantation center (24-hour availability) for specific protocols.
2. Obtain a physician's written order for initiating select protocol in maintaining homeostasis and kidney perfusion to facilitate organ donation.

Complications

Infection
Altered renal perfusion
Acute tubular necrosis

REFERENCES

AMA 1980 Interim Meeting Report: Organ donation and transplantation. J. Tenn. Med. Assoc., 74:7, 507–515, 1981.
Davis, F.D.: Current strategies in the procurement of cadaveric kidneys for transplantation. Nurs. Clin. North Am., 16:565–571, 1981.
Romeo, K.C., and Abbott, N.K.: Facilitating organ donation. J. Emerg. Nurs., 4:35–36, (July-Aug.), 1978.
Stuart, F.P., Veith, F.J., and Cranford, R.E.: Brain death laws and patterns of consent to remove organs for transplantation from cadavers in the United States and 28 other countries. Transplantation, 31:238–244, (Apr.), 1981.

ORGAN PREPARATION _____

Objectives

1. To continue oxygenation and perfusion of the organ.
2. To anticipate and provide medications that may be necessary in organ preparation for subsequent donation.

Special Equipment

Portable oxygen tank
Portable ventilator

Bag/mask
Phenoxybenzamine hydrochloride (Dibenzyline), 100
   mg. (if available)
Methylprednisolone (Solu-Medrol), 1 gram
Heparin, 10,000 units

Procedure

ACTION	RATIONALE
1. Ascertain that donor has been pronounced dead according to neurologic criteria.	
2. Continue to maintain cadaver by ventilatory and blood pressure support until actual moment of organ removal.	2. Kidneys perfused and oxygenated until the moment of organ removal have less chance of developing acute tubular necrosis due to ischemia.
3. Prepare the following medications for anticipated use: A. Methylprednisolone (Solu-Medrol), 1 gram. B. Heparin, 10,000 units. C. Phenoxybenzamine hydrochloride (Dibenzylene), 100 mg. (if available).	3. Pretreatment of donors with select medications may have a subsequent beneficial effect on the transplanted kidney.
4. Optional: Once kidneys are removed from a donor, they may be placed on a perfusion machine on which they can be kept viable for up to 72 hours.	
5. Institute cardiopulmonary resuscitation and prepare for emergency surgery if donor suffers cardiac arrest while waiting for operation.	5. Every effort must be made to prevent warm ischemia.

Precautions

Obtain selected protocols, pharmacologic therapy, and plan of care for organ preparation from local transplant bank.

Related Care

If cardiac arrest should occur during the organ preparation phase, begin cardiopulmonary resuscitation immediately, transport donor to operating room, and assist in facilitating emergency nephrectomy.

Complications

Cardiac arrest
Infection
Tubular necrosis

REFERENCES

AMA 1980 Interim Meeting Report: Organ donation and transplantation. J. Tenn. Med. Assoc., 74:7 507–515, 1981.

Davis, F.D.: Current strategies in the procurement of cadaveric kidneys for transplantation. Nurs. Clin. North Am., 16:565–571, 1981.

Romeo, K.C., and Abbott, N.K.: Facilitating organ donation. J. Emerg. Nurs. 4:35–36 (July-Aug.), 1978.

Stuart, F.P., Veith, F.J., and Cranford, R.E.: Brain death laws and patterns of consent to remove organs for transplantation from cadavers in the United States and 28 other countries. Transplantation. 31:238–244, (Apr.), 1981.

APPENDIX: SAMPLE FLOW SHEETS AND LOGS

Appendix

MGH RESPIRATORY SURGICAL ICU

TUBE INFO.
TYPE: _____
SIZE: _____
Date Inserted: _____
Date To Change: ___

CXR READING

CULTURES
BLOOD ___ __ ____
SPUTUM ____ ____
URINE ____ ____
OTHER ____

MISC. CHEM.

Line	Vent	Cuff Pressure cc. in Cuff	Position of Pt.	Vent. Tidal Volume	Resp. Rate	Peak I.P.	PEEP	T.V. Spon / I.F. / V.C.	FIO₂	PaO₂	PaCO₂	PH	Na / K	Hgb / Hct.	Blood Sugar	Tp. / Osm	Bun / Creat	CA.	Pt. / Con-trol	Ptt. / Plt. ×1000	WBC	Time	Temp.
A																							
B																							
C																							
D																							
E																							
F																							
G																							
H																							
I																							
J																							
K																							
L																							
M																							
N																							
O																							
P																							
Q																							
R																							
S																							
T																							
U																							
V																							
W																							
X																							
Y																							
Z																							

Appendix A. Respiratory Surgical Intensive Care Unit Flow Sheet. (Printed with permission of the Department of Nursing, Massachusetts General Hospital, Boston, MA.)

Illustration continues on the following page.

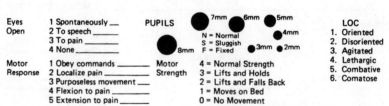

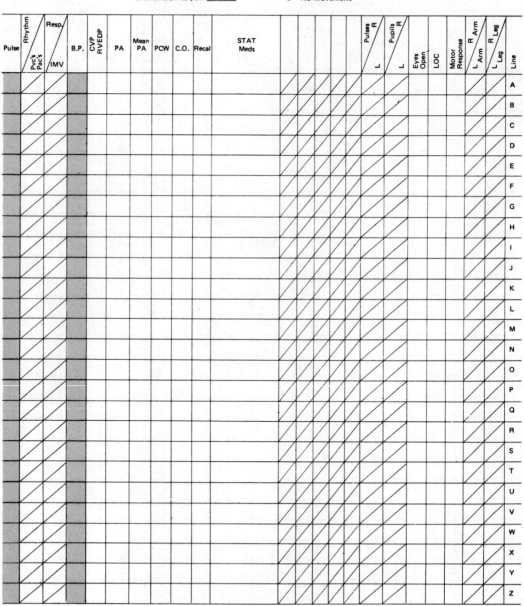

Appendix A.   *Continued*

Lines	Date inserted	Position

Today's Date: _____

Diagnosis:

Admission Date _____ / Op Date

Allergies:

ADDRESSOGRAPH PLATE

INTAKE

Line	SITE:	SITE:	SITE:	SITE:	CC's I.V. Meds.	Blood	Colloid	Flushes	Tube Feed ings	ASP.	P.O.	INTAKE TOTAL
A												
B												
C												
D												
E												
F												
G												
H												
I												
J												
K												
L												
M												
N												
O												
P												
Q												
R												
S												
T												
U												
V												
W												
X												
Y												
Z												

Appendix A. *Continued*

Illustration continues on the following page.

Total Intake   Total Output

2 P.M. _____   _____

10 P.M. _____   _____

6 A.M. _____   _____

OUTPUT

Time	OUTPUT TOTAL	Urine Total	Sugar / Acetone	Urine lytes NA / K	OSM / Sp.Gr.	Chest Tube #1	#2	#3	N.G. Tube				Admission Data Nursing Observations

Appendix A. *Concluded*

NS-2729 Rev. 8/81 (page 1)
(side 1)

THE WILLIAMSPORT HOSPITAL
INTENSIVE CARE UNIT FLOW SHEET

BEGINNING DATE:_____

POST-OPERATIVE DAY#_____

HOSPITAL DAY:_____

INTAKE-OUTPUT RECORD

INTAKE	7 - 3	3 - 11	11 - 7	24 HR. TOTAL	COMMENTS
IV FLUIDS:					
ORAL					
TUBE FEEDING					
IRRIGATION					
TOTAL					
OUTPUT					
URINE					
EMESIS					
N / G DRAINAGE					
CHEST DRAINAGE					
TOTAL					
STOOL					

TREAT MENTS	7 A	8 A	9 A	10 A	11 A	12 N	1 P	2 P	3 P	4 P	5 P	6 P	7 P	8 P	9 P	10 P	11 P	12 MN	1 A	2 A	3 A	4 A	5 A	6 A

SPECIFIC CARE/ACTIVITY	SUGAR/ ACETONE		OCCULT BLOOD				URINE SPECIFIC GRAVITY	
				7-3	3-11	11-7		
			URINE				7-3	
			BM				3-11	
			EMESIS				11-7	
			N/G					
							Wt: _____ Kg.	

Appendix B. Intensive care unit flow sheet. (Printed with permission of the Department of Nursing, The Williamsport Hospital, Williamsport, PA.)

Illustration continues on the following page.

NS-2729 Rev. 8/81 (page 1)
(side 2)

TIME	TEMP	PULSE	RESP	RHYTHM	CUFF BP	ART BP/ ART MEAN	PA SYST/ DIAS.	RA MEAN	AVO$_2$/ C.O.	URINE OUTPUT	CHEST DRAIN

Appendix B. *Continued*

NS-2729 Rev. 8/81 (page 2)

TIME	PUPILS		MOVEMENT OF EXTREMITIES				THE WILLIAMSPORT HOSPITAL DATE			IV INFUSIONS			
	R	L	RA	RL	LA	LL	Level of Consciousness	ICP	Ventric Drainage	TIME			

Appendix B.   *Continued*

Illustration continues on the following page.

NS-2729 Rev. 8/81 (page 3)
(side 1)

THE WILLIAMSPORT HOSPITAL
NURSES NOTES

DATE:_____

TIME		TIME	

Appendix B.   *Continued*

NURSES NOTES

NS-2729 Rev. 8/81 (page 3)
(side 2)

TIME		TIME			
		7-3			
		3-11			
		11-7			

Appendix B. *Concluded*

FORM NO. NR 1680 Rev. 11/80

MONTEFIORE HOSPITAL AND MEDICAL CENTER

CRITICAL CARE NURSING FLOW SHEET

DATE

DIAGNOSIS

DATE OF PROCEDURE

DRUG ALLERGY

R.N.'s NAME 7 A.M.

R.N.'s NAME 3 P.M.

R.N.'s NAME 11 P.M.

TIME	8 AM	9 AM	10 AM	11 AM	12 PM	1 PM	2 PM	3 PM	4 PM	5 PM	6 PM	7 PM	8 PM	9 PM	10 PM	11 PM	12 AM	1 AM	2 AM	3 AM	4 AM	5 AM	6 AM	7 AM
TEMP.																								
AP																								
RHYTHM/ PVC APC																								

BLOOD PRESSURE — 240, 230, 220, 210, 200, 190, 180, 170, 160, 150, 140, 130, 120, 110, 100, 90, 80, 70, 60, 50, 40, 30

RESP. RATE

CVP

PA PRESS

PCWP

IABP RATIO

CALIBRATION

gtts/mg

gtts/mcg

gtts/mcg

gtts/mcg

Hct

Appendix C. Critical care nursing flow sheet. (Printed with permission of the Department of Nursing, Moses Division, Montefiore Medical Center, Bronx, N.Y.)

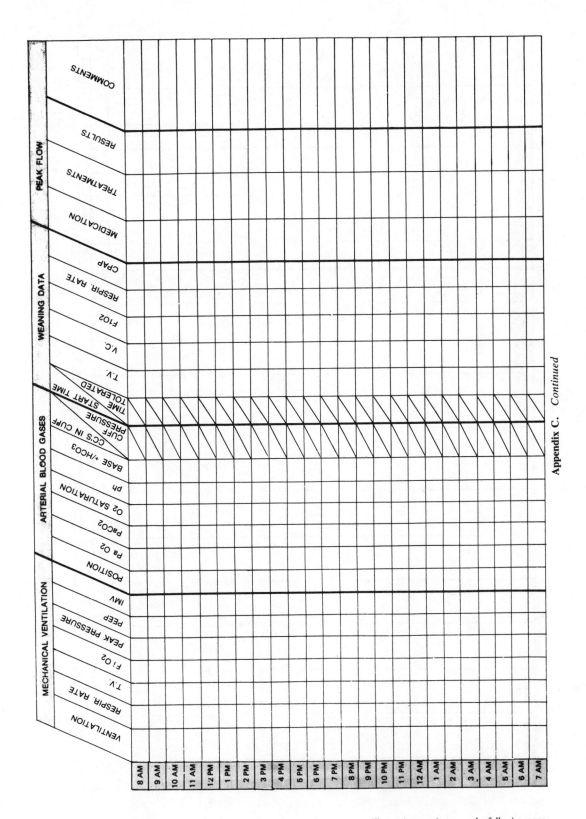

Appendix C.   *Continued*

Illustration continues on the following page.

INTAKE								OUTPUT											
								URINE					DRAINS / TUBES						
TIME	LIQUID P.O	SOLID P.O.				ALBUMIN / BLOOD	TOTAL	DIURETICS	HRLY	SPEC. GRAV.	G & A	Insulin							TOTAL
8 AM																			
9 AM																			
10 AM																			
11 AM																			
12 PM																			
1 PM																			
2 PM																			
3 PM																			
4 PM																			
5 PM																			
6 PM																			
7 PM																			
8 PM																			
9 PM																			
10 PM																			
11 PM																			
12 AM																			
1 AM																			
2 AM																			
3 AM																			
4 AM																			
5 AM																			
6 AM																			
7 AM																			

24 HOUR TOTAL				24 HOUR TOTAL		
TOTAL PARENTERAL	TOTAL BLOOD	TOTAL ORAL INTAKE	TOTAL INTAKE	TOTAL URINE OUTPUT	TOTAL DRAIN OUTPUT	TOTAL OUTPUT

Appendix C. *Continued*

EKG RHYTHM _____ LEAD _____ TIME _____

EKG RHYTHM _____ LEAD _____ TIME _____

EKG RHYTHM _____ LEAD _____ TIME _____

LABORATORY DATA

TIME

TIME →												
TEST NAME →	RESULTS											
HGB												
HCT												
WBC												
PLATELETS												
P.T.												
SODIUM												
POTASSIUM												
CHLORIDE												
BICARB. (CO2)												
GLUCOSE												
BUN												
CREATININE												
T. PROTEIN												
SGOT												
SGPT												
LDH												
CPK												
ALK. PHOSPH.												
AMYLASE												
CALCIUM												

Appendix C. *Concluded*

THE WILLIAMSPORT HOSPITAL
CRITICAL CARE FLOW SHEET

8 HR. TOTALS	INTAKE		OUTPUT				WEIGHT	
	P.O.	I.V.	URINE	N.G.	OTHER	STOOL	Yesterday	Today

DATE		TIME																Time	NURSE'S NOTES

VITAL SIGNS
- TEMP
- PULSE
- RESP
- CUFF BP
- ART BP
- ART MEAN

HEMODYNAMIC
- PA Sys / Dias
- PA MEAN
- RA MEAN
- AVO_2/CO

I.V. INTAKE
- ORAL
- GRAND TOTAL

OUTPUT
- URINE
- Specific Gravity
- Sugar and Acetone
- N/G Drainage
- STOOL
- OTHER
- TOTAL

MEDS

VENT
- FIO_2
- Tidal Volume
- RATE
- PEEP
- Inflation Pressure

LAB DATA

PO_2	O_2 Sat
PCO_2	PH
Bicarb	Hgb
K	CL
NA	BS
Bun	Creat

CARE NURSE SIGNATURE

Appendix D. Critical care flow sheet. (Printed with permission of the Department of Nursing, The Williamsport Hospital, Williamsport, PA.)

ST. JOSEPH'S HOSPITAL
5000 West Chambers Street
Milwaukee, Wisconsin 53210

ICU
LAB WORK SHEET

Date																								
Time																								
Glucose 65-110																								
Bun 10-20																								
Na 135-145																								
Cl 95-105																								
CO_2 24-32																								
Kt 3.5-5																								
Creatinine 0.4-1.5																								
Calcium 8.5-10.5																								
Phosphorous 2.5-4.9																								
Magnesium 1.8-2.4																								
Total Protein 6-8																								
Albumin 3.5-5																								
CPK 50-160																								
Ldh 100-225																								
Hgb/Hct 11.5-15.5/35-47																								
Wbc 5-10																								
Platelets $150-400 \times 10^9$																								
Digoxin 0.9-2.0																								
Theophylline 10-20																								

NOT A PERMANENT PART OF THE CHART
ICU LAB WORK SHEET

Appendix E.   Laboratory Work Sheet. (Printed with permission of the Department of Nursing, St. Joseph's Hospital, Milwaukee, WI.)

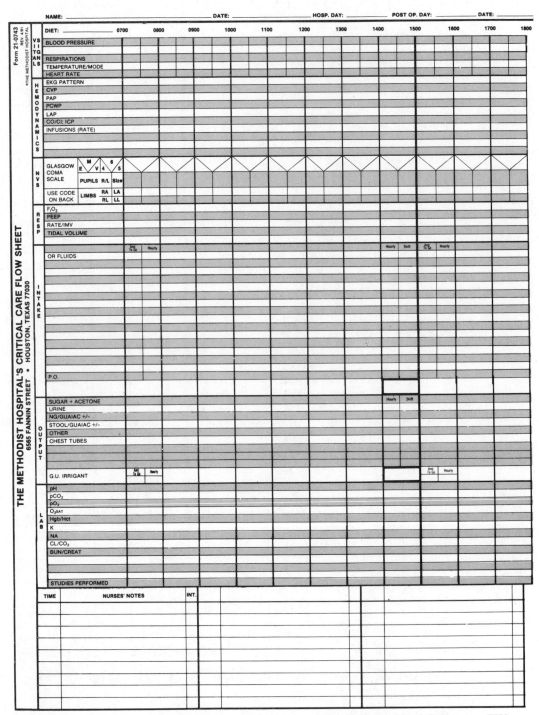

Appendix F.   Critical care flow sheet. (Printed with permission of The Methodist Hospital, Houston, TX.)

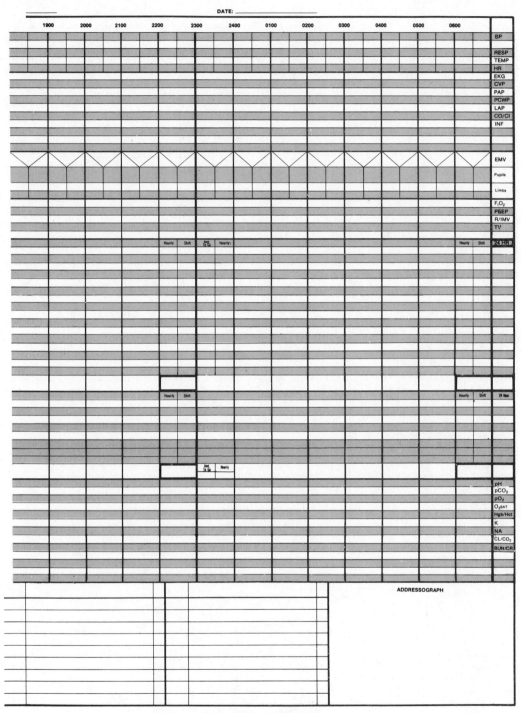

Appendix F. *Continued*

Illustration continues on the following page.

NAME: _____ DATE: _____

TIME	NURSES' NOTES	INT.	TIME	NURSES' NOTES	INT.	TIME	NURSES' NOTES	INT.

Appendix F. *Continued*

DATE: _____   ALLERGIES: _____

MEDICATIONS	7-3	3-11	11-7	NEURO STATUS

PUPILS

+ Reactive   – Nonreactive   ± Sluggish

PUPIL GAUGE (MM)
2 3 4 5 6 7 8 9

GLASGOW COMA SCALE

Eyes	Open	Spontaneously	4
		To verbal command	3
		To pain	2
	No response		1
Best motor response	To verbal command	Obeys	6
	To painful stimulus*	Localizes pain	5
		Flexion—withdrawal	4
		Flexion—abnormal (decorticate rigidity)	3
		Extension (decerebrate rigidity)	2
		No response	1
Best verbal response**		Oriented and converses	5
		Disoriented and converses	4
		Inappropriate words	3
		Incomprehensible sounds	2
		No response	1
Total			3-15

CHARTING CODE: EXTREMITIES

MOVEMENT	ABBREVIATIONS	STRENGTH
Voluntary	V	+ Strong
Command	C	– Weak
Stim (Purposeful)	S	Ø Absent
Withdraws	W	
None	Ø	
Decorticate	Decor.	
Decerebrate	Decer.	

INT.	FULL SIGNATURE	TITLE

TREATMENTS / **TREATMENTS**

ARTERIAL SITE CARE
PRESSURE MONITORING SOLUTION CHANGED
PRESSURE MONITORING SYSTEM CHANGED
BATH
I.D. BAND
IV SITE CARE
IV SYSTEM CHANGE
ORAL HYGIENE
PULMONARY PT.
BAG & SUCTION
IPPB/USM
ENDOTRACHEAL TUBE POSITION CHANGE
FOLEY CATH. CARE
G.U. IRRIGANT SYSTEM CHANGE
POSITION CHANGE
BED GROUNDED/WHEELS LOCKED
SUCTION CANISTER & TUBING CHANGE
SUCTION CANISTER WASH
HYPERTHERMIA BLANKET

ADDRESSOGRAPH

Appendix F. *Concluded*

ICU HEMODYNAMIC ASSESSMENT FLOW SHEET
PART A

ST. JOSEPH'S HOSPITAL
5000 West Chambers Street
Milwaukee Wisconsin 53210

DATE		15	30	45		15	30	45		15	30	45		15	30	45		15	30	45		15	30	45		15	30	45		15	30	45

SYSTOLIC V
DIASTOLIC ∧
PULSE ●

GLASGOW COMA
SCALE AND
NEURO KEY ON BACK
RN SIGNATURE

(Graph grid range: 250, 240, 230, 220, 210, 200, 190, 180, 170, 160, 150, 140, 130, 120, 110, 100, 90, 80, 70, 60, 50, 40, 30, 20, 10)

MEDICATIONS
(CONTINUOUS
INFUSION)

TEMPERATURE

RESPIRATIONS

VENTILATOR SETTINGS	F_IO_2%
	TIDAL VOLUME/MODE
	RATE/PEEP

PRESSURES	CVP
	PAS PAD
	PAM PCW
	CARDIAC OUTPUT
	MABP
	ICP
	CPP

NEURO-LOGICAL STATUS	LOC
	ORIENTATION
	PUPIL — SIZE R
	PUPIL — REACTION R
	PUPIL — SIZE L
	PUPIL — REACTION L

MOTOR FUNCTION	RUE
	RLE
	LUE
	LLE

GLASGOW

FORM 1817X 7/83

ICU HEMODYNAMIC ASSESSMENT FLOWSHEET - PART A

Appendix G. Hemodynamic assessment flow sheet. (Printed with permission of the Department of Nursing, St. Joseph's Hospital, Milwaukee, WI.)

<u>Neurological Check Code</u>

Pupil Size:	1mm	2mm	3mm	4mm	5mm	6mm	7mm	8mm

Pupil Reaction: + Reactive   o Non-Reactive   S Sluggish

Level of Consciousness:

      A – Alert: Normal
      D – Drowsy: Follows commands correctly when aroused,
                  intermittently
      S – Stuporous: Arouses to painfull stimuli
      C – Comatose: No response to pain or commands

Orientation:

      O: Patient is oriented to person, place and time.
      P: Patient is oriented to person.
      P1: Patient is oriented to place.
      T: Patient is oriented to time.
      D: Patient is disoriented to person, place and time.

Motor Function: 6 – Spontaneous   5 – Command   4 – Appropriate withdrawal
                  3 – Flexor   2 – Extensor   1 – None

<u>Glasgow Coma Scale</u>

<u>Key</u>

Eyes Open
    4 Spontaneously   c – eyes closed by
    3 To speech   swelling
    2 To Pain
    1 None

Best Verbal Response
    5 Oriented & converses   T – e.t. tube/trach tube
    4 Disoriented & converses
    3 Inappropriate words
    2 Incomprehensible sounds
    1 None

Best Motor Response

To verbal command: 6 Obeys commands
To painful stimulus: 5 Localizes pain
                    4 Flexion – withdrawal
                    3 Flexion – abnormal (decorticate rigidity)
                    2 Extension (decerebrate rigidity)
                    1 None

Appendix G.   *Continued*

Illustration continues on the following page.

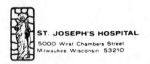

ST. JOSEPH'S HOSPITAL
5000 West Chambers Street
Milwaukee, Wisconsin 53210

ICU HEMODYNAMIC ASSESSMENT FLOW SHEET
PART B

USE BLANK SPACES FOR ADDITIONAL ASSESSMENTS

DATE		TIME	TIME	HOUR								
				ORAL								
		DESCRIBE	DESCRIBE	TOTAL								
NEURO MENTAL STATUS				NG								
				TOTAL								

CARDIOVASCULAR STATUS	RHYTHM					
	HEART SOUNDS			IV's		AMOUNT INFUSED
	NECK VEINS					
	RADIAL PULSES					
	PEDAL PULSES					
	CAPILLARY REFILL TIME					8 HR. SUBTOTAL
	CALF TENDERNESS			BLOOD PRODUCTS		AMOUNT INFUSED
	COLOR/TEMP					
	EDEMA					
						8 HR. SUBTOTAL

PULMONARY	RESP. PATTERN			HOUR								
				URINE								
	BREATH SOUNDS			TOTAL								
				CHEST T								
	SPUTUM			TOTAL								
				CHEST T								
				TOTAL								
				NG								
				TOTAL								

GI	ABDOMEN			DRAIN								
				TOTAL								
	BOWEL SOUNDS			DRAIN								
	NG			TOTAL								
	APPETITE											
				24 HR. INTAKE SUBTOTALS				24 HR. OUTPUT SUBTOTALS				

GU	URINE			
	SPECIFIC GRAVITY			

INTEGUMENTARY	INTEGRITY			
	INCISIONS			SPECIMENS
	DRESSING			SIGNATURE OF RN

FORM 1818X 7/83

ICU HEMODYNAMIC ASSESSMENT FLOW SHEET - PART B

Appendix G. *Concluded*

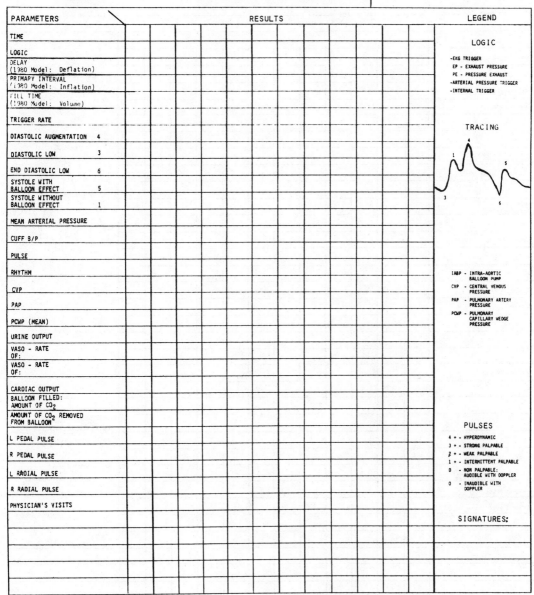

D-8   INTRA·AORTIC BALLOON PUMP FLOW SHEET

Appendix H.   Intra-aortic balloon pump flow sheet. (Printed with permission of the Department of Nursing, St. Luke's Hospital, Cedar Rapids, IA.)

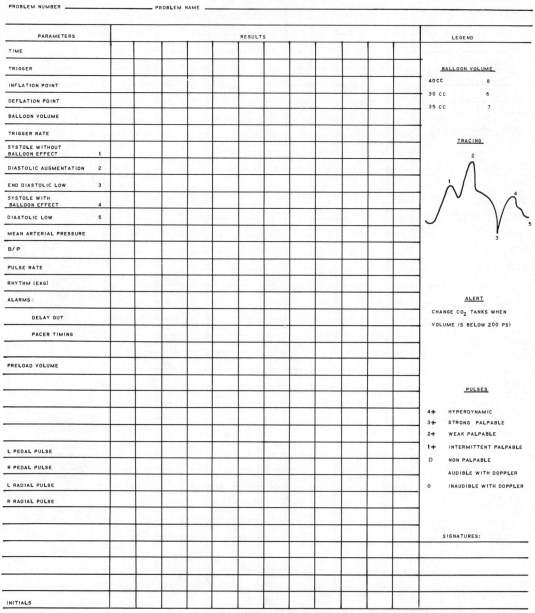

Appendix I.   Intra-aortic balloon pump flow sheet. (Printed with permission of the Department of Nursing, St. Joseph's Hospital, Milwaukee, WI.)

Date   :_____.

Surgeon:_____

Doctor :_____

IABP
FLOW SHEET

MERCY HEALTH CENTER
Dubuque, Iowa

00412

Insertion Date:_____   Removal Date:_____

Insertion Time:_____   Removal Time:_____

Insertion Site:_____   Balloon Size:_____

Time	Pump On/Auto	Trigger	Assist Interval	Rate	Art. Pressure Syst/Dias Mean	CVP	Urine	Meds	Comments/Alarms

Appendix J. Intra-aortic balloon pump flow sheet. (Printed with permission of Mercy Health Center, Dubuque, IA.)

ST. LUKE'S HOSPITAL
Cedar Rapids, Iowa

HEMODIALYSIS FLOWSHEET

Date_____   Treatment #_____   Dialysis_____   Ultrafiltration_____

Last Weight_____   Current Weight_____   Post Dialysis Weight_____

Pre HD Vitals_____   Post HD Vitals_____   Post Lab 508_____

Net Fluid Removal_____   Total Heparinization_____

Access_____   Bath K_____   Ca_____   Additives_____

Dialyzer_____   DFR_____   Cartridge_____

TIME	BP	P/R	BFR	AP	VP/DP	UF	FLUIDS	HEPARIN	ACT	COMMENTS

SIGNATURE:_____

Appendix K. Hemodialysis flow sheet. (Printed with permission of the Department of Nursing, St. Luke's Hospital, Cedar Rapids, IA.)

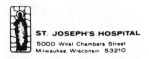

ST. JOSEPH'S HOSPITAL
5000 West Chambers Street
Milwaukee, Wisconsin 53210

HEMODIALYSIS
RECORD

DATE _____

HEMO RUN #	PRIME		DIALYZER				HEPARINIZATION		BATH	

MACHINE CHECKS

BLOOD LEAK	AIR DETECT	TEMP	CONDUCTIVITY	DFR	REJ RATE		WEIGHT PRE	WEIGHT POST	TIME ON	TIME OFF

TIME	BP	P	I/O	+	-	TMP	UF	BFR	SNA/V	HEPARIN	ACT	REMARKS

FORM 1498X REV. 9/82

HEMODIALYSIS RECORD

Appendix L.   Hemodialysis record. (Printed with permission of the Department of Nursing, St. Joseph's Hospital, Milwaukee, WI.)

METABOLIC ACIDOSIS FLOW SHEET

Diagnosis _____

Hourly Intake	0800	0900	1000	1100	1200	1300	1400	1500	8°	1600	1700	1800	1900	2000	2100	2200	2300	8°	2400	0100	0200	0300	0400	0500	0600	0700	8°
PO																											
Intravenous																											
8° Total Intake																											
Insulin																											
HCO₃																											
Output																											
Osmolarity																											
Urine Sugar																											
Acetone																											
Sp. Gr.																											
Na																											
K																											
Cl																											
CO²																											
Sugar																											
pH																											
Laboratory Tests BUN																											
Acetone																											
Lactic Level																											
Serum Osm.																											
Lac. Pyro Ratio																											
C.V.P.																											
Misc. Levin																											

24 Hour Intake   24 Hour Output

Nurse ☐   ☐

49-10-36   **D-5 METABOLIC ACIDOSIS FLOW SHEET**   070636

Appendix M.   Metabolic Acidosis flow sheet. (Printed with permission of the Department of Nursing, Mercy Hospital, Cedar Rapids, IA.)

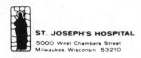

ST. JOSEPH'S HOSPITAL
5000 West Chambers Street
Milwaukee, Wisconsin 53210

PERITONEAL DIALYSIS FLOW SHEET

DIAGNOSIS 1			DIAGNOSIS 2				ABD. GIRTH	WEIGHT	DATE	

BOTTLE NO.	%	MEDICATION ADDED	TIMES SOLUTION IN			TIMES SOLUTION OUT			PATIENT VOLUME		OTHER REMARKS	INIT.
			START	FINISH	VOLUME	START	FINISH	VOLUME	+ OR −	CUM.		

INIT.	SIGNATURE	INIT.	SIGNATURE	INIT.	SIGNATURE

FORM 1313X REV. 9/80

PERITONEAL DIALYSIS FLOW SHEET

Appendix N.   Peritoneal dialysis flow sheet. (Printed with permission of the Department of Nursing, St. Joseph's Hospital, Milwaukee, WI.)

MERCY HEALTH CENTER

PERITONEAL DIALYSIS RECORD

DATE	SOLUTION TYPE	MEDICATIONS ADDED	SOLUTION IN			SOLUTION OUT			DIFFER-ENCE PLUS OR MINUS	COMULA-TIVE DIFFER-ENCE
			START-ING TIME	FIN-ISH TIME	VOLUME	START-ING TIME	FIN-ISH TIME	VOLUME		

Appendix O.   Peritoneal dialysis record. (Printed with permission of Mercy Health Center, Dubuque, IA.)

Patient Identification

MERCY HOSPITAL NEUROLOGICAL ASSESSMENT

mercy
HOSPITAL

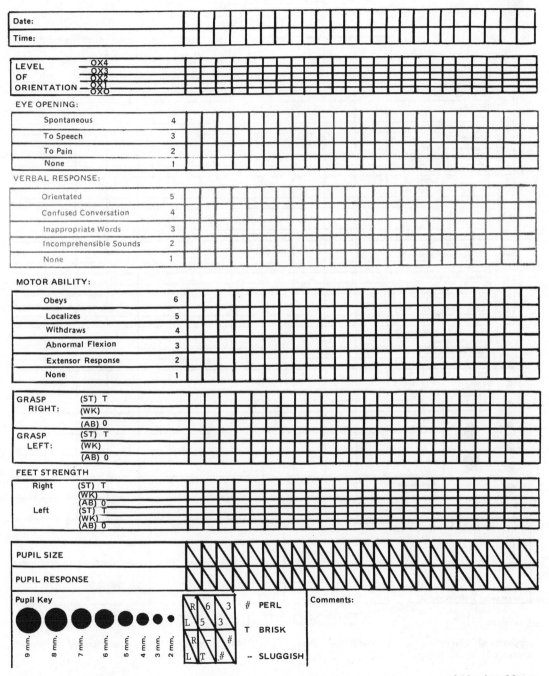

Date:	
Time:	

LEVEL OF ORIENTATION
OX4
OX3
OX2
OX1
OXO

EYE OPENING:

Spontaneous	4
To Speech	3
To Pain	2
None	1

VERBAL RESPONSE:

Orientated	5
Confused Conversation	4
Inappropriate Words	3
Incomprehensible Sounds	2
None	1

MOTOR ABILITY:

Obeys	6
Localizes	5
Withdraws	4
Abnormal Flexion	3
Extensor Response	2
None	1

GRASP RIGHT:	(ST) T
	(WK)
	(AB) 0
GRASP LEFT:	(ST) T
	(WK)
	(AB) 0

FEET STRENGTH

Right	(ST) T
	(WK)
	(AB) 0
Left	(ST) T
	(WK)
	(AB) 0

PUPIL SIZE	
PUPIL RESPONSE	

Pupil Key

9 mm. 8 mm. 7 mm. 6 mm. 5 mm. 4 mm. 3 mm. 2 mm.

R	6	3	# PERL
L	5	3	T BRISK
R	–	#	
L	T	#	– SLUGGISH

Comments:

Appendix P. Neurological assessment form. (Printed with permission of the Department of Nursing, Mercy Hospital, Cedar Rapids, IA.)

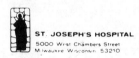

ST. JOSEPH'S HOSPITAL
5000 West Chambers Street
Milwaukee Wisconsin 53210

NEUROLOGICAL ASSESSMENT FLOW SHEET

			DATE	DATE	DATE	DATE	DATE	DATE	DATE	DATE	DATE	DATE	DATE	DATE
			TIME	TIME	TIME	TIME	TIME	TIME	TIME	TIME	TIME	TIME	TIME	TIME
INSTRUCTIONS ON BACK OF FLOW SHEET															
LEVEL OF CONSCIOUSNESS	**EYE OPENING**	SPONTANEOUSLY												
		TO SPEECH												
		TO PAIN												
		NONE												
	VERBAL RESPONSE	ANSWERS APPROPRIATELY												
		CONFUSED CONVERSATION												
		INAPPROPRIATE WORDS												
		INCOMPREHENSIBLE SOUNDS												
		NO VERBAL RESPONSE												
	MOTOR RESPONSE'	PURPOSEFUL — OBEYS												
		PURPOSEFUL — LOCALIZES												
		SEMI-PURPOSEFUL												
		DECORTICATE												
		DECEREBRATE												
		FLACCID												
STRENGTH OF EXTREMITIES (VOLUNTARY)	**ARMS**	NORMAL POWER												
		CAN OVERCOME RESISTANCE												
		CANNOT OVERCOME RESISTANCE												
		OVERCOMES GRAVITY												
		FLICKER OF MUSCLE												
		NONE												
	LEGS	NORMAL POWER												
		CAN OVERCOME RESISTANCE												
		CANNOT OVERCOME RESISTANCE												
		OVERCOMES GRAVITY												
		FLICKER OF MUSCLE												
		NONE												

PUPILS
+ REACTS
± IMPAIRED REACTION
− NO REACTION

	R SIZE												
	R REACTION												
	L SIZE												
	L REACTION												
	BLOOD PRESSURE												
	PULSE												
	RESPIRATION												
	TEMPERATURE												

PUPIL SCALE (MM)

	INITIALS												

INITIAL	SIGNATURE	INITIAL	SIGNATURE	INITIAL	SIGNATURE
INITIAL	SIGNATURE	INITIAL	SIGNATURE	INITIAL	SIGNATURE
INITIAL	SIGNATURE	INITIAL	SIGNATURE	INITIAL	SIGNATURE
INITIAL	SIGNATURE	INITIAL	SIGNATURE	INITIAL	SIGNATURE

DECEREBRATE   DECORTICATE

FORM 1178X 7/83

NEUROLOGICAL ASSESSMENT FLOW SHEET

Appendix Q. Neurological assessment flow sheet. (Printed with permission of the Department of Nursing, St. Joseph's Hospital, Milwaukee, WI.)

I.D. Bracelet ☐
Addressograph ☐

Massachusetts General Hospital
RECOVERY ROOM RECORD

Name: _____ Age: _____
Unit #: _____ Ward: _____
Date: _____
Anesthetic Agent: _____

ALLERGIES: _____

Pre-existing problems: _____
_____
_____

Relaxants: _____ Reversed ☐
Intubated ☐ _____
Intra-op problems: _____

Pre-op Med. _____

Intra-op medications: _____
_____

EBL: _____ Procedure: _____
_____

Time
AP
Cardiac Regularity/Rhythm
Cardiac Arrhythmias
IV Drugs gtts/mgm or mcg:
CSM
CVP
Spinal Level
Resp. Rate
Temp.
Dressing X or D
Dressing X or D
State of Airway
State of Consciousness

Dressing Code
D = Dry   X = See Note

State of Airway Code
1 clear   2 NP Airway
3 OP Airway   4 Endo-tube
5 Guarded   6 Trach

State of Consciousness
1. Awake & oriented
2. Awake & disoriented
3. Arousable
4. Unresponsive

BLOOD PRESSURE
240
200
190
180
170
160
150
140
130
120
110
100
90
80
70
60
50
40

NEURO

Eyes	1 Spontaneously
Open	2 To speech
	3 To pain
	4 None
Motor Response	
1. Obeys commands	
2. No response to commands	
3. Responds to painful stimuli	
4. Purposeless movement	
5. Decorticate	
6. Decerebrate	

Motor Strength
4 = Normal Strength   L arm
3 = Lifts and Holds   L leg
2 = Lifts and Falls Back   R arm
1 = Moves on Bed   R leg
0 = No Movement

PUPILS
7mm 6mm 5mm
8mm   4mm
N=Normal 3mm
S=Sluggish
F=Fixed 2mm
Ⓛ
Ⓡ

Appendix R. Recovery room record. (Printed with permission of the Department of Nursing, Massachusetts General Hospital, Boston, MA.)

Illustration continues on the following page.

Time	Ventilator Settings			Spontaneous Mechanics		Anesthesia Lab										Chemistry Lab					Hematology Lab (Baker)		
	PEEP	Resp Rate	Tidal Volume	Insp. Force	T.V./V.C.	FiO₂	pO₂	pCO₂	pH	Na	K	Hct.	TP/OSM	B.S.	BUN/Creat	NA/K	B.S.	Hct.	PT/PTT	PLAT/WBC

OTHER BLOOD WORK:

Time	X-ray Results	Time	EKG Result

Time	MEDICATIONS	Signature

PROGRESS NOTES

Appendix R. *Continued*

PROGRESS NOTES

Appendix R.   *Continued*

Illustration continues on the following page.

Date_____

Blood Bank Sample_____

Units Set Up _____

Massachusetts General Hospital

WHITE RECOVERY ROOM FLUID BALANCE RECORD

INTAKE

Time/Amt.	Parenteral Fluid	Abs.	Time/Amt.	Blood Prod.	Abs.

| Operating Room and Recovery Room TOTAL | | | Operating Room and Recovery Room TOTAL | | |

| MURPHY DRIP | | | | URINE | | | | DTV_____ | TUBES | |

Time	Amt.	In	Out	Time	Hrly	Cum	Diuretics S & A, Sp. Gr.	Time	Drainage	Chest

TOTAL INTAKE:_____ TOTAL URINE:_____ TOTAL OUTPUT:_____

TOTAL DRAINAGE TUBES:_____

Appendix R. *Concluded*

ST. LUKE'S METHODIST HOSPITAL
CEDAR RAPIDS, IOWA 52402

CODE BLUE FLOW SHEET

DATE: _____ TIME: _____ LOCATION: _____

ADMISSION DIAGNOSIS: _____ PERTINENT HISTORY: _____

TYPE OF ARREST: (√ ALL APPROPRIATE)

☐ RESPIRATORY　　☐ CARDIAC　　☐ ECG MONITORED　　RECOGNIZED BY:

　　　　　　　　☐ VENTRICULAR TACHYCARDIA　　☐ WITNESSED　　TIME:

　　　　　　　　☐ VENTRICULAR FIBRILLATION　　☐ UNWITNESSED　　TIME OF TEAM ARRIVAL:

　　　　　　　　☐ ASYSTOLE

PHYSICIANS IN ATTENDANCE: _____

NURSES IN ATTENDANCE: _____

SUPPORT SERVICES: _____

Time	Resp: A - Assisted S - Spontaneous FIO$_2$	Pupils	B/P	Pulse	Monitor Pattern	Defib	Blood Gases	Na H CO$_3$	Epine-phrine	Lido-caine	Atropine	Calcium	Dopamine		COMMENTS: INTUBATION FAMILY NOTIFIED

RESULT OF RESUSCITATION MEASURES: _____　　RECORDER: _____

D-4 CODE BLUE FLOW SHEET

CODE BLUE CHARGE RN: _____

EVALUATION OF CODE BLUE EFFORTS

SUCCESSFUL: ☐　　UNSUCCESSFUL: ☐

CARDIAC STATUS: _____　　SILENT CODE: ☐ (FOR MONITORED AREAS ONLY)

RESPIRATORY STATUS: _____　　EQUIPMENT PERFORMANCE:

NEURO STATUS: _____

OTHER: _____

EVALUATION OF TEAM EFFORTS

D-4 CODE BLUE FLOW SHEET

Appendix S. Code blue flow sheet. (Printed with permission of the Department of Nursing, St. Luke's Hospital, Cedar Rapids, IA.)

Mercy Health Center
St. Joseph's—St. Mary's
CODE 4 FLOW SHEET

Date:_____Time:_____   CPR Initiated by_____
Location of Arrest:_____   Pre-Cordial Thump by _____
Recognized by:_____   Pre-Arrest Diagnosis_____
_____

Staff Nurses Responding _____
_____

Type of Arrest:	Initial Assessment:_____ Time:_____	Team Responding to Code Intubated by:_____ Time:_____

Type of Arrest:
[ ] Respiratory
[ ] Cardiac
[ ] Witnessed
[ ] Unwitnessed

Initial Assessment:_____ Time:_____

Respiration	Pulse-carotid	Pupils
[ ] Present	[ ] Present	[ ] Reactive
[ ] Absent	[ ] Absent	[ ] Non-reactive

Team Responding to Code

Doctors/Time	Nurse—iCU / ER / Time	Respiratory/Time
_____	_____	_____
_____	_____	_____
_____	_____	_____

TIME	AIRWAY Oral–ET F₁O₂	RESPIRATIONS A – Assisted S – Spontaneous	PULSE P – Pulse PWC–Pulse With CPR	RHYTHM/RATE Record strip on back of white copy	CPR M – Maintained S – Stopped	PUPILS	BP	DEFIBRILLATED Watt/Sec.	NA BICARB 50meq/50cc, 1meq/Kg*	EPINEPHRINE 1/10,000 – 1mg/10ml 5cc*	LIDOCAINE 100mg/5ml 1mgm/Kg*	Ca CHLORIDE 1gm/10cc 5ml – 10% Solution*	ATROPINE 1mg/10ml .5–1mg initially*	BRETYLIUM 50mg/ml 5mg/Kg*		DOPAMINE DRIP 400mg/250cc D₅W 5–10mcg/Kg/min*	LIDOCAINE DRIP 2gm/500cc D₅W*	ISUPREL 1mg/250cc D₅W 2–20mcg/min*	

[ ] IV Present   [ ] IV Started   Order to Stop Code 4 Given By: Signatures:
_____   Nurse—Med _____

Needle	Site	Solution	By Whom

Other IV Solution _____   Family Notified/Time_____   Recorder _____
ABG's/Time_____   Pastoral Care Notified/Time_____   Doctor _____
00515

*ACLS Recommended Adult Dose   White, Chart – Yellow, Pharmacy – Pink, Education

Appendix T.   Code 4 flow sheet. (Printed with permission of Mercy Health Center, Dubuque, IA.)

INDEX

Page numbers in *italics* refer to figures; page numbers followed by t refer to tables.

621